ROCKEFELLER MONEY, THE LABORATORY, AND MEDICINE IN EDINBURGH 1919–1930

T0260573

Rochester Studies in Medical History

Senior Editor: Theodore M. Brown
Professor of History and Preventive Medicine
University of Rochester

ISSN 1526–2715

ROCKEFELLER MONEY, THE LABORATORY, AND MEDICINE IN EDINBURGH 1919–1930

New Science and Old Country

Christopher Lawrence

R UNIVERSITY OF ROCHESTER PRESS

Copyright © 2005 Christopher Lawrence

All Rights Reserved. Except as permitted under current legislation,
no part of this work may be photocopied, stored in a retrieval system,
published, performed in public, adapted, broadcast, transmitted,
recorded, or reproduced in any form or by any means,
without the prior permission of the copyright owner.

First published 2005
Reprinted in paperback 2013

University of Rochester Press
668 Mt. Hope Avenue, Rochester, NY 14620, USA
www.urpress.com
and Boydell & Brewer Limited
PO Box 9, Woodbridge, Suffolk IP12 3DF, UK
www.boydellandbrewer.com

ISSN: 1526-2715
hardcover ISBN: 978-1-58046-195-5
paperback ISBN: 978-1-58046-456-7

Library of Congress Cataloging-in-Publication Data

Lawrence, Christopher, 1947-
    Rockefeller money, the laboratory, and medicine in Edinburgh, 1919-1930 : new
science in an old country / Christopher Lawrence.
        p. ; cm. – (Rochester studies in medical history, ISSN 1526-2715 ; 5)
    Includes bibliographical references and index.
    ISBN 1-58046-195-6 (hardcover : alk. paper)
    1. Rockefeller Foundation–History. 2. University of Edinburgh Faculty of Medicine–
History. 3. Medicine–Scotland–Edinburgh–History–20th century. 4. Medical colleges–
Scotland–Edinburgh–History–20th century. 5. Medical education–Scotland–Edinburgh–
History–20th century. 6. Medical education–Scotland–Edinburgh–Endowments–
History–20th century. 7. Medicine–Research–Scotland–Edinburgh–History–20th centu-
ry. 8. Medicine–Research–Scotland–Edinburgh–Endowments–History–20th century. 9.
Medical laboratories–Scotland–Edinburgh–History–20th century.
    [DNLM: 1. Rockefeller Foundation. 2. Royal Infirmary of Edinburgh. 3. University
of Edinburgh. Faculty of Medicine. 4. Hospitals, University–history–Scotland. 5.
Schools, Medical–history–Scotland. 6. Foundations–history–Scotland. 7. History, 20th
Century–Scotland. 8. Laboratories, Hospital–history–Scotland. 9. Social Change–
history–Scotland. WX 28 FS2 L419r 2005] I.Title. II. Series.
    R497.E34L39 2005
    610'.71'14134–dc22

                                                                            2005010469

A catalogue record for this title is available from the British Library.

This publication is printed on acid-free paper.
Printed in the United States of America

CONTENTS

v

FIGURES AND GRAPHS

Figures

Graphs

ACKNOWLEDGMENTS

To three people I owe major debts. I have talked endlessly to Mike Barfoot and Steve Sturdy who know this material as well as (and a lot of it better than) I do. They have been tireless critics and good friends. We by no means agree on all the interpretations that follow, for which I take responsibility, but I could not have arrived at them without their engagement. I owe immeasurable thanks to Helen Coyle who was research assistant on this project for two years. Helen was both an assiduous researcher when directed but also had tremendous initiative and could turn up new sources with ease. She was also a wonderfully organized record keeper (as I continue to discover as I look through the files).

For reading and commenting on the manuscript or individual chapters I am grateful to Andrew Doig, Bill Bynum, Harry Marks, George Weisz and two anonymous referees. I presented some of what follows at a seminar at the Wellcome Centre for the History of Medicine where the now late Roy Porter made a characteristically off-the-cuff remark that prompted me to think about this material in a new way. Thanks to Martin Edwards for useful discussions about control and to Stephen Casper for being provocative and for alerting me to Edwin Bramwell's diaries.

A great number of people assisted with research in various ways. Some of the following may be surprised to find themselves here. I did not meet them but Helen Coyle found their help invaluable. Thanks to Mr Ian Milne, Librarian, and all the library staff at Royal College of Physicians of Edinburgh; Mr Arnott Wilson, Archivist, University of Edinburgh Library, Special Collections; Dr Murray Simpson, Miss Jean Archibald, and staff at the Special Collections Department, University of Edinburgh Library; Julie Hutton, John Simmons and Mike Barfoot,

Lothian Health Services Archive, Special Collections, University of Edinburgh; National Archives of Scotland, Edinburgh; Mrs Sheila Mackenzie, Research Assistant, Manuscripts Division, National Library of Scotland, Edinburgh; Mrs Elspeth Shields, Secretary to Professor Webb, Department of Clinical Pharmacology, Western General Hospital, Edinburgh; Professor David Webb, Christison Chair of Therapeutics, Department of Clinical Pharmacology, Western General Hospital, Edinburgh; Harold Averill and Garron Wells, and the staff of the University of Toronto Archives; Pamela Miller and the staff of the Osler Library for the History of Medicine, McGill University, Montreal; Dr Henry Adam (interview); Dr Rae L. Lyon (interview); Dr Andrew Doig (interview); Dr Ernest Jellinek (interview); Elliot Simpson, Biochemistry Department, Monklands Hospital, Airdrie; Robert McMaster, Biochemist, Royal Infirmary of Edinburgh; Professor Jonathan L. Meakins and wife Dr Jacqueline McClaran; Mr Ian McIntyre, Consultant Surgeon, Department of General Surgery, Western General Hospital, Edinburgh; Walter Hawkins, senior technician in the Lister Laboratories, Royal Infirmary of Edinburgh; Professor Sir Patrick Forrest; Darwin Stapleton and the staff of the Rockefeller Archive Center; Jim Proffit, Chief Medical Laboratory Scientific Officer, Royal Infirmary of Edinburgh; the staff of the Wellcome Trust Library for the History and Understanding of Medicine; Chris Carter, photographer at the Wellcome Trust; Professor David Bloor and the Science Studies Unit, University of Edinburgh (for accommodating Helen Coyle), Carole Tansley, also of the Unit, for all sorts of support; at the Wellcome Centre for the History of Medicine, University College London, Emma Ford for word processing and Sharon Messenger and Caroline Overy for research. Two generous grants were received from the Wellcome Trust to support Helen Coyle for two years.

For permission to quote from manuscripts I am grateful to The Royal College of Physicians of Edinburgh; Lothian Health Services Archive; the University of Edinburgh Archives, by courtesy of Edinburgh University Library; Medical Research Council; Osler Library of the History of Medicine, Montreal, Quebec, Canada (McGill University); University of Toronto Archives; the Rockefeller Archive Center. For permission to quote from the private papers of Edwin Bramwell I am grateful to Hilda McKendrick.

ABBREVIATIONS

EUA   Edinburgh University Archives
EUL   Edinburgh University Library
LHSA   Lothian Health Services Archive
MRC   Medical Research Council (material held at the PRO)
OLHM Osler Library of the History of Medicine (McGill University)
PRO   Public Record Office
RAC   Rockefeller Archive Center
RCPE   The Royal College of Physicians of Edinburgh
RFA   Rockefeller Foundation Archives (material held at the RAC)
RIE   Royal Infirmary of Edinburgh
UE   University of Edinburgh
UTA   University of Toronto Archives

1

INTRODUCTION: MEDICAL CULTURES

In 1933 an officer of the Rockefeller Foundation (RF) of New York, R. A. Lambert, visited the Edinburgh Medical Faculty, into which his institution had poured a great deal of money over the previous ten years. He was struck by the fact that, "For a generation at least, the School has obviously lived to a considerable extent on its reputation and its policies have been determined largely by tradition." He catalogued what he considered Edinburgh's shortcomings and the changes that might give his paymasters cause for hope that the sort of medicine they wished to see in Scotland was being instituted. One of the sources of optimism was a weakening of the "old individualism."[1] Lambert could hardly have been plainer: in some medical quarters in Edinburgh, tradition and individualism were highly prized and the RF found them an obstacle to its vision of medical reform.

This is a story of the encounter of two cultures. First a relatively old one, that of a large section of the professional middle class in Scotland, particularly Edinburgh. Much, but by no means all, of this culture was shared with a counterpart in the south of England. Second, a new one which characterized parts of North America (and Britain). It is a history of their striving to harmonize but also of their misunderstandings and mutual manipulation. At times it is a tale of a radical clash between wider historical and moral assumptions. This is the general story but it is one that can be told through the specific meeting (by no means always eye to eye) of two types of medicine. The specific narrative centres on attempts to introduce new medical practices and new ideas about science into old institutions. The general story is more formless, harder to grasp and pin down. The new accounts of medicine and science, however, did not simply detail better ideas and technologies for curing the sick. They challenged older cherished models of the social order. They embodied conceptions of health—well-being—and its relation to social organization. They prescribed a premier place for science in social planning and the management of modern society. Indeed they redefined what constituted a healthy society and who should bring it about and how. Somewhere between the very specific and the very general lies a linkage, a middle level of explanation. Here I demonstrate how wider assumptions were built into the everyday workings of familiar institutions. For example, by reading the lines as written, and sometimes between them, it is possible to show that part-time professorships were not simply supported for monetary ends (for the private practice they permitted) but had built into them the values that sustained the voluntary hospital system. Controversies over part-time versus full-time chairs were controversies about cultural values and the social order in which they were embedded.

There are many institutional players and many actors in this history but for the purposes of an introduction they can be reduced to twelve: seven institutions and five individuals. The first two institutions are the medical Royal Colleges of Edinburgh, that of the Physicians and that of the Surgeons. They will not get a great deal of mention in these pages but their power, especially as licensing and validating bodies, must not be forgotten. Little occurred in the medical politics of Edinburgh without their governing bodies knowing and without their approval. The Colleges had a long historical and ongoing involvement with the University of Edinburgh and the Royal Infirmary of Edinburgh (RIE), both formally and informally. Formally two Fellows from each of the Colleges were members of the Board of Management of the Infirmary. There was always a Medical Faculty member of the University Court and this representative would invariably have been a Fellow of one or other of the Colleges. The Colleges were very much involved politically in the organization and promotion of medical teaching, research, and patient management in Edinburgh. This involvement was almost incomprehensible (as well as unacceptable) to the Americans. The University (especially its Faculty of Medicine) and the RIE are the next two institutions in the "old country." Steeped in traditions, of which they were very proud, they were keen to preserve the best of the received ways of doing things yet also sought to be modern and forward-looking. Yet, and this is a major medical theme of the 1920s, what it meant to be modern and forward-looking was heard differently in different ears and in different places. The Department of Therapeutics of the Medical Faculty and its Biochemical Laboratory (later Clinical Laboratory) in the Infirmary jointly constitute my fifth institution. Together they were, to some extent, a Trojan horse of medical change in Edinburgh. Across the Atlantic, in New York, and this is my sixth institution, was the headquarters of the RF. This building was home to very distinct ideas of what modern medicine should look like. These ideas were shared in Great Britain by the powers that ran my final, crucial institution, the Medical Research Council (MRC). The MRC and the RF constitute most of the "new" of my subtitle, which is to say that medical innovation and novel ideas about medical science were British as well as American in origin.

In terms of human actors, Richard Pearce, Director of the RF's Division of Medical Education and Walter Morley Fletcher, Secretary of the MRC, were major champions of the new, who were, as they saw it, endeavouring to drag Edinburgh medicine from a past of antiquated practices into the modern world. Their principal agent was Jonathan Meakins, a Canadian who was appointed the first Christison Professor of Therapeutics in Edinburgh in 1919. Meakins was an apostle of the modern in medicine. He left Edinburgh somewhat disillusioned in 1924. His successor was David Murray Lyon, a man firmly in an older Edinburgh tradition and a source of disappointment to Pearce and Fletcher. Although modern minded in his own way and a loyal servant of the University and Infirmary, his ideas for creating a modern medical department did not conform to those of the RF and the MRC. The last of my major players was Edwin Bramwell, Professor of Clinical Medicine, and again, although a distinguished neurologist, perhaps a man more on the side of the old than the new. A host of other characters will also appear in this book variously aligned by me with the innovative or the traditional. It should not be thought I am making stark contrasts between old and new. Positions were nuanced and varied with context but, none the less, traditional and modern ways of carrying out substantive medical activities, notably teaching, research, and simply practising clinical medicine can be discerned. Elaborate historical and "philosophical" arguments defending why these things should be done in particular ways were also much in evidence.

A major site of the encounter between Edinburgh and the new medicine was the RIE's Biochemical Laboratory, which opened in 1921. This was to a great extent Meakins's creation; it was his fiefdom—the seat of his research and the home of diagnostic testing for the whole hospital. It was, for some observers, a true symbol of modernity. I analyse its place in the life of the hospital and the University over a ten-year period. Obviously 1919 and 1930 are arbitrary years to start and finish. British and North American archives are so rich, however, the book would never have been completed had it strayed in to the 1930s. In spite of their arbitrariness, the dates were distinct turning points in Edinburgh's medical history. Serious consideration of the restructuring of teaching and research that had been considered before the Great War was only implemented in earnest after it, notably with the appointment of Meakins. The Division of Medical Education was created at the RF in 1919 with Pearce at its head. At the other end of the decade, George E. Vincent, President of the RF since 1917, retired in December 1929, the same year a comprehensive plan to reorganize RF programmes and policies had been approved. Pearce died in 1930, the year marking the end of serious Rockefeller involvement in Edinburgh medicine of the sort described here. Fletcher died in 1933. The year 1930 virtually saw the disappearance of the last of the team of researchers that Meakins had built around himself. The end of the decade witnessed major physical reconstruction of the Medical School. Ten years allows me to contrast roughly five years of Meakins's reign with five years of Murray Lyon's. A decade of laboratory life is also enough to see the main trends in routine clinical testing and in research.

There are two sub-plots that I explore, principally in chapters 7–9. Both relate to things now taken for granted in medicine that were still being established in the 1920s. They are closely related to each other. First was the creation of the category "metabolic disease." The Edinburgh Biochemical Laboratory workers were a small number of local figures in a wider community who were important in recasting clinical disorders, for example diabetes and Graves' disease (thyrotoxicosis), in biochemical terms. The laboratory was not simply an ancillary to bedside medicine: it was used as an agent of conceptual change. Symptoms, diseases, disorders, and syndromes were framed anew in biochemical language and their pathology embedded in biochemical tests (as indeed was the concept of the "normal"). Clinicians on the wards of the Infirmary were asked by the inhabitants of the Department of Therapeutics to rethink traditional categories. My second sub-plot is the beginning of a distinction between routine and research in clinical work. Ethical and other considerations make these activities relatively distinct today. This was not so, for the most part, in the 1920s. Clinicians recognized a difference but admitted to it being hard to make in practice. It was no more obvious in 1930 than it was in 1920, but that there was a difference was being discussed. Arguably the disappearance of charitable care after the Second World War was a major factor in establishing clearer cut categories.

Because of the centrality of the Biochemical Laboratory to this book the RF appears as a major player in the reform of British and particularly Edinburgh medicine. It is important to place the RF input in a broader context. Huge and powerful though it was, it should be borne in mind that reform of medical organization, research, and education were high on the domestic agenda. In the 1920s medical schools and national medical bodies in Britain were actively debating reform regardless of the RF. To take a specific example: it is clear from a recent history of medical education at St. Bartholomew's Hospital, which was richly supported by the RF and other charities, that national and local forces were generating a great deal of debate and change at the hospital. These factors were far more important than philanthropic input, which was confined to quite localized schemes.[2]

The 1920s have been widely reckoned to be years of crisis. The word was in frequent use at the time in political, cultural, social, and economic spheres.[3] Historians often resort to the term to describe various features of the era. It does not seem to have been commonly employed by the Edinburgh medical community but it is clear that many in the 1920s, both within and without Edinburgh, considered that the Medical School had somehow seen better days and had now lost its way and that reinvigoration was needed. There was some measurable truth in this, as well as subjective perceptions. Before the Great War, the only serious competitors to Edinburgh as large medical educational institutions were Glasgow and London. After the war new, so-called redbrick, universities began to flourish in the English provinces and their medical schools started to attract students who would have once made the trek to the North. Overall between the wars, says one observer, higher education in Scotland "fared badly . . . the number of full-time students at the four universities fell from 10,400 in 1924 to 9,900 in 1937, while the English Universities registered a rise of nearly 19 per cent."[4]

A key feature of the Edinburgh clinical school was its inbreeding. The staff of the Infirmary (and therefore the clinical teachers) was almost invariably recruited from the ranks of Edinburgh graduates. There were some that found this unhealthy and wanted what they called "fresh blood" from outside to reinvigorate the school. There were others who took great pride in this tradition and saw it as essential to the maintenance of Edinburgh's eminence or, with careful future selection of staff, to its regeneration. The tension between demands for fresh blood and the desire to keep the Edinburgh stock pure was present in a number of aspects of University and, particularly, Infirmary life.

Trying to describe this book in conversation, I have many times been struck by how taken for granted is the essential "correctness" of modern medicine, the feeling of its inevitable rise and triumph because of its "rightness." In outlining my themes to anyone inclined to listen I tried to be fair to all sides, to talk on the one hand about Edinburgh, its traditions, and those who defended them and on the other of the proponents of the new in medicine. In many instances I have been met with the response: "Well, they [the moderns] were right of course." The assumption was made instantly that medicine today shows that reformers were midwives to good (read "modern") medicine and any questioning of this must have been made by fuddy-duddies, nostalgic obstructionists, born in the wrong age, and more interested in private patients than corporate medical advance. I have hung out for symmetry of understanding in the book.

As historians know all too well it *is* much harder to present the losers' case. I think they had one. None the less as regards elite Edinburgh culture as a whole the imperative to suspend judgement is tempered by the feeling that this was a Juggernaut, laden with the freight of the Enlightenment, shuddering to a halt. The reader, I hope, will understand my sentiments when encountering, albeit fleetingly, the imago of modernity in the form of Dorothy Meakins dancing in Edinburgh.

The new medicine was not an unqualified success. A glance today at, for example, the discussions in medical journals, the criticisms made by alternative and complementary medical groups or patient-powered lobbies, the findings of committees on medical educational reform, or perhaps, especially, the reports of medico-legal cases will reveal one of the new medicine's legacies. All this paperwork is riddled with concerns about the relation between bedside medical skills and the data of the laboratory. Are doctors losing touch with their patients by over-reliance on the laboratory, or are they failing to investigate their patients thoroughly and neglecting laboratory testing? Is objective data taking the place of the patient's subjective guide to sickness? Are the nuances of illness that can be understood by the experienced clinician who is immersed in the clinical art lost by the blunderbuss approach of the laboratory? One could start addressing these issues anywhere in the past but for specific and general reasons I have focused on the 1920s. Although there are pre-World War I antecedents it was in the 1920s that doctors and others began to produce a substantial literature on this subject, because the laboratory was being introduced into medical care on a large scale along with a wholesale reorganization of hospital practice and education. I have sought to understand the sentiments of those who were suspicious of such moves and to show in detail how they turned to clinical skills when, by the standards of some of their contemporaries (and certainly by today's), a laboratory test could or should have been employed. I am not an idealist. These men did not adopt this position solely from a love of the clinical art and an appreciation of its values that they deemed irreplaceable by laboratory knowledge. They had real material and ideological interests which are hard to disentangle: a devotion to private practice, a commitment to charitable care, a love of clinical and political individualism, a bourgeois sense of their rightful place in Caledonian society, and a earnest Edinburgh-centred, cultural, Scottish nationalism.

One methodological point: my interests have long been in questions of scientific and medical knowledge—how they are made, what work they are put to, how they are used to transform conceptions of the natural order, and how changes of social order are brought about (or not) with the creation of new knowledge, and vice versa. This interest remains at the core of this book. A number of readers have remarked (perhaps not all entirely approvingly) on the detail I have gone into in reporting a great deal of correspondence which might broadly be called political. I have done this in order to help elucidate clinical and research work. Whether I have done this well or badly I leave the reader to judge but for me the shaping of the knowledge made in the lab and on the ward lies in the detail. What has made this study so enjoyable has been the opportunity to reconstruct the life of an early twentieth-century lab on many levels and to show, perhaps, that a conversation over a cup of tea taken by Principal Ewing of the University of Edinburgh and Walter Fletcher of the MRC at the Athenaeum (a gentlemen's club in London) had a bearing on the sort of knowledge made in the Department of Therapeutics just as so obviously did the intellectual power and scientific skills of Jonathan Meakins. Harry Marks has said something similar about his study of therapeutic evaluation. "My approach," he records, "is premised on the convictions that ideas can best be studied in context, and that the administrative memo can reveal as much about the intellectual history of an era as the more formal treatises sometimes favored by intellectual historians."[5]

On a definitional point I have made frequent use of the words "culture" and "myth" in this book and in the former case, totally, and in the latter, almost completely, I have not made the faintest attempt at definition. To do so would have added yards of text and footnotes in order to have set out approximations that would not please everyone and might possibly satisfy no one. I hope my meanings are clear from the way I have used these words, two of the historian's most useful friends.

This is a book about Edinburgh and its most famous hospital in the 1920s. Each year, literally thousands of patients were treated there. For the most part they were the relatively poor of the city and the surrounding areas. Of their lives before they entered the Infirmary we know almost nothing. Of what became of them afterwards we know even less. To their sufferings we have only meagre access through medical records. Of the effect of their illnesses on them and their families we have been given scarcely the remotest clue. Anyone looking in this book for a reconstruction of the lives of the patients mentioned here will search long for little return, although no reader can miss the poignancy of some of the brief histories I report. A project on the medical experiences and lives of patients in hospital in Scotland in the 1920s is an enterprise entirely different to the present one. The current history, however, is not unrelated to the lives of patients. At the bedsides of those who are named in this book, almost certainly unknown to them, a struggle over medical knowledge and authority was being enacted. This was a struggle, I think, that extended far beyond the confines of medicine. The struggle (by no means over) would change the medical experiences and lives of all of the patients who followed.

I have organized my chapters by themes and within the chapters by chronology. The mass and diversity of material would have made impossible an overall chronological approach. I first look at medical research and education in Britain, particularly in London. I describe American attitudes to them. I follow this with an account of the organization of medical teaching and education in Edinburgh and the staffing structure of the RIE. I go into some detail over various medical modernizing projects proposed in the city and describe the circumstances of Meakins's appointment and the creation of a biochemistry laboratory in an obsolete isolation hospital at the RIE. I then look at American attitudes to Edinburgh medicine. I follow this with an account of the RF's negotiations with Edinburgh to fund a new, purpose-built biochemistry laboratory. Entwined in this story is the departure of Meakins. I then explore the RF's relatively successful efforts to transform the surgical teaching and research on North American lines and its failed attempts to reform the Medical Departments by trying to establish the long-standing, prestigious Chair of Medicine on a full-time basis. In the final three substantive chapters I look at the work of the lab and the extent of the impact it made on the hospital and the medical world more broadly. In the first I look at the growth of routine testing and Meakins's attempts to import a new style of medical thinking into the Infirmary. I then examine the scientific research done in the lab. Chapter 9 takes a look at selected case notes of Edwin Bramwell in an attempt to see how a rather traditional physician used the lab as a diagnostic resource. I also examine surgical case notes and the insulin trials carried out in the hospital. In Chapter 10

I briefly look at what happened to clinical medicine in Edinburgh in the 1930s and finally I take a brief stab at what I think all this adds up to.

Notes

1. R. A. Lambert, "Edinburgh Medical Faculty—Impressions of a Visit July 6–8, 1933," July 18, 1933, folder 18, box 2, series 405, RG 1.1, Rockefeller Foundation Archives, RAC. Lambert was a pathologist who joined the RF in 1928.

2. Keir Waddington, *Medical Education at St Bartholomew's Hospital 1123–1995* (Woodbridge, Suffolk: The Boydell Press, 2003). St Mary's Hospital, Paddington, which undertook medical educational reform between the wars, relied almost entirely on local benefactions. See E. A. Heaman, *St. Mary's: The History of a London Teaching Hospital* (Montreal & Kingston, London, Ithaca: Liverpool University Press, McGill–Queen's University Press, 2003).

3. R. J. Overy, *The Inter-War Crisis 1919–1939* (Harlow: Pearson Education Limited, 1994).

4. Christopher Harvie, *No Gods and Precious Few Heroes: Twentieth-Century Scotland*, 3rd ed. (Edinburgh: Edinburgh University Press, 1998), 78.

5. Harry M. Marks, *The Progress of Experiment: Science and Therapeutic Reform in the United States, 1900–1990* (Cambridge: Cambridge University Press, 1997), 10.

2

MEDICAL REVOLUTIONS

The Edinburgh Medical School was founded in 1726 and the RIE in 1729. Two hundred years later medicine could be said to have undergone one revolution and to be undergoing another. These revolutions are best described in terms of ideal types, for the spectrum of theories, assumptions, practices, and institutions that they embraced varied widely. The first revolution, often called hospital medicine, occurred in the early nineteenth century and involved the gradual transformation of a medicine based largely on the patient's narrative to one based on physical examination and the use instruments, famously the stethoscope. Clinicians, on hospital wards and in the post-mortem room, largely created this new medicine. By 1900 the method of examining patients employed within this "clinico-pathological" approach had been thoroughly systematized. Indeed an Edinburgh physician, Harry Rainy, practising at the RIE in the early 1920s was co-author of what was possibly *the* standard British manual of physical examination.[1]

Of course this change in medical knowledge and practice did not come alone. There were changes in institutions, organization, social relations, and attitudes that were integral to it. First, hospital practice

11

expanded enormously. Almost invariably hospitals were institutions dedicated to the treatment of the poor although this began to change in the early twentieth century as members of the middle classes began to be admitted to them. By the end of the nineteenth century, the hospital was regarded as the necessary site for the student, under the eye of a senior physician, to learn the ritual of clinical examination. Second, morbid anatomy was held to be *the* science that underpinned the new medicine. It was institutionalized academically in pathology departments in university medical schools and practically in hospital departments where the pathologist reported on specimens and performed post-mortems. Morbid anatomy, both gross and histological, became an integral part of the medical curriculum. In hospitals, ambitious young hospital doctors would seek assistantships in pathology departments and carry out hours of post-mortem work (often unpaid) that would ensure, they hoped, that they had impeccable credentials for promotion to more senior positions and thus the kudos to attract private patients outside of the hospital. Pathological anatomy and bedside observation were regarded as forms of natural history and were seen as the most promising way to advance medical knowledge. Besides the study of normal and diseased bodies, observing the natural history of flora and fauna was a common hobby among medical practitioners.

The new medicine also bred something subtler than method: it bred assumptions, although these were in many ways developments of much older attitudes. In the nineteenth and early twentieth centuries, elite doctors (patrician medical men) valued clinical experience coupled with morbid anatomical knowledge as central to the most important part of medicine: diagnosis. Medical experience, some said, could not always be put into words and the manner in which a skilled clinician arrived at a judgement was often regarded as incommunicable.[2] Clinical practice, individual judgement, and individualism in a broader sense were seen as entwined and were highly prized. Medical values were inextricably bound to broader social and political ones. Doctors at the great hospitals held the best clinical practice to be based not only on medical learning but also on all-round knowledge. Distinguished clinicians in Britain and parts of North America saw themselves as cultured gentlemen. Their devotion to private medical practice and resistance to full-time university chairs of medicine might be explained glibly by pecuniary motives.

There was much more to it than that however. Elite doctors were like many Victorian "men of letters." These were individuals—Matthew Arnold might be the quintessential example—mainly in the law, the Church, the civil service, and the literary professions who had time to support themselves in the manner appropriate to their station and also to pursue in their leisure hours interests in such things as oriental languages, political thought, and history. They were "public moralists."[3]

Patrician doctors then did not regard their learning and lifestyle simply as accomplishments necessary for the discerning exercise of medical skill, they saw them as essential to the maintenance of existing social relations and values. More generally this was an example of an attitude among the middle classes in Britain that Richard Shannon has characterized as the professional service version of *noblesse oblige*. It was an attitude that served to maintain the "traditional social and political forms of the ruling class."[4] This characterization perfectly captures why these men treated the poor in hospital gratis and why they valued private practice so highly. These attitudes were still prevalent in the 1920s. In London and Edinburgh, however, practitioners subscribed to slightly different accounts and historical myths of these "traditional social and political forms." In both cases the accounts and myths prescribed the doctor's place and role within the social order. In both instances too, ideas of the social order implicitly and sometimes explicitly embodied conceptions of the health of the people in the broadest sense—their well-being perhaps.

The methods, organization, and assumptions brought about by the first medical revolution were all to be challenged by a second one. This revolution centred on the creation of what is perhaps best termed, for current purposes, academic medicine.[5] Like hospital medicine it had its methods of producing knowledge as well as its pedagogical, institutional, and attitudinal dimensions. Its origins are usually traced to Germany but in the 1920s, west of continental Europe, the big players were North America, London, and Cambridge. The first and perhaps earliest constituent of academic medicine was the establishment of the view that experimental laboratory sciences should be the basis of medical practice and education and the means of new knowledge production. Of course in some ways this view can be traced back way beyond the nineteenth century but to do this would be to conjure antecedents without appreciating the new shapes of nineteenth-century scientific disciplines. By the late nineteenth century in many places, and by the 1920s pretty well everywhere, the basic medical sciences, especially physiology, were taught by men, and latterly also women, who were employed by universities and medical schools as full-time professional scientists. When they were not teaching they worked in their labs on experimental research. Such a development was unprecedented. Now these scientists were not solely the servants of medicine even though that rhetorical posture sometimes helped them shoehorn their disciplines into medical schools. Although these professionals preached the gospel that research in the basic sciences was the soundest means of teaching aspiring doctors and advancing medical practice they also had their own professional agendas.

Those clinicians who enthusiastically approved of this new medicine endeavoured to bring ideas, methods, and technologies from the basic sciences, notably physiology, to the bedside. Many of them bemoaned the older stress on morbid anatomy to the detriment of physiological or what was sometimes called "dynamic" thinking about disease. Experimentally-minded clinicians did indeed transform medicine in this period. They took physiological concepts derived from laboratory experiments and used them to create new accounts of disease and medical specialities. For example, the physiological idea of the heart's innate rhythmic activity, a concept generated in the physiological laboratories of Cambridge University, was used as the basis of a "new cardiology" based on function. This new approach, in turn, was employed to create a medical speciality.[6] Technologies such as the electrocardiograph, the sphygmomanometer, and the X-ray, derived from the basic biological and physical sciences, increasingly appeared in the hospital in this period. The laboratory entered medicine in another way too. As modern germ theory was accepted, bacteriology chairs were established in universities and bacteriological laboratories were set up in hospitals (usually beginning as subsidiaries of pathology departments). In these labs diagnostic tests were performed, increasingly under the eye of specialist bacteriologists. In the 1920s biochemistry labs that were seats of research and diagnosis also began to appear in hospitals.

The second constituent of academic medicine was the increasing prominence of university staff in the teaching and practice of clinical subjects. The ideal model, for many, was to have medicine based around clinical professors who, with assistants, were to be paid to teach, practise, and carry out research full time in university hospitals. Enthusiasts for this view favoured disbanding voluntary service and forbidding professors having access to private practice. Such professors were to have autonomous control of all the medical or surgical beds in a hospital. They were also to have the right to nominate their juniors on merit rather than have them appointed by seniority and by lay people, practices that prevailed in Britain. This new model was intimately linked to the rise of the new basic laboratory sciences. All those who promoted the full-time system expected the new professors to conduct research in their wards in conjunction with laboratory experiments, training their students and potential researchers in laboratory and clinical work simultaneously. This mode of research came to be known as clinical science. Clinical research, of course, could be undertaken within the framework of the older clinico-pathological model. In this instance the orientation was usually to the natural historical description of disease, the reporting of one or more case histories, and the discoveries made at post-mortem of morbid anatomical change. In the new clinical science, on the other hand, the focus was on physiological problem solving applied to disease. Always in the background were the norms of the laboratory. For example, knowing the oxygen saturation levels of normal venous blood, the clinical challenge was to discover to what degree it was changed in, say, pneumonia (and possibly determine what practical value this knowledge might have). A preference for either the clinico-pathological approach or the physiological one (with all their corollaries) sometimes created tensions among hospital staff which were displayed in competition for funding or appointments.

Besides their new approach to the study of health and disease, academic physicians also had their own ideas about the social organization necessary for medical problem solving. Many distrusted individual clinical experience and held that only a team comprising clinicians and laboratory workers (perhaps from several institutions) could arrive at sound knowledge of, say, the therapeutic efficacy of a new drug.[7] In this respect, allegiance to academic medicine and its reward system might rank higher than loyalty to a particular institution.

Thus, by the 1920s the laboratory had become prominent in medicine in three areas: first in pre-clinical and clinical teaching, second as a site of research, and third, especially in the case of bacteriology and clinical pathology, as a place for the routine testing and examination of specimens taken from the sick. For the most part, because historians have concentrated on the creation of scientific disciplines and "pure" scientists in this period, an important feature of the growth of laboratory science has been neglected. Workers attempting to organize new subjects in universities, experimental physiology or biochemistry for instance (although the physical sciences also provide many examples), often stressed the "pureness" of their disciplines. That is, they claimed disinterested research in the pursuit of knowledge was the highest good. Although such knowledge, it was frequently said, might one day have a practical pay-off, the so-called "applied sciences" were often looked down on by students of the "pure" ones. Walter Morley Fletcher took this "purist" view of physiology. What many historians have overlooked is the sizeable move in this period to create practical laboratory disciplines that would serve local communities. Medicine exemplifies this trend well, although other professions could be chosen. During the inter-war years many university laboratories forged links with hospitals, local practitioners, and public health officials to carry out tests and monitor the health of communities.[8] The Biochemical Laboratory at the RIE, which was devoted to research *and* patient management, is an example. However, not everyone agreed that university laboratories should be involved in community activities. In 1923 the *Lancet* criticized the Pathology Department of the University of Leeds for its public health work since it was "weakening the ideals of higher education."[9] Another aspect of this rise of "practical" academic medicine at this time was the forging of links with industry, especially the pharmaceutical industry. One case study of American medicine has shown that the disease pernicious anaemia was reconceptualized in this period in terms of the therapeutic efficiency of a mass-produced pharmaceutical preparation.[10]

Partly as a consequence of the growth of the laboratory sciences, medical specialization increasingly appeared in the inter-war years. The laboratory sciences were one of the resources (there were others, childbirth for example) that potential specialists used to demarcate new areas of expertise. The pathologist had set pattern for this, but the early twentieth century saw the appearance of bacteriologists, clinical pathologists, radiologists, cardiologists (a speciality as noted based on laboratory physiology) and others. In university hospitals specialist chairs were established.

As might be appreciated the assumptions of academic medicine were not universally shared, notably in Britain. Many clinicians, especially in London with its hospital-based medical schools, distrusted the power of universities. Many valued private practice, voluntary service in hospitals, and a system of appointment to hospital posts by seniority. Hospital managers, too, often resented attempted incursions of academic power into their strongholds. Although no doctor drilled in the older methods of clinical medicine repudiated the new sciences, many felt that they occupied too much time in the medical curriculum and that the most ardent supporters of these sciences ignored the contributions that clinical experience could make to medical advance. Voicing a related concern some clinicians said that the use of laboratory diagnostic testing was excessive and was usurping clinical skill. Many doctors saw their clinical experience being discounted. The trend towards specialization was deplored by many clinicians in the name of the virtues of generalism, meaning a rounded education and a broad knowledge of disease. Specialists, such critics said, could not see the whole picture. If some within the profession worried about the increasing dominance of the laboratory sciences, outside the profession there were groups militantly opposed to them. For antivivisectionists, medical laboratories were synonymous with animal experiment, organized protest against which was present throughout the 1920s. Hospital governors and managers had particular cause to fear this movement since any suggestion that a voluntarily-supported hospital was harbouring animal experiments could result in the withdrawal of the patronage of the wealthy, whose donations were essential to the running of many of these institutions.

Suspicion of academic medicine ran deeper than worry about its challenges to day-to-day medical practices and organization. Like the medicine it was supplanting, academic medicine was part of a real and realizable social order. In its promotion its supporters aspired to establish new "social and political forms." Science, and especially scientific research, was seen as a premier instrument for analysing social problems and providing solutions to them. The ideal social order was perceived as professional and technocratic. The organization and the maximization of the efficiency of work were seen as major social goals that would bring about a stable society. Like the clinical order it threatened, academic medicine had its implicit and explicit accounts of a healthy nation.

As indicated, the professional medical sciences and academic medicine originated in Germany but their large-scale institutionalization occurred in North America, and later in Britain. But why, how, and by whom were these disciplines institutionalized? There is currently a substantial historical literature on the rise of academic medicine and introduction of laboratory sciences into medical education and practice.[11] Although there is no consensus as to why this occurred there are powerful arguments to suggest it was part of a wholesale reorganization of medicine and a reorientation of its relation to society. In the long run it was part of the growth of the hierarchical, corporately-organized delivery of health care to industrial societies. These changes were not confined to medicine. Education, industry, and commerce underwent similar revolutions. Concerns with scientific management, order, and efficiency helped drive these things. Businesslike models of organization came to dominate medicine much as they did many other walks of life. In America some doctors approvingly likened the best hospitals to businesses, even factories.[12] In 1916 an article appeared in the American journal *Modern Hospital* entitled "The Modern Hospital as a Health Factory."[13] None of this is to suggest that the new laboratory sciences were an ideological front with no medical efficacy, rather it is to argue that ideas of efficacy were bound to a wholly new world of medical organization. Not surprisingly then, clinicians who were cautious about the extent to which the laboratory sciences were becoming part of medical education and clinical practice voiced concerns about new modes of medical organization. It is quite clear that in the inter-war years these concerns were not just about medicine but about the modernization of culture at large: about mass production, mass consumption (particularly of newspapers, radio programmes, and movies), and about the perceived decline of intellectual elites. For many in Britain, America was the source of these decadent invaders.

If, briefly, these are some of the reasons for the transformations in medicine in the early twentieth century, how did this modernization occur and who promoted it? In North America the answer is clear. Around the turn of the nineteenth and twentieth centuries the United States had undergone massive population growth, urbanization, and industrialization. In the process vast fortunes were made by men such as Meyer and Daniel Guggenheim, John Pierpont Morgan, Andrew Carnegie, and John D. Rockefeller, Sr. Such men sought to use their money during their lifetimes and after for public purposes, education particularly, but also for the founding of hospitals, the building of parks, concert halls, art galleries etc. They did this on a lavish scale. Many of America's most prestigious higher education institutions, particularly scientific institutions, were founded or supported by philanthropic money in this period. These included, among many, the universities of Johns Hopkins, Columbia, Chicago, Brown, Vanderbilt, and the Massachusetts Institute of Technology. Harvard did particularly well out of philanthropic money. In this way philanthropy, "The Gospel of Wealth" as it was also known, was seen as a major factor in stabilizing a volatile society.[14] Equally, through higher education, supporters of philanthropy promoted the doctrines of efficiency and of science as the instruments of progress.

For present purposes the most important of the American philanthropists were the Rockefellers (John D., Sr. and Jr.). Between the wars Rockefeller funding of clinical medicine in Britain, and Edinburgh in particular, was the tip of an iceberg of money given to medical projects all over the world, notably projects in tropical medicine. John D. Rockefeller, Sr. began giving money to various causes in a large and chaotic fashion in the 1860s. In 1891 a Baptist minister, Frederick T. Gates, took charge of Rockefeller's philanthropic affairs. In 1901, with the support of John D. Rockefeller, Jr., Gates established the General Education Board, an administrative channel for directing Rockefeller money to deserving causes, notably black schools in the South, the Board's remit being limited to the United States. At some point in the 1890s Gates considered that giving money to medicine would promote health and social harmony, an idea he said that crystallized after reading William Osler's *Principles and Practice of Medicine* in 1897. Osler's book at the time was perhaps the most accessible guide to the new scientific medicine, embracing as it did germ theory, the latter being seen as one of the great triumphs of laboratory-based medicine. Osler was one of the leading teachers of medicine in North America and Britain in the first two decades of the twentieth century. He was well known, well connected, widely admired, and very influential. He was appointed Regius

Professor of Medicine at Oxford in 1904. He died in 1919. Anyhow, apparently on account of reading Osler, Gates was taken by the notion of creating an institute for the promotion of scientific medicine. In 1901 the Rockefeller Institute for Medical Research was incorporated in New York to give grants to medical researchers. For various reasons this was not satisfactory to those involved, especially Gates. The upshot was a bricks and mortar solution. The Rockefeller Institute laboratories were officially dedicated in 1906. In 1910 the Institute acquired its own hospital where research fellows from all over the world came to learn clinical science. They were not permitted to carry out private practice. The Institute was also home to a periodical whose name proclaimed its programme, the *Journal of Experimental Medicine*.[15]

Postgraduate researchers staffed the Rockefeller Institute and no attention was paid to undergraduate medical training. Philanthropic money touched this, however, and in a big way. In Baltimore, the Johns Hopkins Hospital, which opened in 1889, and the University Medical School, which was inaugurated in 1893, combined to form an educational and research centre that was the envy of all who strove to establish academic medicine. Here full-time basic scientists taught the pre-clinical courses whereas, at this time in most American schools and many British ones such courses were still given by practising clinicians. However, the clinical professors at Hopkins, such as Osler who went there in 1889, resisted the full-time system, preferring their lucrative private practices, and claiming they were the better teachers for their wider experience. The clinical full-time issue was to be a contentious one over the years not only in America but also in Britain.[16] With Gates in control of the funds, Rockefeller monies were channelled into Hopkins and institutions that promised to model themselves on Hopkins-like lines. Some time towards the end of the first decade of the twentieth century Rockefeller and Gates turned their sights to the world stage. The institution for funnelling funds abroad was the RF, incorporated in 1913.

Besides the RF many other sources of philanthropic funding shaped American medicine in the twentieth century. The Carnegie Foundation for the Advancement of Teaching also had a major input. In 1908 the Foundation commissioned an educationalist, Abraham Flexner, to conduct an investigation into North American medical education. In 1910 the famous Flexner report appeared.[17] Taking Hopkins as his yardstick,

Flexner exposed what he saw as the comparatively dreadful standards in many American schools and he came out firmly in favour of academic medicine and the importance of the laboratory sciences in training and research.

The scale of American philanthropy should not obscure how important charitable giving was in promoting science and medicine in British universities and other institutions. Money was donated to these causes to promote British industry, to improve the education of the disadvantaged, to foster health, and "for the general good."[18] Science and medicine were also seen as valuable in running the Empire. For example, the School of Tropical Medicine at University College, Liverpool was founded on philanthropic money. The most significant domestic source of philanthropic funds invested in Edinburgh medicine in this period derived from the estate of Sir William Dunn. This was managed by trustees who consulted Walter Morley Fletcher of the MRC at every turn. Besides being directed towards Edinburgh, on Fletcher's advice Dunn money was used to establish an Institute of Biochemistry at Cambridge and an Institute of Pathology at Oxford.[19] Dunn money, however, did not compare with the Rockefeller coffers. Fletcher was the trusted advisor of the Rockefeller disbursement in Britain.

Unlike America, in Britain the state, threatened by Germany's economic and industrial growth, began to inject money into science through universities and other institutions. Colonial concerns were also a stimulus to state and philanthropic funding. Imperial College, London (the name speaks its horizons) opened in 1908 in order to furnish the Empire with scientists and engineers. In medicine too, state intervention was an agent of change. Before the First World War nothing quite like the Johns Hopkins model existed in Britain. The medical schools at the Universities of Cambridge (until 1909), Edinburgh, and University College, London with their nearby or associated hospitals might have claimed to be nearest to it. Forces were at work, however, pushing British medicine in the academic direction. In 1909 a Royal Commission under Lord Haldane was appointed to inquire into university education in London. Its first report was published in 1910 and its final report in 1913.[20] London University was an umbrella institution which, after 1900, covered all ten of the London hospital schools such as Guy's, St. Bartholomew's and St. Thomas's. These schools, however, largely acted independently of the

University. The Haldane Commission heard evidence from Abraham Flexner, who was surveying medicine in Europe. Flexner approved of the "practical" bias of British medical education but condemned its resistance to the "scientific attitude" and to "modern methods of investigation."[21] He called for a breaking of the seniority system in hospitals.[22] Nearly fifteen years later he was still commenting on how the "Briton prides himself on being 'practical'."[23]

The Haldane Commission recommended the creation of hospital units controlled by clinical professors with assistants all paid for by the University. There were to be beds under professorial control and a laboratory in close proximity to them for diagnosis and research. There was to be "some opportunity for private practice."[24] War interrupted implementation of the recommendations but in 1919–20 a combined total of nine medical and surgical units were created at four London hospitals. Further units were established in the 1920s. Unit Directors often had trouble convincing their consultant colleagues of their academic mission. Directors who were in control of diagnostic laboratories sometimes found clinicians dismissive of laboratory research and testing. The units, however, were a sign of the British state's somewhat reluctant but increasing support of medical research and teaching.

Also at work in the state promotion of academic medicine in Britain was the Medical Research Committee, founded in 1911. In 1920 it became the Council (MRC). Established to study tuberculosis, it was steered by its managing committee to fund all sorts of medical research.[25] From 1914 and throughout the 1920s, Walter Morley Fletcher was the powerful secretary of Committee and Council. Fletcher was a Cambridge-trained experimental physiologist and physician. He saw the future of medicine in the professorial system and in laboratory science, both clinical and pre-clinical, and had rather obvious contempt for older attitudes. Fletcher effectively controlled the MRC's purse strings and had a massive, and very often final, say in the way government and domestic and foreign philanthropic organizations disbursed their money in academic medicine in Britain. By the 1920s a coterie of supporters of academic medicine with Fletcher at its hub had established itself in the United Kingdom. Academic doctors often kept in close contact with each other and besides their scientific interests saw themselves promoting a medicine vital to social stability and progress. Devotion to physiology was a particularly important entrance card into this club. To have studied science at Cambridge University, England, also helped, although neither requirement was indispensable.

Notes

1. Robert Hutchison and Harry Rainy, *Clinical Methods: A Guide to the Practical Study of Medicine* (London: Cassell, 1897). There were many subsequent editions; the last co-authored by Rainy was the 8th. It appeared in 1924.

2. Christopher Lawrence, "Incommunicable Knowledge: Science, Technology and the Clinical Art in Britain 1850–1914," *Journal of Contemporary History* 20 (1985): 503–20.

3. Stephan Collini, *Public Moralists: Political Thought and Intellectual Life in Britain 1850–1930* (Oxford: Clarendon Press, 1991).

4. Richard Shannon, *The Crisis of Imperialism 1865–1915* (Frogmore: Paladin, 1976), 216.

5. I could call it scientific medicine as did many of its practitioners, but this loses the sense of those who saw the university as its institutional base.

6. Christopher Lawrence, "Moderns and Ancients: The New Cardiology in Britain 1800–1930," in *The Emergence of Modern Cardiology*, ed. W. F. Bynum, Christopher Lawrence, and V. Nutton, *Medical History*, Supplement 5 (1985): 1–33.

7. Harry M. Marks, *The Progress of Experiment: Science and Therapeutic Reform in the United States, 1900–1990* (Cambridge: Cambridge University Press, 1997).

8. An important protagonist of this revisionism has been Steve Sturdy. See his "Medical Chemistry and Clinical Medicine: Academics and the Scientisation of Medical Practice in Britain, 1900–1925," in *Medicine and Change: Historical and Sociological Studies of Medical Innovation*, ed. Ilana Löwy (Paris: Montrouge, 1993), 371–93. For his case study based on this model see "The Political Economy of Scientific Medicine: Science, Education and the Transformation of Medical Practice in Sheffield, 1890–1922," *Medical History* 36 (1992): 125–59.

9. "Pathological Departments," *The Lancet* 2 (1923): 522.

10. Keith Wailoo, *Drawing Blood: Technology and Disease Identity in Twentieth-Century America* (Baltimore: The Johns Hopkins University Press, 1997), Chapter 4.

11. The literature, too large to cite here, mostly pertains to North America. For this see, Joel D. Howell, *Technology in the Hospital: Transforming Patient Care in the Early Twentieth Century* (Baltimore: The Johns Hopkins University Press, 1995). For British material and an important interpretation see Steve Sturdy and Roger Cooter, "Science, Scientific Management and the Transformation of Medicine in Britain c.1870–1950," *History of Science* 36 (1998): 421–66. Harry Marks doubts the dating of the changes Sturdy and Cooter describe. He considers they are largely post 1900 phenomena and the 1870 date is misleading. Personal letter to author, undated.

12. On hospitals as factories see Christopher Crenner, "Organisational Reform and Professional Dissent in the Careers of Richard Cabot and Ernest Amory Codman," *Journal of the History of Medicine and Allied Sciences* 56 (2001): 211–37.

13. Cited in Howard S. Berliner, *A System of Scientific Medicine: Philanthropic Foundations in the Flexner Era* (New York: Tavistock, 1985), 136.

14. Andrew Carnegie, "The Gospel of Wealth," *North American Review*, 1889, cited in Raymond B. Fosdick, *The Story of the Rockefeller Foundation* (New York: Harper and Brothers, 1952), 5. See also Andrew Carnegie, *The Gospel of Wealth and other Timely Essays* (New York: Doubleday, Page & Co., 1905).

15. There are far too many articles and books on the relation of Rockefeller philanthropic institutions and medicine to cite here. The subject is also very contentious. Fosdick's *The Story of the Rockefeller Foundation* is an insider's version (he was President of the RF for twelve years) By contrast a Marxist version can be found in (among others) E. Richard Brown, *Rockefeller Medical Men: Medicine and Capitalism in America* (Berkeley: University of California Press, 1979).

16. For full-time chairs in North American and British universities in 1925 see, Abraham Flexner, *Medical Education. A Comparative Study* (New York: The Macmillan Company, 1925), 48–51. For a study of the changes in medical education in this period see, Thomas Neville Bonner, *Becoming a Physician: Medical Education in Britain, France, Germany, and the United States, 1750–1945* (New York: Oxford University Press, 1995).

17. Abraham Flexner, *Medical Education in the United States and Canada*, Bulletin no. 4 (New York: Carnegie Foundation for the Advancement of Teaching, 1910).

18. Peter Alter, *The Reluctant Patron: Science and the State in Britain 1850–1920* (Oxford: Berg, 1987), 53.

19. Sir William Dunn was a Scottish-born banker and London Alderman who died in 1912 and left his fortune to charity. It was managed by trustees. See Robert E. Kohler, "Walter Fletcher, F. G. Hopkins, and the Dunn Institute of Biochemistry: A Case Study in the Patronage of Science," *Isis* 69 (1978): 331–35.

20. Royal Commission on University Education in London, *Final Report*, 1913 (Cd. 6718), Parliamentary Papers, vol. xxiii: 543.

21. Abraham Flexner, *Medical Education in Europe*, Bulletin no. 6 (New York: Carnegie Foundation for the Advancement of Teaching, 1912), 66.

22. George Graham, "The Formation of the Medical and Surgical Professorial Units in the London Teaching Hospitals," *Annals of Science* 26 (1970): 1–22. Flexner on seniority at 3.

23. Flexner, *Medical Education. A Comparative Study*, 242.

24. Graham, "The Formation of the Medical and Surgical Professorial Units," 9.

25. See the essays in *Historical Perspectives on the Role of the MRC: Essays in the History of the Medical Research Council of the United Kingdom and its Predecessor, the Medical Research Committee, 1913–1953*, ed. Joan Austoker and Linda Bryder (New York: Oxford University Press 1989).

3

THE ROCKEFELLER FOUNDATION AND THE CULTURE OF BRITISH MEDICINE

RF perceptions of Britain require understanding within two wider frameworks, one encompassing the other. First is RF global policy and strategy. Perceptions of, and interventions in, British medicine were not simply local but very much a part of a panoramic view. Second, RF global policy itself needs situating within America's social, political, economic, and cultural relations with Europe, and indeed much of the world, in the first decades of the twentieth century. To deal with the latter first: in a valuable corrective to the thesis of American exceptionalism, Daniel T. Rodgers has argued that in areas of social policy (poor relief, housing, town planning, workmen's insurance etc.) from the 1870s Americans were deeply interested in European ideas and practices.[1] Indeed, before 1914 the arrow of what was deemed progressive change ran largely from Europe to America. American interest in European ideas continued during and after the war. However, matters were different. After 1918 (and a little before), on both sides of the Atlantic, the word "reconstruction" was on everyone's lips. Americans were concerned to reconstruct at home and later they pressed to be involved in the reconstruction of Europe. After the armistice, American intervention in Europe was devoted to relief; for example the American Red Cross was involved in picking up the pieces in war-torn France. Later, however, relief turned to reconstruction and, to take the example of France again, attempts were made to rebuild villages and towns in conformity with the Europe of the American imagination.[2] But, as is well known, the 1920s also saw a changed relationship with America, notably in the importation into Europe of American engineering techniques and mass-produced consumer goods. This development was identified by many as an aspect of modernism. "Fordism," the assembly line production of standardized goods, was a key term of the decade. America's mass production economy, which was seen to serve the needs of the many rather than the few, was welcomed by progressives in Europe as an important post-war development and a milestone in economic and social growth. Technology and organization were seen jointly as the key to "an orderly community of abundance."[3] Conservatives, however, saw in the transatlantic commodity invasion a destruction of traditional European culture. "The fear of American influence," writes Siân Nicholas, "was one of the most striking features of British cultural discourse in the interwar years."[4]

American medicine replicates several of the themes noted above. Before the war American doctors and educationalists were anxious to take from Europeans, particularly the Germans, ideas they could implement at home. Gradually in these years the reconstruction of American medicine was begun. This was pushed ahead after 1918 but now with little reference to contemporary European ideas. American doctors who favoured reconstruction saw themselves as the bearers of modernity. After the war the flow of medical ideas and practices was largely from America to Europe. Just as American aid to Europe after the war was at first confined to general relief measures, so too the RF was at first involved in the giving of medical aid to assist the victims of epidemics and malnutrition. Such valuable assistance helped ameliorate distress but was unlikely to change medical thinking, institutions, and practice. Fairly quickly the RF's strategy, which had already been formulated and which bore all the American hallmarks of standardization and uniformity, was worked out in practice as a way of reconstructing medicine on a world scale. There was, it could be said, a "Fordism" in the RF's approach to medicine. And just as there was a European suspicion of the new American culture at large so there was also resistance to the RF's strategies and goals. To some extent resistances to modernism (identified with America) and to modernism in medicine (identified with academic medicine and by implication often the RF) were part of a common ideology although they were not inseparable.

A number of historiographical points about the RF's programme merit mention. It is well known that the RF launched a massive international scientific and medical programme between the wars.[5] In less developed countries the main thrust of that programme was in public health and in particular the eradication of diseases such as hookworm and yellow fever. In western Europe millions of Rockefeller dollars went into medical education and in attempts to create university clinics on the Johns Hopkins model. Useful as the distinction is between public health and medical education (for it was embodied in two different administrative sections of the RF) it obscures the common approach shared wherever Rockefeller money went (including rural and urban America). The medical education strategy that was to be so important in Edinburgh was governed by the same philosophy that ruled the public health programme. Public health and medical education reform went hand in hand. Disease eradication campaigns were not confined to non-western countries. Malaria was targeted in Italy and tuberculosis (TB) in France, for example. One of the first post-war initiatives combined medical education reform and public health programmes in a very obvious way. In the 1920s Rockefeller money was used to establish the London School of Hygiene and Tropical Medicine, a postgraduate school within the University of London.[6] Conversely the restructuring of medical education was not a goal limited to Europe. The RF established or helped promote its vision of the modern medical school in, for example, Beirut, Sao Paulo, Hong Kong, Singapore, Bangkok and Peking (now Beijing). Laboratory science was central to both the public health and medical education enterprises. However, Rockefeller solutions were by no means seen (except on 61 Broadway—the RF headquarters) as appropriate, timeless, objective interventions. Everywhere they encountered resistance based on alternative, local ways of problem solving. In this respect Edinburgh was no different from Fiji. These resistances were not simply responses to American medicine but were sometimes responses to what was perceived as American cultural imperialism in general.

The two names that most frequently crop up in connection with the RF and medical education in the 1920s are George E. Vincent, President of the Foundation after 1917, and Richard M. Pearce, Director, from the beginning, of the Division of Medical Education established in December 1919. He remained there until his death in 1930. Pearce had formerly been Professor of Pathology and Research Medicine at the University of Pennsylvania. Also important was Alan Gregg, Pearce's right-hand man, who became Director of the new Division of Medical Sciences after Pearce's death. Pearce strove for a single global policy. In 1925 he was lamenting the hotchpotch he had inherited and that he had been unable to "work out" a "consistent program" for, and he gave as examples, Brazil, Siam (now Thailand), the Far East, Brussels and Copenhagen.[7]

Analysis of RF strategy in non-western countries between the wars brings into sharp focus assumptions which were also at work in medical education in the western world. RF international intervention also merits attention because it shows how there was an attempt to solve national problems by applying what were seen as universal answers based on science: in other words American technocratic solutions. The Foundation's overall aim, it has been argued, "was rationalization and homogenization: of populations, of scientific approaches, and of scientific methods."[8] In 1913, the newly-established Foundation created an International Health Commission, which became a Board in 1916 and a Division in 1927. After becoming President of the Foundation, Vincent immediately launched a massive, integrated global programme in public health and medical education.[9] The scale of Rockefeller international intervention is staggering. Practically every country in the world received some form of assistance although those with strong colonial governments were touched least.

The RF's stated intentions were always the promotion of the cause of human betterment through science and education. In Foundation policy the physician and scientist were favoured over, say, the economist or urban planner as the agents of change. The technology of the vaccine or the insecticide efficiently administered was seen as the most progressive of social forces. Disease was construed as *the* major obstacle to improvement. Poverty in Rockefeller eyes was largely a consequence of rather than a cause of disease. This was evident in the justification of the hookworm programme in Mexico. The Mexican freed of debilitating hookworm disease, it was said by a Rockefeller officer in 1925, would have "more money in his pocket with which to buy better food, better clothes, better homes and better schools. With better schools there will come enlightenment. Intelligence will displace ignorance, and with intelligence there will come a true social revolution."[10] Such a goal, however, was not based upon the promotion of local tradition. The Foundation was keen to show that "the American 'way of health' was an especially efficient way to advance goals such as modernization or increased economic efficiency."[11] Generally, and certainly in the Edinburgh case, the word "tradition" was anathema to the Foundation. It is not too far-fetched to describe the Foundation's ideology as religious, indeed messianic. In 1923 Pearce, writing of the prospects of change in Edinburgh, observed, "I think we can do valuable missionary work [here]."[12] The RF possibly also saw itself as waging war (perhaps a holy one) for the cause of academic medicine. In 1923 Pearce thanked Walter Fletcher for supplying "ammunition in connection with my present program for Great Britain."[13] Fletcher's language, too, was suffused with military and imperial metaphors, and visions of mastery. The advance of modern medicine was owing to its "great army of workers."[14] Unlike experimental enquiry, he said, the clinical art had failed to "bring any essentially new powers of dominion over the natural processes of disease and recovery."[15]

The RF public health programme largely targeted diseases with relatively well-defined incidence, obvious injurious socio-economic effects, and an etiological agent that was known or whose mode of transmission was known. By and large these diseases were susceptible to laboratory investigation and were eradicable by some combination of vaccines, straightforward public health measures, and education. Hookworm, yellow fever, and malaria roughly fulfilled these criteria. Leprosy and TB, in which there was clearly some extremely complicated relation to the socio-economic causes of poverty, did not. Except for the slightly odd case of France, TB was never the focus of a major programme. The Foundation consistently refused to get involved with TB in Mexico, a country to which it paid a great deal of attention and where a successful yellow fever eradication programme had been organized.[16]

The RF was inflexible, obsessive almost, about the methods and standards it approved of and funded. Public health schools were supported by the Foundation when they conformed to the model of the School of Hygiene and Public Health at the Johns Hopkins University. The Foundation had funded this institution, which opened in 1918, to train public health experts who worked throughout the world. In the field only the best qualified and up-to-date experts were countenanced and only what were seen as the most scientific of methods were approved. Organization was a high priority. The Foundation aimed at what it deemed were universal, stateless solutions to public health matters. The tropical medicine programme, which largely began by instituting prophylactic and therapeutic measures, increasingly incorporated laboratory investigations, especially at the Rockefeller Institute in New York, until then largely concerned with the diseases of industrial society.

Not surprisingly Foundation policy ran into enormous local difficulties. On the one hand Rockefeller intervention was seen as part of sinister American imperialism, on the other it simply did not work because it ignored (frequently deliberately) local practices. Problems were encountered with cultures that apparently shared enthusiasm for modern scientific approaches. The French TB programme looked, even to observers at the time, like a dialogue of the deaf.[17] RF support for French medical education quickly conflicted with Gallic approaches.[18] The Irish programme stumbled over a number of factors, principally because the Irish made the common mistake of thinking the RF would dole out money regardless of any scheme proposed. Second, medicine in Dublin, like Edinburgh, was then controlled by several different bodies, not just a university, something the RF found hard to deal with. Rockefeller men (in one unfortunate case, Gregg), conversely, occasionally showed a crass understanding of Irish politics and sometimes treated the country as though it were part of England.[19] RF confidence in its own programmes and lack of sensibility to national sentiments is indicated by Pearce's confession that he "didn't know Europe."[20] Its single-mindedness was well illustrated in Fiji. Sylvester M. Lambert was a Rockefeller representative in the South Pacific where hookworm, yaws, and malaria were endemic and western medical practitioners were few. Lambert campaigned to train local practitioners to a minimal level. They understood local customs and would therefore, the argument ran, be able to dispense basic public health advice. He reported that his plan gave Pearce and the New York office "almost physical nausea." Pearce insisted that Rockefeller "must stick to the policy of aiding only Class A schools."[21] This tone will be heard again in relation to Edinburgh. The RF in New York thus sometimes strained relations with its own local agents, medical organizations of all sorts, and also foreign governments. India supplies a case history of the latter sort of tension; in this case the government was the British one.[22]

In every sphere RF strategy was to identify what it saw as far-sighted institutions and individuals whose leadership, research, and teaching could be expected, with encouragement, to follow American lines. In public health the Foundation granted fellowships, supported travel, created experts, arranged international meetings, and established institutes and clinics. A scheme for training statisticians began in the early 1920s, indicating the Foundation's awareness of the importance of creating international uniformity as a road to political stability (it also contributed generously to the League of Nations to which the USA did not belong). In the medical education division, Pearce targeted particular schools that looked the most likely to reform themselves on lines the Foundation approved. He then dealt with hand-picked individuals within those institutions. Promising researchers were awarded fellowships to travel to America and study, mainly at Hopkins and the Rockefeller Institute. Always, laboratory research and education were to be entwined in any institution the Foundation aided.

The question obviously arises: to what extent was the Foundation an instrument of American interests? The answer is that it was, but not in any obvious way. RF employees saw themselves as furthering social progress by employing universal approaches based on objective science. None the less these approaches, however universal they were proclaimed to be, were the modern American way of doing things and were seen as such by many both at home and abroad. The word "Rockefeller" was not held in high regard in many corners of American government nor by many members of the US public. The RF itself was seen by some as anti-American, as a charitable cover for furthering industrial strategies. In the midst of the philanthropic public health programmes there was a strike of mine workers in Colorado where the Rockefellers had interests that culminated in the "Ludlow massacre" of 1914 in which many were killed. This did the Rockefeller name little good.

American commercial and economic interests did, knowingly or not, follow Rockefeller enterprises. This was particularly true of South America. Sometimes Rockefeller officials were more forthcoming than they knew about their policies. As one observed in 1917: "Dispensaries and physicians have of late been peacefully penetrating areas of the Philippine islands and demonstrating the fact that for the purposes of placating primitive and suspicious peoples medicine has some advantages over machine guns."[23] Political considerations and American interests were ever present but not often crudely visible. Generosity did not flow equably. The Soviets were denied aid even for famine and typhus relief in 1921. Yet the Foundation's position with regard to Russia looks less like anti-Communist dogma than recognition of the impossibility of running things in that country in the way it preferred.[24]

In Europe Rockefeller officials walked a delicate tightrope between intervening in the affairs of nation states and promoting peace and international collaboration by the alleviation of ill health. As noted, soon after the war the Foundation's international strategy was shorn of short-term relief measures, such as feeding programmes, and directed towards long-term goals. A great deal of its energy was aimed at modernizing public health in politically unstable areas, notably Poland and what it called Central (otherwise Eastern) Europe. Yugoslavia was a major beneficiary of this programme. A State School of Hygiene was established in Poland in 1926 on the Hopkins model, half funded by Rockefeller and half by the Polish state. Such intervention, whether designed as political or not, served American (and western European interests). These regions were literally and metaphorically a cordon sanitaire—a buffer against invasions of both armed forces and epidemic diseases.[25] Thus local measures had wider ends built into them. Equally, in post-war Britain and the Empire, RF largesse besides effecting immediate medical reform was intended to help bring stability and to deliver conditions for the growth of the "community of abundance." It was certainly seen in this way by the donors and some of the recipients even if was not always formulated in those terms.

Pearce's division began its dealings with Britain after the war. Although Rockefeller observers occasionally made distinctions between the north and south of Britain, by and large they viewed the island as having a common (including a common medical) culture. To natives, however, there were important differences depending on which side of the Anglo-Caledonian border you were standing. In line with their view of Britain as homogeneous, Americans often used the words British and English (or Britain and England) synonymously, so when the words are used it is not always easy to know if Scotland is included or not. Usually it should be assumed that it is. To be fair this conflation of national identities was a habit the Americans had picked up from the British themselves (and not only the English). Bonar Law, half Scottish and half Canadian by birth, called himself "Prime Minister of England."[26]

London, as capital of the British Empire, was one of Rockefeller's principal targets for medical reform. Edinburgh was another since its medical school turned out so many doctors who served the Empire.[27] In Britain, as elsewhere, the Foundation employed a policy as good as carved in stone: it negotiated only with universities and, if essential, government, and it only funded or founded institutions within a university. Equally noteworthy about the way the Foundation operated is that the individuals that it targeted and worked with often had greater allegiance to academic medicine at large than to their domestic institutions.

First I explore RF perceptions of British medicine in general, surveying changing attitudes and policy towards Oxford, Cambridge, and London in the 1920s. The Oxbridge and London context is essential for understanding the attitudes of Fletcher, who felt at home in the rarefied scientific atmosphere of Cambridge. In London he circulated among academic clinicians and basic scientists but he was often locked in conflict with the medical elite of the hospitals and the Royal College of Physicians and that of the Surgeons.[28] His diplomatic skills should not be forgotten, however. He could smooth the ruffled feathers of crusty surgeons, such as Sir Berkeley Moynihan, with relative ease.[29] A crucial part of the story of Rockefeller intervention in Britain was the close links that were forged between the RF and the MRC. Pearce and Fletcher obviously had high regard for each other. Like Fletcher, Pearce was a canny administrator (and something of a cold fish). He saw eye to eye with Fletcher on most matters and used him as his confidante in all questions of Rockefeller disbursement in Britain. Conventions are important for decoding levels of confidence and friendship in correspondence in this period. When correspondents write, "Dear Fletcher," "Dear Meakins," "Dear Pearce," or whoever, a level of intimacy beyond the formal can be assumed.

Much communication that is beyond the historian's reach is going on elsewhere (often in London clubs, especially the Athenaeum). On the other hand correspondence beginning, "Dear Dr. Fletcher," "Dear Professor Murray Lyon," conveys that relations are being maintained at a formal level.

American academic clinicians associated with the RF did not think much of British medical education, staffing structures, the organization of research, and hospital administration. In September 1922 the Foundation sent two distinguished academic practitioners to Britain for over two months to report on medical education in its universities and hospital medical schools. Evarts Graham was Professor of Surgery at St. Louis and David Edsall was a physician and Dean of Harvard. Their stay, said Edsall, was "Thundering hard work."[30] Their reports were wide-ranging and paid close attention to the relations between the basic sciences, particularly physiology and biochemistry, and bedside medicine.

The tone of Graham's report might be judged from the comments of President Vincent, who saw Graham on his return in December 1922. Vincent wrote: "Graham, of St. Louis, turned up the other day and gave a most unfavorable description of medical education in England. One got the impression that he regarded it in all respects as inferior to our system."[31] Graham's report did indeed paint a dismal picture of British medical education if compared with the American academic ideal. Indeed a contrast with America was frequently made in his report. He began: "The American visitor to the London schools is impressed [i.e. shocked] at once by the fact that the clinical teaching is much more casual than in the better of the American schools. The students are apparently instructed less and are allowed to shift for themselves more than is the case in America." The fragmentation of medical care disappointed him. He noted: "The American and German custom of having a more or less autocratic head in charge of a clinical department does not exist in the British schools." The description "autocratic" held no fears for him as it did for some British practitioners. He lamented that: "The result of this system is that in each hospital there are several units more or less completely isolated from each other, and the quality of the work done by one unit may be distinctly inferior to that of another in contiguous wards."[32] In a report on medical education of 1925, Abraham Flexner made a similar criticism. Under conditions of isolation, he wrote, "university ideals and activities are on the clinical side impossible."[33] A consequence of this seemingly fragmented system was soon apparent to Graham: "One striking difference between the British and American schools which results from the relatively small size of the British staffs is the tendency towards less specialization than is the case in many of the American schools." He was astonished to discover that "a chief of service [not a British term] is expected to have equal interest and skill in treating a case of brain tumor, a prostatic obstruction, a lung suppuration or club feet." For Graham this was a criticism, for many Britons it would have been a compliment. He pointed to the expressed preference for generalism among British consultants: "Many of the leaders of British surgery decry the American tendency of what they call over-specialization. They argue that an individual who confines his work to one field must of necessity become narrow and constricted in his point of view and that many patients entrusted to his care will suffer accordingly." Poor organization of care, Graham thought, ran to poor administration: "The records made by the dressers, and even the permanent records of the hospitals, are very much inferior to the records in American hospitals." Such record keeping precluded "*systematic study.*" Graham also noted the paternalism fostered by the staff of the famous hospitals: "The great age of many of the hospitals (800 years, for example, in the case of St. Bartholomew's and more than 700 years in the case of St. Thomas') has created a traditional halo of reverence for the institution among the poor of the neighborhood which is practically unknown in America."[34] "Reverence" from the poor was expected by many patricians (although some were shocked by it). It was the reciprocal obligation entailed by *noblesse oblige*.

Graham then turned to what he saw as the cause of neglect of physiological science on British wards: the stress that was laid on morbid anatomy. "The British surgeon," Graham wrote, "is at his best when confronted with the problem of the diagnosis and operative relief of a purely anatomical lesion. He shows himself less favorable when confronted with a physiological problem." The British trained surgeon, he added, "seems to think almost solely in terms of anatomical lesions and tends to disregard functional defects. He is less of a philosopher and more of a craftsman." Many British surgeons might not have demurred, seeing their "craft" as analogous to the physicians' "art". Graham observed: "In spite of the fact that the British physiologists lead the world, they seem to have had but little influence on the surgeons." This absence of a physiological point of view was, he said, "shown very strikingly in a variety of ways." Notably insofar as "Functional tests and the newer blood chemistry which are so commonly used in America, especially with reference to the kidney, seem to be almost unknown to the British surgeons." This he identified as part of a general attitude: "Except in the case of routine examinations of the urine, laboratory methods are used in the minority of cases. Many patients, even the majority in some hospitals, do not even have a blood examination of any kind. Patients who are obviously anemic are allowed to spend weeks in a hospital without even a single examination of the hemoglobin content or a count of the red blood cells." He went on: "The more complicated blood examinations, such as the Wassermann test, the determination of the blood urea or the non-protein nitrogen, the estimation of the blood sugar, etc., are performed in only exceptional instances." In general, he thought, "There seems to exist among the surgeons a feeling that laboratory examinations are unnecessary."[35]

Some British clinicians would, of course, have found this position acceptable for a number of reasons. Graham explained:

> The teachers in the medical schools defend their lack of emphasis on lab-oratory aids and special procedures in diagnosis on the ground that their function is to train general practitioners and men who will go to remote corners of the British Empire to practice surgery. They state that these men must depend very largely upon ordinary methods of physical exam-ination for their diagnoses because complicated laboratory facilities will not be available.

There was a second reason:

> They declare also that they think Americans are going to extremes in their excessive use of laboratory methods, often, they imply to the exclusion of the sound and well-tried methods of inspection, palpation, percussion and auscultation. They hold the opinion that the American student is prone to accept a diagnosis based on laboratory methods even when such a diagnosis is contradicted by the plain clinical facts, that he is therefore liable often to be needlessly in error or hopelessly confused and that without elaborate laboratory paraphernalia he is at sea.

Graham's disappointment did not only extend to the routine use of science on the ward. He complained: "There is little of any surgical research being done in Great Britain which is experimental and which is likely to contribute any new knowledge to the question of function, in other words to the subject of physiology."[36]

David Edsall, who spent the months from October 1922 to January 1923 visiting Britain, was only slightly more complimentary than Graham. Before he had finished his trip to London, Edsall had formed a poor impression. He understood "pretty clearly" after three weeks why London physicians "have contributed so little to clinical medicine" and "how little they comprehend (those that have been over here) our methods and standards." He was "quite clear" in his mind "that we are producing a better product clinically and especially a more broadly and soundly trained man." Edsall felt too, "we [also] produce many more of the advanced fine type."[37] In his final report, like Graham, he bemoaned the lack of a physiological approach to disease in Britain. The rot started early on: "Most of the students seem to me to know their physiology when they come into clinical medicine distinctly less well than our students and to have little comprehension of the clinical applications of physiology." He had no doubt where the problem originated. It was "in considerable part due to a fact that . . . British clinicians, as a class, devote much less attention to physiology in their teaching and in the work in the wards than do a large group of clinical teachers at present active in this country, particularly the younger group of clinicians." Edsall found it "strange that the physiological aspects of disease—the living aspects—receive so little attention in most British clinics (with a few exceptions) when so many British clinical teachers have passed through an exceptionally fine physiological atmosphere in their early training." His suggestion as to the cause of this was that "clinical investigative interests have remained largely [confined to] descriptive pathology." Edsall found a further reason for neglect of physiology on the ward, which was, paradoxically, "the magnificent progress of English physiology as a science." It was "abstruse and more separated from the problems of the patient."[38]

Like Graham, Edsall encountered suspicion of laboratory tests. He recorded that "It is a common feeling apparently among London clinicians in particular, but also elsewhere, that it is even rather foolish and unwise to teach students skill in, and real comprehension of the effective laboratory methods of clinical diagnosis, as they will not use them." Americans, of course, did things differently: "I have had some of the most distinguished British clinicians express surprise and obvious doubt when I told them that these things were done either by themselves or by technicians employed by them, in a large portion of cases amongst the good general practitioners in this country." When British students did learn clinical testing, Edsall deplored the fact that they learnt the practices away from the ward and patients. He noted: "In the English hospitals a very customary method is to have the clinical laboratory work done by the pathological service and in such instances the students have a period of time devoted to pathological clerking and part of this period is spent in learning and practicing these methods, the students doing the simpler clinical laboratory examinations under the supervision of the pathologist, while the pathologist does the more difficult ones."

The result was that, "In such instances the clinical service does not make these examinations at all, unless some individual happens to care to do so in his cases, but sends requests for all blood examinations and the like to the pathological service and gets reports back." This method of teaching, he observed, "wholly detaches the matter . . . from its natural place in clinical work and robs both the students and the clinical staff of the constant practice in doing these things and in interpreting the significance of the findings in individual cases."[39]

For rather different reasons many senior British physicians also deplored this practice and insisted on performing all their own tests. This was done, however, in the name of clinical individualism. For example, Thomas (Tommy), Lord Horder, a St. Bartholomew's Hospital physician, the man considered the greatest diagnostician of the age, considered the clinician who carried out his own tests was "independent of his surroundings."[40] On one occasion he recounted how, very recently "a patient told me that an eminent specialist in tropical diseases kept him waiting more than two hours whilst his blood, sputum and stools were searched [by the specialist] for parasites."[41] But it was not only the organization of testing that irritated Edsall for, he wrote, "Nearly everywhere I found a feeling that we teach students in this country, and do ourselves, an actually undesirable amount of clinical laboratory work, and I was repeatedly told with some satisfaction that they [British teachers] minimized the clinical laboratory and its results deliberately in the students' minds and advised them not to depend upon it."[42]

Edsall used the word "utilitarian" pejoratively several times to describe many aspects of British medicine, by which he seemed to indicate practical or pragmatic and lacking in theory. For example, he recorded that, "I have not emphasized . . . as much as I feel disposed to do, the utilitarian spirit that is often very prominent, in some of the pathological departments especially, and I think it is important to make emphatic a very curiously disappointing utilitarian spirit that pervades a great deal of the medical teaching in a considerable proportion of the schools that I visited, most of all in the clinical work." His contempt for this system manifested itself in his estimation of the product: "The English student often impressed me as a courageous bluffer."[43]

Graham and Edsall were specific as well as general in their criticisms. In December 1922 on Graham's return, President Vincent wrote to Pearce: "Graham spoke of University College as the worst school he visited." Graham thought C. C. Choyce, Director of the Surgical Unit, "mediocre and unimaginative" and the pathologist A. E. Boycott "indifferent to teaching and lacking interest in students." Graham considered Thomas Lewis, without doubt the most distinguished British clinical scientist of the day, "so absorbed in research as almost to resent the presence of students." Generally he found "all the personnel doing little reading and showing slight familiarity with current developments in scientific medicine and educational methods."[44] In spite of all this the Foundation had great expectations that University College London (UCL) and University College Hospital (UCH) would be the flagships of academic medicine. First, because UCH was the only hospital in London built to provide a university faculty with teaching facilities. Second, T. R. Elliott, Director of the Medical Unit, had been invested with most of the hopes for bringing the new medicine to London. Elliott was a personal friend of Fletcher's and like him a graduate of Trinity College, Cambridge, rigorously trained in physiology. To be fair too, Pearce did not agree with "the Graham analysis of the University College group."[45] None the less, Vincent had told Pearce, "the situation calls for your most diplomatic and ingenious methods of analysis, suggestion, and redirection."[46]

A few weeks later, still backing investment in UCL and UCH, Vincent described how tradition governed the speed of the wheels of change in the Old World. He wrote to Pearce: "One quite understands that growth, especially in Britain, cannot take place very rapidly. Your experience in China will give you patience."[47] Two days after this Pearce recorded in his diary that his British allies were sympathetic to his goals. Of Elliott and Fletcher, Pearce recorded that "both admit the accuracy of his [Edsall's] criticism and are grateful to him for his many suggestions." Graham they found "not very helpful" but his criticisms "essentially correct."[48] Edsall was, indeed, the more optimistic of the two observers. Just before his return he wrote to Vincent that although he was "greatly disappointed in the actual clinical methods and the product," he thought "valuable suggestions can be got" from British training in schools and the early stages of medical education.[49]

In February 1923, Alan Gregg, Pearce's right-hand man since 1922 and eventual successor, reported the comments of "Dr. Rose" on Edsall's impressions.[50] Gregg thought Rose's account "explained in a way the impression which I had from working with the Englishmen during the war. They seemed to have ability to think on any subject as well as they reasoned in the field of medicine." At first sight English doctors might have taken this as a compliment. It seemed to indicate medical reasoning was not distinct from that all-round mental acuity which they valued so highly. Gregg's gloss on his remark, however, was that: "Their work in the wards had a curious lack of desire to observe closely and to be as definite and complete in working up a case as was possible. I attributed that to the effect of three years of war, and it may be indeed that war was the cause of their clinical attitude . . . their training may have had a good deal to do with it." "They seemed," he went on, "to be quite unconscious, or better careless, of the fact that rare conditions exist more frequently than they are recognized." He said, "There was also a great deal of talk of passing of examinations." There was also, he observed, probably accurately, "a very strong professional solidarity against the laity, together with a very strict sense of the proprieties within the profession and an amazing bitterness against confreres who broke with this tradition." He concluded, "I had the impression that I wouldn't mind being sick in England if it could only be a common disease."[51]

In February 1923 Edsall sent Pearce what he had "thus far written of the report." Edsall summed up what he thought of British medicine. He complained of the students' "lack of knowledge of the tools of physical diagnosis and clinical laboratory work when they begin medicine." He criticized the British for devoting "a disproportionate amount of time to gross morbid anatomy" while in the clinic they neglected physiology and "living dynamic pathology." He thought British final year students had "an attitude toward medicine and a knowledge of it" not very different to Americans finishing their third year.[52] Not every American academic clinician took this point of view. Harvey Cushing, perhaps America's most distinguished surgeon and virtual creator of neurosurgery as a speciality, condemned the new emphasis on the pre-clinical sciences and favoured lots of practical clinical work.[53]

Unlike Edsall, Graham seems to have delivered only a preliminary verbal report and he apologized to Pearce in July 1923 for not having sent a full written version.[54] However, Edsall's final document had not yet been delivered either. Graham's was being typed up in October when he reported that Sir George Newman, Chief Medical Officer of the Ministry of Health, and the Edinburgh surgeon, Sir Harold Stiles, were anxious to see it. Pearce received the final report in the same month.[55] By mid-November Edsall was apologizing for his tardiness. By the end of that month Pearce had read Graham's report and had given him permission to send copies to Newman and Stiles.[56] Edsall's report was not sent to Pearce until mid December.[57] Pearce artfully suggested the reports be sent to Elliott and Newman so that if they were published "we could state that the criticism of English authorities had been considered and if necessary they could be included as footnotes."[58] It is not surprising that Edsall's report was sent to Fletcher and even less surprising is that Fletcher was "very enthusiastic," in the sense that he agreed with its criticisms and it supported his position.[59]

Meanwhile, anticipating a negative response from Sir George Newman, Edsall sought to query Newman's credentials. Edsall wrote to Pearce that the "main question I have is whether Newman really knows enough about education, which I somewhat seriously question from my conversations with him."[60] Newman, in fact, took a keen interest in medical education but, although a reformer in some ways, he was a great admirer of an English clinical tradition.[61] He did not see eye to eye with Fletcher on research and valued natural history in the ward as much as animal experimentation in the lab.[62] Newman sent his comments in January 1924. Among many observations his principal one was that the

American method "seems to me to have all the advantages if you are going to make Professors and Specialists of all your men, but it is less good for making [general] practitioners."[63] After seeing this comment and similar ones Edsall wrote to Pearce: "Nor do I think they [the British] get at all the fact that we are teaching them [medical students] science, not in order to make scientists of them, but to make better clinicians of them."[64]

Elliott, like Fletcher, was enthusiastic about Edsall's survey. His comments were virtually the reverse of those of the British clinicians cited in the report. His praise for America was for its educating large numbers of all-round competent practitioners. His condemnation of British education was based on its concentration on producing an elite, highly-skilled few. His political language is revealing. In our educational methods he wrote to Edsall, "we were only thinking of chances for the best men. And we cared little about the average crowd. Aristocracy and democracy again!" Combining this with another British analogy he went on, "your demands in democratic America are different: you ask for the highest standard of all, knowing that a rigid discipline by unyielding high standards can raise an ordinary body of men to such a great height of courage and efficiency as is shown by every man in a regiment of our guards."[65]

While all this was going on Pearce was labouring away at what he called his "program" for medical reform in Britain. This centred on Oxford, Cambridge, London, Cardiff, and Edinburgh. Elite scientific opinion in the inter-war years regarded Oxbridge as different from universities elsewhere. This sentiment was concisely expressed in a letter from the Trinity graduate, Fletcher, to Pearce in 1923. Fletcher told Pearce: "It is not realised easily in other countries that Oxford and Cambridge are not merely the two senior Universities among others, but occupy a wholly special position." Fletcher explained that this was because "Their ancient endowments, and the special glamour of their reputations and of the amenities of life within them, tend to draw to them the ablest brains among all classes of the community from the very poorest upwards, and from all parts of the United Kingdom." Stressing to an American his perception of what he saw as the meritocratic nature of these institutions (which was only true to a limited extent) Fletcher described how "The ablest young students in London compete for scholarships at Oxford and Cambridge, and so do very numerous boys from Scotland, as well as young graduates of the Scottish Universities." "The significance of this," he said,

> is well illustrated by the example of the Physiology Department of the University College, London, of which the reputation under Starling and Bayliss has been so high for a quarter of a century. In the whole of that time Starling has never produced a valuable research worker, or even his own demonstrators, from among London students. His best men have always been those coming to him from Oxford or Cambridge, chiefly the latter, or from abroad.

Fletcher felt the same about pathology. This he saw as an "independent science" just like physiology. He lamented its "subservience within hospitals": that is, its morbid anatomical approach and control by clinicians rather than its having an experimental orientation and a place in basic science departments. Pathology, he believed, "suffers chiefly from the fact that it enjoys little or no effective recruitment to the subject at Oxford and Cambridge."[66] Fletcher had his generally low opinion of British medicine confirmed by Edsall's report. He told Edsall he was "perfectly right . . . in detecting the two classes here into which medical students here are divided,—the small group of really well educated men, chiefly from Oxford and Cambridge, and the other much larger group."[67]

Following a British trip in 1923 Pearce returned home in "good form" since, on the boat, "alcohol supplies ran out early." Pearce thought Fletcher's account of Oxbridge would be invaluable in promoting reform.[68] There was no certainty the RF programme would succeed, however; indeed there was the possibility of complete reversal in some areas. In 1924 Vincent had heard that it was "reported that all the surgical units in Great Britain will be abandoned except the one at University College, which will be maintained because of our gift to that center."[69]

Although in London RF assistance centred primarily on UCL and UCH, other hospitals where there were professorial units, St. Bartholomew's, the London, and St. Thomas's also received grants. At the London Hospital, Rockefeller money helped rationalize laboratory space. Perhaps signalling his secular missionary zeal, Pearce reported to Vincent in 1923 that, "wonderful to relate, an old chapel is to be encroached upon in order to make modern laboratory space."[70] By 1925, Pearce was apparently developing confidence that his programme for British medicine might be coming to fruition. Revealing his plans and achievements to Gregg he indicated the importance of the British Empire in his vision. Although his projects were framed solely in medical terms, Pearce no doubt saw medicine as promoting political stability in the inter-war world. He said that in the light of his "knowledge of conditions in a number of the dominions and colonies, I studied in England, Scotland and Wales the laboratories and clinics which should in the long run influence medical work in the empire."[71]

Fletcher too saw medical advance based on experimental science as crucial to the health, prosperity, and stability of the Empire. In a radio broadcast he said that failure of government to take "full account of the science of living things" had meant that "we have been handicapped as a nation in the past, and are to-day being heavily handicapped, both in our government at home and in the administration of India and other parts of our Empire overseas."[72] "There can be no right government of any part of our Empire," he wrote, "and no true advance of the industries and people within it except in the light of truth . . . in the fundamental matters of human life, [and] of animal and vegetable life."[73] In his writings on Empire, Fletcher was especially fond of substituting English for British, and England for Britain. This was ironic considering how particularly prominent the Scots had been and were in imperial expansion and administration.

Of his endeavours on behalf of British domestic and imperial medicine, Pearce wrote, perhaps immodestly:

> *I* have been able to work a program, which *I* considered wise for the empire, the dominions and colonies . . . *I* decided that an outstanding institute of anatomy serving the empire should be established, and this was established at University College. *I* decided that there must be a similar center for pathology, and this is being established at Cambridge. *I* decided . . . it was advisable to supplement this by a center for physiological chemistry at Oxford. This is under way . . . Again, in London *I* decided that the . . . academic chair[s] in clinical subjects should be supported. This idea you'll be pleased to hear has been put in force by aiding to establish a well-rounded school at University College.[74]

A year later Rockefeller minutes recorded: "The main effort is in University College Hospital Medical School and the Faculty of Medical Sciences of University College, to which considerable sums have been given to aid them in a joint effort to develop a complete medical school in London."[75] There was one thing at least that did not need Rockefeller aid. In 1925 Pearce had written: "After studying physiology it seemed unnecessary to do anything as English physiology is the best in the world, the laboratories well equipped, plenty of men going into the subject, and its future secure." He thought, he told Gregg, "it may serve as a model for anything of this kind."[76] Pearce's optimism, however, could wax and wane. Earlier in the same year he had a request for assistance for the London Hospital from Lord Knutsford (Sydney Holland, Second Viscount Knutsford, Fletcher's uncle on his wife's side). Pearce replied that the outcome of Rockefeller investment in Great Britain was "doubtful." This was, he observed, "largely on account of the peculiar point of view concerning medical education" held in that country.[77]

None the less, nearly a year later, minutes of the Foundation were rather more sanguine about the policy for medicine in Great Britain and what the Foundation considered had been achieved:

> The program of the Division of Medical Education in Great Britain has for its object the encouragement of two distinct efforts in medicine.
>
> (a) Aid for the development of the laboratory side of medicine. This aim has been accomplished by assisting in the establishment of a center for anatomy at University College, for pathology in Cambridge, and towards the cultivation of biochemistry at Oxford in order to supplement the present effort at Cambridge.
>
> (b) The stimulation of the development of academic clinics in medicine, surgery, and obstetrics, the most important aid in this regard being our large contribution to University College for the aid of these subjects in operation with government grants.[78]

Pearce's relations with the British are exemplified in his dealings with St. Thomas's Hospital. These merit brief attention since the full-time Professor and Director of the University Unit there since 1920, Hugh MacLean, had a particular interest in clinical biochemistry. MacLean was an Aberdeen medical graduate with extensive post-graduate experience in physiology and biochemistry. He had studied in Berlin. Besides his research, MacLean was endeavouring to set up a diagnostic laboratory service for the hospital's clinicians. There are, then, strong similarities with Edinburgh here. In January 1923 Pearce was in London. MacLean wrote to him anticipating a visit. He thanked Pearce for his support noting: "In the face of a certain amount of opposition to newer methods and ideals, it is naturally very stimulating and helpful to have one's methods approved of." His ambition at St. Thomas's was "to correlate as thoroughly as possible the clinical and laboratory sides of medicine." Sadly, he said, the laboratory lacked facilities for students to study cases under their care on the wards (the American ideal). "At the present time," he told Pearce, "we are doing the best we can with an old military hut." MacLean sketched out for Pearce plans for reform.[79] Shortly after this Pearce visited St Thomas's. He reported to Vincent that when the unit was first established the hospital "believed in the principle of Units for Research only and not for Clinical work or teaching." Indeed the hospital authorities had tried to recruit the "pure" physiologist, E.H. Starling, who did no clinical work whatsoever. Starling declined and MacLean was appointed. Against "great opposition" MacLean insisted on three principles:

> 1st—That he and his immediate full time Staff, have active charge of patients.
> 2nd—That all Students pass through the Unit and receive the benefit of the methods of the Unit.
> 3rd—That all Students be instructed thoroughly in both Clinical and Laboratory methods by the Unit.

In these endeavours Pearce reported that MacLean had been "wonderfully successful."[80] Pertinent here is that MacLean offered his laboratory's facilities to the St. Thomas's surgeons, notably insisting that they perform renal function tests before operations on the prostate. Surgeons did not welcome this innovation. Certainly, when diagnostic laboratories first appeared in hospitals, surgeons could be quite hostile. An American surgeon, J. Chalmers DaCosta, in an address in 1907, complained, "The world is being ruled by shallow men." Too many surgeons, he said, "give a great deal of attention to laboratory methods of supposed precision, and very little to absolute bedside acquaintance with disease." "A great peril of the present day," he warned, was "the decay of individualism."[81] Pearce reported in 1923 that at St. Thomas's: "At first the Surgeons did not conform [to MacLean's wishes] and insisted that they could tell clinically whether a patient would stand the operation [prostatectomy]. After, however, MacLean's prognostication as to the outcome had proved true in several instances, it became routine to do the proper test."[82]

Excited about MacLean's work, Pearce had wondered about the possibility of a gift of $50,000 "to bring about the necessary changes he [MacLean] desired."[83] In February 1926 the Rockefeller Trustees appropriated £15,000 to create a new laboratory.[84] However, as with every other initiative the RF backed, MacLean had also to raise money from other sources. St. Thomas's was a success story but there was no inevitability about it. It had crucially depended, so the RF considered, on backing the right man. Pearce, perhaps unwittingly, revealed to MacLean a general as well as a specific truth about Rockefeller politics when he told him in 1926 that "you would not have had my moral support and of course you would not have had any assistance from the Foundation if you had not developed the right sort of attitude in regard to the modern teaching of medicine."[85] "Attitude" was a key word in the Rockefeller vocabulary.

The enthusiastic reports of MacLean and Pearce need to be treated with caution. In Edinburgh, Meakins's modern professorial department and its laboratory were peripheral to the hospital's main concerns. In 1925 MacLean had told Pearce: "Up to last year, it was not certain whether the Unit system would become permanent at St. Thomas'."[86] Hostility to academic medicine was real enough. At St. Bartholomew's some of the voluntary staff regarded the medical unit with contempt and saw it as marginal to patient management and, more important, proper clinical research.[87] Richard Armstrong, a consultant there, wrote in 1930 of a serum therapy trial: "Be damned to [medical] Professors—say I— they are apt to scoop the credit and spare the pains."[88] Fletcher's daughter, presumably reporting Fletcher's less formal views, recorded that he had found "fighting . . . for better team-work," and establishing professorial units, "uphill work." It was, she said, "often disliked by the big men in the profession." Either she or Fletcher glossed this by saying that the "big men" were "not always quite big enough to put the nation's health before their individual interests."[89] This possibly meant that the unit system, with paid staff, was seen as the thin end of the wedge of state medicine. London consultants largely resisted this move. Opposition was deeply enfolded in an ideology of freedom of choice, the idea of the doctor as the leisured man of letters, and material fears of loss of income coupled with the political belief that the free market was the best way to deliver health care. It is surely not irrelevant to an understanding of Fletcher's poor relations with the "big men" that he promoted state medicine. "I have always been inclined to believe," he said, "that the ideal policy for the profession is to aim at the abolition of the individual fee in favour of salaries."[90] Indeed, Fletcher considered the advance of science and the rise of state medicine were inextricably linked.

Today, academic medicine has been so thoroughly adopted in Britain that it seems like the best way of doing things. With hindsight its adoption looks inevitable and those who were suspicious of it in the inter-war years appear as backwoodsmen: a crusty old guard, benighted and hostile to the new. However, the sentiments of those doctors who were less than enthusiastic for the wholesale importation of transatlantic medicine suggest that their worries were grounded not only in their local, immediate interests but also in wider cultural concerns about modernity and its perceived threat to older, idealized, perhaps mythical, ways of life.[91] A debate had been going on in Britain over the relative value of laboratory and clinical knowledge well before RF involvement was visible. This debate furnished a number of assumptions on which post-war arguments by clinicians for resistance to academic medicine were elaborated.[92] It was not, of course, the case that the whole medical elite in Britain was united in its suspicion of American medicine any more than all inter-war intellectuals were suspicious of Hollywood and the Charleston (although many were). Most of my general conclusions apply to selected members of the elite in London and in Edinburgh. In both places there were doubts about an all-encompassing move to academic medicine (no one disputed the value of selective adoption). However, the views of some Edinburgh doctors, although strikingly similar to those of their London counterparts, were grounded in different perceptions of the medical man's place in society (and nature). The reasons for this were historical and pertained to the different cultures of the two nations.

To some extent the responses of a small number of London doctors to academic medicine were shaped by a myth of the ideal doctor practising single-handedly in a rural world and having a rightful place in a hierarchy topped by the gentry and aristocracy (with the doctor just below) and stretching down to the honest labourer. Of course, none of these clinicians chose to *practise* in the countryside. The myth served to describe the doctor's position and role in an ideal face-to-face society of patronage and mutual obligation. At this time, in the great old London hospitals, almost all consultant work was part time and on a voluntary basis. State medicine struck right at the heart of the world of the "Distinguished Clinicians," the "infallible augurs," as Gowland Hopkins called them sarcastically in a letter to Fletcher.[93] The charitable medical services offered by consultants to hospitals were not just acts of Christian benevolence, they embodied a world of social relations that had existed in various forms in Britain for a good many centuries and were given their recognizably modern shape in the Enlightenment. Democracy and rights to health care were killing them off.

Hospital work was carried out by men who took pride in charitable service. For the most part these men had no strong loyalties to London University (although they might have to Oxford or Cambridge, where many studied basic science as undergraduates). In America (and Scotland) the university was central to what was deemed the best medical education whereas in London it was relatively marginal. Fletcher, not surprisingly perhaps, took the American view of the place of the university in medical education. "[The] school of medicine," he wrote, "should continue always to be . . . an integral and organic part of the university."[94] This was definitely not the relationship between the old hospital schools of London and its University.

In the 1920s there were various differences in the perception of the place of medicine and the doctor in modern society. To caricature for the sake of contrast: these differences can be seen by comparing the ethos of the Harley Street world of London, where medicine was a vocation for gentlemen, with that of progressive institutions in America, where it was profession for the scientific expert (the technocrat perhaps). In Britain, among "Distinguished Clinicians" a preferred model of medical practice was that of the single-handed individual. In the US, among academics, teamwork was favoured and industry and business were the analogues (Fletcher, remember, had found introducing teamwork a struggle). In their private practices, London patricians served a plutocratic clientele including royalty, the aristocracy, and the gentry. London consultants were themselves wealthy and lived in a style not unlike that of their patients. They enjoyed genteel leisure activities, such as dining well, gardening (with a suitable number of under-gardeners), motoring, and in some cases hunting and shooting. Tommy Horder, for example, had a Harley Street home, an estate in Sussex, several gardeners, and a Rolls Royce.[95] These doctors cultivated the role of gentlemen, moral advisors, and custodians of culture. They valued all-round clinical experience as the highest medical good. There is an irony here, for although many London consultants were general practitioners among their private patients, becoming a GP in the usual sense of the term was regarded as having become a failure. Lord Moran, Dean of St. Mary's Medical School, famously regarded GPs as consultants who had fallen to the lower rung of the medical ladder.[96]

"Distinguished Clinicians" did not, of course, have a monopoly among professionals of love of the genteel life (or tradition). Oxbridge dons relished it too. Fletcher came from a devout, Nonconformist, middle class family. He was educated at University College School and at Trinity College, Cambridge, and studied clinical medicine at St. Bartholomew's Hospital. Outside of his family, two things dominated his life: the promotion of basic science and the donnish world of Trinity College, where he was a Fellow. The aquiline Fletcher loved natural history, book and antique collecting, gardening, fly-fishing, fine wines, and perhaps most of all, deer-stalking in Scotland. He was not averse to plugging the occasional Indian crocodile either. The skin could always be used to make him a cigar case or "a little bag" for his wife to use.[97] His bookshelves at home were overhung with mounted antlers. He was punctilious and a stickler for knowledge of the classics. "To Walter," wrote Maisie Fletcher (his daughter), "the solidarity of tradition always counted for so much that was of supreme value."[98] Fletcher also loved America and he loved dancing. He moved easily in elevated (mainly Liberal, Cambridge connected) circles—Wedgwoods, Hollands, Darwins, Barlows, Cecils were always around. He had a "happy relationship" with A. J. Balfour, the senior Conservative politician and former Prime Minister who was also a serious student of philosophy and a countryside-lover.[99] The "happy relationship" extended further than philosophy and the landscape (Fletcher was close enough to Balfour to stay at his country estate in Whittinghame, Scotland). As Chairman of the Committee of the Privy Council for Medical Research, 1920–22, 1925–29, Balfour was on two occasions Fletcher's boss. Fletcher was always likely to get his way in Edinburgh or at least prevent others getting theirs—Balfour was Chancellor of the University, 1891–1930.

Fletcher cherished many of the things that were moulded by the clinical elite into an account of the past that was medically conservative. But for Fletcher these same things were the pleasures of a Cambridge don, they were not shaped into a vision of English society as organic, deferential, and rural. Health, for Fletcher, was not constituted by social relations but by productive work. Fletcher was a thorough modern. He was convinced that basic scientific enquiry and scientific planning were the most powerful tools for acquiring natural knowledge and engineering rational social change. The nation's great failure was its inability to grasp the role that science alone could play in the solution to its problems.

Fletcher represented the ills of modern industrial society in terms of technical solutions ascertainable by scientific research. "The Industrial Revolution," he wrote, "changed the face of the country . . . It raised countless problems which were really problems of physiology." During the Industrial Revolution the "bodies of men, women and children . . . were brought into contact with unresting machinery. They were exposed to the heat of furnaces, they were exposed to the products of chemical processes, and many were exposed to the conditions of deep mining." However, "If ever there was a time when knowledge of the laws of life and of the human machinery, and its sympathetic application, were needed it was then." Experts had been employed to "keep in easy and effectual use . . . lifeless machinery," yet no one considered it "worth while to have expert advice in the proper selection and the proper care of human machinery." He saw as a key moment the creation of the Industrial Fatigue Research Board, founded in 1918 to study the productivity of munitions workers. This Board, he wrote, had made possible "sustained progress" in "finding the right task for the right worker and of discovering the conditions of work that give the optimum of ease and efficiency in its performance." We "all agree," he said, "the proper test of the health of a nation is the number of vigorous young men and women able to do the work of the country."[100] One of the assumptions underlying the acceptance and spectacular achievements of physiology at the turn of the century was that the discipline could investigate the body as a machine for converting energy. Correctly understood in this way, the laws of physiology might then be applied to make the labouring body an efficient motor. This is one of the ways in which Fletcher construed physiology while patricians—on the ward at least—stressed the body's irreducible, holistic, characteristics.[101] He would have been apoplectic on hearing Thomas Horder say: "Our ancestors didn't follow any scientific methods. To tell the truth, Nature taught man how to be healthy long before science discovered the laws of health."[102] "[L]et us keep ourselves physically fit," was Horder's injunction, "but let physical fitness be for some purpose."[103]

For Fletcher there was nothing in the way of material disadvantage that could not be solved by research. Never one to retreat publicly into nostalgia and ever the realist he saw the greatest problems facing humankind were to be found in the wretched lives of the inhabitants of "industrial cities." A man has "no eyes," he wrote, if "he does not have a sinking heart at the numbers of stunted figures, poor physiques, and bad teeth" he sees among factory workers or spectators "at a cup-tie match."[104] In the hands of science lay the solution to these evils. Fletcher never hinted at a political analysis of industrialization or a political solution to its effects. It is not that Fletcher had not seen or was unaware of the extremes of privilege. During the Great War he visited France while working for the MRC and trying to get the government to see the value of science to victory. He wrote: "I am in extremely comfortable . . . in very good quarters . . . rather like staying at Eton or Cambridge and being entertained by the Eton beaks or by dons." Another night he dined "in a small French hotel—excellent dinner and good red Burgundy wine."[105]

He may have ignored or avoided politics in the widest sense but he did denounce answers to the ills of modern life that were not provided by scientific research. Notably, throughout his career Fletcher railed against common sense as a guide to solving human problems. Common sense was the enemy of science. It was, of course, or could be, the enemy of elitism. On one occasion Fletcher recollected he had met a government minister who said to him, "well doctor I don't hold with research. If we want to stop disease we must give the people better grub and less dirt." Fletcher agreed but added that he wished the minister "could tell me what better grub was and what less dirt was—for I knew no way of finding out those two things except by persistent scientific research work."[106] Tommy Horder, on the other hand, although by no means opposed to research, considered: "Look after the accessibility of food and nutrition will look after itself."[107] Fletcher's views were quite compatible with an appreciation of the past and were as socially exclusive as those of the patricians. Fletcher's elite, however, was not constituted by bedside doctors. Fletcher's new priesthood (clinicians sometimes explicitly described themselves in this way) was composed of research scientists. "Progress is only made in scientific work," he said, "by men and women of long training and having exceptional ability and imagination."[108] This was a bid to establish a new medical and scientific elite. It is no wonder that his view that those doctors who treated patients should be salaried state servants stuck in a few throats.

The world view of the patricians conformed to their view of the organization of medical practice and their account of the body. As doctors they were committed to clinical individualism. On the ward they summoned up organic ideals of the body, emphasized the importance of the healing power of nature and the centrality of clinical observation as a source of medical knowledge. Fletcher thought studying individual patients brought "sterility" to scientific progress.[109] Patricians were not opposed to science, far from it, but their anxieties appeared as concerns that the organization of laboratory science was usurping their clinical skill. Specialization in particular was an object of contempt.[110] Even such distinguished clinicians as Archibald Garrod, famed for his work on inborn errors of metabolism, could worry in 1919 about a "tendency to ascribe almost all advances in medicine to the workers in pathological laboratories, and to represent the workers in the clinical branch as merely applying in practice knowledge which has been gained in the laboratories."[111] Similarly Tommy Horder, who welcomed the laboratory sciences, warned of their dangers: "The use of tools in diagnosis detracts nothing from the fundamental importance of examination conducted by the unaided senses. The physician who is tempted to substitute the microscope for a trained eye and an experienced hand stands to lose a good deal by the exchange." "To change the physician for the pathologist," he said, "can but end in disaster."[112] The negative responses to academic medicine were not confined to practising clinicians. Sir George Newman certainly had his reservations about American ways of doing things.[113]

In Chapter 9 I shall hint at an irony in the patricians' ideology. The defence of clinical experience and individualism was closely linked for many of them to the voluntary hospital system. On their ward rounds the great clinicians could and did show off their considerable skills to students and younger staff. Much of their time, however, was spent in private practice, not at the bedside in hospital treating the sick and supervising their juniors. Left to their own devices on the wards there is more than a suspicion that inexperienced staff resorted to the laboratory as a blunderbuss measure for diagnosis and management in a manner that would have appalled their consultants. It is hard to resist the cliché about being hoist by one's own petard.

Challenging though American medicine was, it was part of the more general threat of the modern. Clinicians of this generation had, like a good number of intellectuals who had doubts about modernity, been brought up in the late summer of Victorian liberalism and many retreated after the war to more pessimistic positions.[114] This pessimism was often coupled with condemnations of mass production and mass culture and appeals for the creation of, or a return to, an organic rural village life. If the health of a nation for Fletcher was "the number of vigorous young men and women able to do the work of the country," for the patricians it was something that grew from the way of life of an (for them romanticized) organic, closely-knit society. Their intense worries about academic medicine centred on anxieties about the decline of the individual clinician and this was a focused anxiety about the decline and decadence of civilization in general. Take for instance the St. Bartholomew's Hospital physician Sir Walter Langdon Brown, who complained that "the division of labour in a large factory has reached such a pitch that in many occupations craftsmanship is dead and the workman has become a robot."[115] Tommy Horder lamented that "the large town . . . tends to stultify initiative and resource, which are the very root of genius."[116] Brown considered that "It is one of the drawbacks of . . . vast new suburbs . . . which radiate out like huge tentacles from London, destroying the countryside as they grow, that they offer so few opportunities for communal life."[117] Mass consumption and entertainment (notably the movies), the patrician doctors found equally enervating. "We don't read any more," lamented Horder. "For sport, we watch the professionals play our games for us. For amusement, we crowd into 'the pictures'."[118] Francis Crookshank associated "jazz-bands" with people of the "coarsely sensual kind" and noted of the "kinema" that it was the "greatest enemy of the epoch to intellectual culture." The lower stages of evolution encompassed "the shiftiness of the monkey, the film star and the imbecile."[119]

This patrician model of clinical individualism was embedded in nostalgia and in the countryside. There was, said these doctors, an English tradition in medicine that gave it a down-to-earth, commonsense quality. English medicine for these men was embodied in the late eighteenth-century doctor, Edward Jenner, the discoverer of vaccination. Jenner, they insisted, was the single-handed country practitioner who had saved civilization from a dreadful disease, smallpox, through simple natural historical inquiry. Fletcher, on the other hand, considered Jenner's work "an ingenious practical dodge; it was not more than that."[120] For the patricians Jenner was, they all agreed, a country gentleman who rode to hounds and wrote poetry for recreation. He lived, a family man with his servants, in an organic, rural, patriarchal community where he dutifully did his rounds, serving his patients, who in turn felt and showed gratitude. Finally, he was an inquisitive, acute observer, a great natural historian: a pure empirical mind unfettered by theory. He stood for both the England and the medicine that was being destroyed by modernity.[121] In a different way, Fletcher was not devoid of vestiges of mythologizing the English. Advocating scientific research into nutrition, he observed that the physique of the factory worker was "not a native standard characteristic of England, because we know that there is no racial stock so capable as our own of producing the best types of stature, health and beauty."[122]

The myth of the doctor was strongly rural. Although these doctors practised in (and no doubt loved) London, it was the countryside to which they retreated that was the model for social order, not London. They had been brought up in a world of social change in which the countryside was identified with immemorial (God-given in some instances) order, and stability.[123] In contrast (although not marked), those Edinburgh doctors who were apprehensive about American advances and the importation of academic medicine developed similar responses but from a more autonomous professional, and civic-based, ideology centred on the university.

Notes

1. Daniel T. Rodgers, *Atlantic Crossings: Social Politics in a Progressive Age* (Cambridge, MA: The Belknap Press, 1998).

2. Ibid., 369–70.

3. Charles S. Maier, *Recasting Bourgeois Europe. Stabilization in France, Germany and Italy in the Decade after World War 1* (Princeton: Princeton University Press, 1975), 12.

4. Siân Nicholas, "Being British: Creeds and Cultures," in *The British Isles: 1901–1951*, ed. Keith Robbins (Oxford: Oxford University Press, 2002), 103–35.

5. On science in general see Gerald Jonas, *The Circuit Riders: Rockefeller Money and the Rise of Modern Science* (New York, London: W. W. Norton and Company, 1989). On mathematics see Reinhard Siegmund-Schultz, *Rockefeller, and the Internationalization of Mathematics between the Two World Wars: Documents and Studies for the Social History of Mathematics in the 20th Century*, Science Networks Historical Studies, 25 (Basel: Birkhäuser, 2001).

6. Lise Wilkinson and Anne Hardy, *Prevention and Cure: The London School of Hygiene & Tropical Medicine: A 20th Century Quest for Global Public Health* (London: Kegan Paul, 2001).

7. Pearce to Gregg, December 28, 1925, folder 67, box 5, series 401, RG 1.1, Rockefeller Foundation Archives, RAC.

8. Ilana Löwy and Patrick Zylberman, "Medicine as a Social Instrument: Rockefeller Foundation, 1913–45," *Studies in History and Philosophy of Biological and Biomedical Sciences* 31 (2000): 365–79. The whole volume is a special issue devoted to "The Rockefeller Foundation and the Biomedical Sciences."

9. Raymond B. Fosdick, *The Story of the Rockefeller Foundation* (New York: Harper and Brothers, 1952), 28–29.

10. Cited in Löwy and Zylberman, "Medicine as a Social Instrument," 368.

11. Ibid., 370.

12. Pearce to Edwin Embree, February 25, 1923, folder 32, box 3, series 405, RG 1.1, Rockefeller Foundation Archives, RAC. Embree had joined the RF in 1917 as secretary to the President, George E. Vincent.

13. Pearce to Fletcher, November 14, 1923, folder 67, box 5, series 401, RG 1.1, Rockefeller Foundation Archives, RAC.

14. Walter Morley Fletcher, "An Address on the Scope and Needs of Medical Research," *British Medical Journal* 2 (1932): 42–47.

15. Walter Morley Fletcher, *Medical Research: The Tree and the Fruit*, British Science Guild, The Norman Lockyer Lecture (London: MRC, 1929), 8.

16. Anne-Emanuelle Birn, "Wa(i)ves of Influence: Rockefeller Public Health in Mexico, 1920–50," *Studies in History and Philosophy of Biological and Biomedical Sciences* 31 (2000): 381–95.

17. Lion Murad and Patrick Zylberman, "Seeds for French Health Care: Did the Rockefeller Foundation Plant the Seeds between the Two World Wars?" ibid., 463–75.

18. Jean-François Picard and William H. Schneider, "From the Art of Medicine to Biomedical Science in France: Modernization or Americanization?" in *Rockefeller Philanthropy and Modern Biomedicine: International Initiatives from World War I to the Cold War* ed. William H. Schneider (Bloomington: Indiana University Press, 2002), 106–24.

19. J. B. Lyons, "Irish Medicine's Appeal to Rockefeller," in ibid., 61–86.

20. William H. Schneider, "The Men who Followed Flexner: Richard Pearce, Alan Gregg, and the Rockefeller Foundation Medical Divisions, 1919–1951," in ibid,, 7–60, 21.

21. Cited in Fosdick, *The Story of the Rockefeller Foundation*, 118.

22. Indian resentment at British control developed enormously between the wars and by the late 1920s Congress was demanding complete independence. Through repression and constitutional reform Britain retained the upper hand. Increasingly during this period provincial governments were charged with public health administration but lacked the financial wherewithal to handle it. Preventative medicine was largely for colonials. The RF attempted to introduce disease control programmes, demonstration health units, and the training of public health personnel. The diseases targeted were hookworm and malaria in the Madras presidency in the south. This was after discovery of the high levels of hookworm infestation in migrant labourers. The Foundation got nowhere. Government red tape and indifference stymied active public health measures. See Shirish N. Kavadi, *The Rockefeller Foundation and Public Health in Colonial India 1916–1945. A Narrative History* (Pune/Mumbai: Foundation for Research in Community Health, 1999).

23. Cited in E. Richard Brown, "Public Health in Imperialism: Early Rockefeller Programs at Home and Abroad," in *The Cultural Crisis of Modern Medicine*, ed. John Ehrenreich (London: Monthly Review Press, 1978), 252–70.

24. Susan Gross Solomon, " 'Through a Glass Darkly': the Rockefeller Foundation's International Health Board and Soviet Public Health," *Studies in History and Philosophy of Biological and Biomedical Sciences* 31 (2000): 409–18.

25. Marta Aleksandra Balinska, "The Rockefeller Foundation and the National Institute of Hygiene, Poland, 1918–45," ibid., 419–32; Gábor Palló, "Rescue and Cordon Sanitaire: The Rockefeller Foundation in Hungarian Public Health," ibid., 433–45; Paul Weindling, "Public Health and Political Stabilisation: The Rockefeller Foundation in Central and Eastern Europe between the Two World Wars," *Minerva* 31 (1993): 253–67.

26. François Bédarida, *A Social History of England 1851–1990* (London and New York: Routledge, 2004), xv. Bédarida cites other amusing examples.

27. See Donald Fisher, "The Rockefeller Foundation and the Development of Scientific Medicine in Britain," *Minerva* 16 (1978): 20–41. Fisher concentrates mainly on London and to some extent on Oxbridge. Edinburgh barely gets a mention.

28. See the essays in *Historical Perspectives on the Role of the MRC: Essays in the History of the Medical Research Council of the United Kingdom and its Predecessor, the Medical Research Committee, 1913–1953*, ed. Joan Austoker and Linda Bryder (New York: Oxford University Press 1989).

29. Maisie Fletcher, *The Bright Countenance. A Personal Biography of Walter Morley Fletcher* (London: Hodder and Stoughton, 1957), 270–71.

30. Edsall to Pearce, November 13 , 1922, folder 217, box 16, series 401, RG 1.1, Rockefeller Foundation Archives, RAC.

31. Vincent to Pearce, December 7, 1922, folder 67, box 5, series 401, RG 1.1, Rockefeller Foundation Archives, RAC.

32. Evarts A. Graham, "A Report of an Investigation of the Teaching of Surgery in Representative British Medical Schools, Based on a Visit to Great Britain in 1922 under the Auspices of the Division of Medical Education, Rockefeller Foundation," 1, 2, 2–3, folder 217, box 16, series 401, RG 1.1, Rockefeller Foundation Archives, RAC. It is sometimes unclear whether Graham is describing London or Britain.

33. Abraham Flexner, *Medical Education. A Comparative Study* (New York: The Macmillan Company, 1925), 28. He excepted the London academic units but made it clear the judgement applied to Scotland.

34. Graham, "Report," 4, 25, 8 (emphasis mine), 6.

35. Ibid., 22, 9, 10, 11.

36. Ibid., 24, 10.

37. Edsall to Pearce, November 13, 1922, folder 217, box 16, series 401, RG 1.1, Rockefeller Foundation Archives, RAC.

38. David Edsall, "Comparative Observations of Methods of Education in Clinical Medicine in Great Britain and the United States 1922–3," 21, note 52, folder 217, box 16, series 401, RG 1.1, Rockefeller Foundation Archives, RAC.

39. Ibid., note 2–3, note 40–41.

40. Thomas Horder, *Clinical Pathology in Practice* (London: H. Froude, 1910), 1.

41. Thomas Horder, "Clinical Medicine as an Aid to Pathology: A Criticism," *St. Bartholomew's Hospital Journal* 19 (1911–12): 192–95. The title was intentionally ironic.

42. Edsall, "Comparative Observations," note 41.

43. Ibid., note 64.

44. Vincent to Pearce, December 7, 1922, folder 67, box 5, series 401, RG 1.1, Rockefeller Foundation Archives, RAC.

45. Pearce to Vincent, December 23, 1922, folder 217, box 16, series 401, RG 1.1, Rockefeller Foundation Archives, RAC.

46. Vincent to Pearce, December 7, 1922.

47. Vincent to Pearce, January 12, 1923, folder 217, box 16, series 401, RG 1.1, Rockefeller Foundation Archives, RAC. A comment that lends irony to Tennyson's famous lines: "Better fifty years of Europe than a cycle of Cathay."

48. R. M. Pearce, Diary, January 14, 1923, folder 217, box 16, series 401, RG 1.1, Rockefeller Foundation Archives, RAC.

49. Edsall to Vincent, [early 1923], folder 217, box 16, series 401, RG 1.1, Rockefeller Foundation Archives, RAC.

50. This was Wickliffe Rose, formerly a Professor of Philosophy, Director of the International Health Division of the RF.

51. Gregg to Pearce, February 2, 1923, folder 217, box 16, series 401, RG 1.1, Rockefeller Foundation Archives, RAC.

52. Edsall to Pearce, February 26, 1923, folder 217, box 16, series 401, RG 1.1, Rockefeller Foundation Archives, RAC.

53. John F. Fulton, *Harvey Cushing: A Biography* (Springfield, IL: C. C. Thomas, 1946), 377–84.

54. Graham to Pearce, July 26, 1923, folder 217, box 16, series 401, RG 1.1, Rockefeller Foundation Archives, RAC.

55. Graham to Pearce, October 16, 1923, folder 217, box 16, series 401, RG 1.1, Rockefeller Foundation Archives, RAC; ibid., Gregg to Graham, October 22, 1923.

56. Pearce to Graham, November 27, 1923, folder 217, box 16, series 401, RG 1.1, Rockefeller Foundation Archives, RAC.

57. Edsall to Pearce, December 12, 1923, folder 217, box 16, series 401, RG 1.1, Rockefeller Foundation Archives, RAC.

58. Pearce to Edsall, December 14, 1923, folder 217, box 16, series 401, RG 1.1, Rockefeller Foundation Archives, RAC.

59. R. M. Pearce, Interviews, London, February 23–27, 1924, folder 217, box 16, series 401, RG 1.1, Rockefeller Foundation Archives, RAC.

60. Edsall to Pearce, January 10, 1924, folder 217, box 16, series 401, RG 1.1, Rockefeller Foundation Archives, RAC.

61. On Newman's ambivalence see W. F. Bynum, "Sir George Newman and the American Way," in *The History of Medical Education in Britain*, ed. Vivian Nutton and Roy Porter (Amsterdam: Rodopi, 1994), 37–50.

62. See Steve Sturdy, "Hippocrates and State Medicine: George Newman Outlines the Founding Policy of the Ministry of Health," in *Greater than the Parts: The Holist Turn in Biomedicine 1920–1950*, ed. Christopher Lawrence and George Weisz (New York: Oxford University Press, 1998), 112–34.

63. Newman to Edsall, January 30, 1924, folder 217, box 16, series 401, RG 1.1, Rockefeller Foundation Archives, RAC.

64. Edsall to Pearce, September 26, 1924, folder 217, box 16, series 401, RG 1.1, Rockefeller Foundation Archives, RAC.

65. Elliott to Edsall, March 13, 1924, folder 217, box 16, series 401, RG 1.1, Rockefeller Foundation Archives, RAC.

66. Fletcher to Pearce, October 25, 1923, folder 67, box 5, series 401, RG 1.1, Rockefeller Foundation Archives, RAC. On pathology at Cambridge and the struggles to make it a basic science see Mark W. Weatherall, *Gentlemen, Scientists and Doctors: Medicine at Cambridge 1800–1940* (Woodbridge, Suffolk: The Boydell Press in Association with Cambridge University Library, 2000).

67. Fletcher to Edsall, January 31, 1924, folder 67, box 5, series 401, RG 1.1, Rockefeller Foundation Archives, RAC.

68. Pearce to Fletcher, November 14, 1923, folder 67, box 5, series 401, RG 1.1, Rockefeller Foundation Archives, RAC.

69. Vincent to Simon Flexner, July 2, 1924, folder 14, box 2, series 405, RG 1.1, Rockefeller Foundation Archives, RAC.

70. Pearce to Vincent, January 29, 1923, folder 245, box 18, series 401, RG 1.1, Rockefeller Foundation Archives, RAC.

71. Pearce to Gregg, December 28, 1925, folder 67, box 5, series 401, RG 1.1, Rockefeller Foundation Archives, RAC.

72. Walter Morley Fletcher, *Biology and Statecraft*, The Seventh of the National Lectures Delivered on 23 January 1931 (London: The British Broadcasting Corporation: 1931), 6.

73. Fletcher, *Medical Research*, 22.

74. Pearce to Gregg, December 28, 1925, folder 67, box 5, series 401, RG 1.1, Rockefeller Foundation Archives, RAC. Emphasis mine.

75. Minutes of the Rockefeller Foundation, November 5, 1926, folder 245, box 18, series 401, RG 1.1, Rockefeller Foundation Archives, RAC.

76. Pearce to Gregg, December 28, 1925, folder 67, box 5, series 401, RG 1.1, Rockefeller Foundation Archives, RAC.

77. Pearce to Lord Knutsford, April 16, 1925, folder 245, box 18, series 401, RG 1.1, Rockefeller Foundation Archives, RAC.

78. Minutes of the Rockefeller Foundation, February 24, 1926, folder 333, box 26, series 401A, RG 1.1, Rockefeller Foundation Archives, RAC.

79. MacLean to Pearce, January 26, 1923, folder 333, box 26, series 401A, RG 1.1, Rockefeller Foundation Archives, RAC.

80. Pearce to Vincent, January 28, 1923, folder 333, box 26, series 401A, RG 1.1, Rockefeller Foundation Archives, RAC.

81. J. C. DaCosta, "Address on the Occasion of the Graduation Exercises at the Naval Medical School in Washington," in *Trials and Triumphs of Surgery and other Literary Gems* (Philadelphia: Dorrance, 1907), 394, cited in Keith Wailoo, *Drawing Blood: Technology and Disease Identity in Twentieth-Century America* (Baltimore: The Johns Hopkins University Press, 1997), 64.

82. Pearce to Vincent, January 28, 1923, folder 333, box 26, series 401A, RG 1.1, Rockefeller Foundation Archives, RAC. It was not just the Americans who were shocked by the purported clinical skills of British surgeons. English authors sympathetic to the new medicine equally reported almost with embarrassment surgical claims to experience being a sufficient guide to bedside judgement. Sir Clifford Allbutt, Regius Professor of Physic at Cambridge, noted in 1920 that "older surgeons, naturally relying on their invaluable sagacity and resourcefulness, are disposed to look on biochemistry as a fad." "Modern Therapeutics," *The Practitioner*, September, 1920: 157–63, quote at 162.

83. Ibid.

84. Pearce to MacLean, February 24, 1926, folder 333, box 26, series 401A, RG 1.1, Rockefeller Foundation Archives, RAC.

85. Pearce to MacLean, April 1, 1926, folder 67, box 5, series 401, RG 1.1, Rockefeller Foundation Archives, RAC.

86. MacLean to Pearce, [early December, 1925], folder 333, box 26, series 401A, RG 1.1, Rockefeller Foundation Archives, RAC.

87. See Keir Waddington, *Medical Education at St Bartholomew's Hospital 1123–1995* (Woodbridge, Suffolk: The Boydell Press, 2003), 169, 199.

88. Armstrong to F. H. K. Green, December 5, 1930, FD1/2368, PRO. Cited in Martin Edwards, "Control and the Therapeutic Trial 1918–1948" (M.D. Thesis, University of London, 2005).

89. Fletcher, *The Bright Countenance*, 168.

90. Ibid., 196.

91. My use of myth is illustrated in Chapter 5 in relation to Scottish visions of the past. It is not synonymous with imaginary.

92. The debate was particularly bitter at St Mary's Hospital, Paddington, where American influence was minimal. See E. A. Heaman, *St. Mary's: The History of a London Teaching Hospital* (Montreal & Kingston, London, Ithaca: Liverpool University Press, McGill–Queen's University Press, 2003), 119–201.

93. Fletcher, *The Bright Countenance*, 285.

94. Walter Morley Fletcher, "University Ideals and the Future of Medicine," *JAMA* 19 (1930): 1389–93.

95. Mervyn Horder, *The Little Genius: A Memoir of the First Lord Horder* (London: Gerald Duckworth and Co., 1966).

96. Frank Honigsbaum, *The Division in British Medicine: A History of the Separation of General Practice from Hospital Care 1911–1968* (London: Kogan Page, 1979), 117.

97. Fletcher, *The Bright Countenance*, 205.

98. Ibid., 32.

99. Ibid., 30. Balfour and Fletcher make strange bedfellows at first sight although it is soon apparent that they were filled with similar contradictions. As a young man Balfour wrote a conservative attack on scientific naturalism, yet as a politician he was very supportive of experimental science. Conversely Fletcher the technocrat was very conservative in his friends and recreational tastes. On Balfour as a philosopher see L. S. Jacyna, "Science and Social Order in the Thought of A. J. Balfour," *Isis* 71 (1980): 11–34.

100. Fletcher, *The Bright Countenance*, 236–38.

101. Anson Rabinbach, *The Human Motor: Energy, Fatigue and the Origins of Modernity* (Berkeley: University of California Press, 1992).

102. Thomas Horder, *Health and a Day* (London: J. M. Dent and Sons Ltd., 1937), 105.

103. Ibid., 57.

104. Fletcher, *The Bright Countenance*, 238.

105. Ibid., 129.

106. Ibid., 238, 179.

107. Horder, *Health and a Day*, 152.

108. Fletcher, *The Bright Countenance*, 195.

109. Fletcher, *Medical Research*, 8.

110. Christopher Lawrence, "Still Incommunicable: Clinical Holists and Medical Knowledge in Interwar Britain" in *Greater than the Parts*, 94–111.

111. Archibald E. Garrod, "The Laboratory and the Ward," in *Contributions to Medical and Biological Research Dedicated to Sir William Osler* (New York: Paul B. Hoeber, 1919), 59–69.

112. Horder, *Clinical Pathology in Practice*, 1.

113. Bynum, "Sir George Newman and the American Way"; Sturdy, "Hippocrates and State Medicine." Newman illustrates the problem of lumping and splitting a small number of medical men. He was a proponent of state medicine.

114. These doctors can probably be accommodated to Gramsci's class of "traditional intellectuals." Marginal, diverse, and critical of modernity this class in the 1920s has had a significant place in Marxist discussions of British history in this period. For a good summary of this historiography see Alan O'Shea, "English Subjects of Modernity," in *Modern Times: Reflections on a Century of English Modernity*, ed. Mica Nava and Alan O'Shea (London: Routledge, 1996), 7–37. Note, however, the conflation of England and Britain in this essay and the others in the volume.

115. Walter Langdon-Brown, *Thus We are Men* (London: Kegan Paul, 1938), 27.

116. Horder, *Health and a Day*, 70. On Horder and Brown see Christopher Lawrence, "A Tale of Two Sciences: Bench and Bedside in Twentieth-Century Britain," *Medical History* 43 (1999): 421–49.

117. Brown, *Thus We are Men*, 13.

118. Horder, *Health and a Day*, 69.

119. Francis Crookshank, *The Mongol in our Midst*, 3rd ed. (London: Kegan Paul, Trench, Trubner, 1931), 107, 179.

120. Fletcher, *Medical Research*, 6.

121. Christopher Lawrence, "Edward Jenner's Jockey Boots and the Great Tradition in English Medicine 1918–1939," in *Regenerating England: Science, Medicine and Culture in Inter-War Britain*, ed. Christopher Lawrence and Anna-K. Mayer (Amsterdam: Rodopi, 2000), 45–66. For a study the nostalgia for a lost rural England in the 1920s see Alun Howkins, *The Death of Rural England: A Social History of the Countryside since 1900* (London: Routledge, 2003); Michael Bartholomew, *In Search of H. V. Morton* (London: Methuen, 2004).

122. Fletcher, *The Bright Countenance*, 238.

123. Bédarida, *A Social History of England 1851–1990*, 29.

4

THE ORGANIZATION AND ETHOS OF EDINBURGH MEDICINE

In London most of the medical schools had been created within the great old hospitals and were based in them. Qualification was traditionally achieved not by university degree but by examination at the Royal Colleges of Physicians and of the Surgeons, or the Society of Apothecaries. London University was a relatively late addition to medical education in the capital and, even in the 1920s, still not regarded as important in some quarters. London University was an umbrella organization: administering, degree awarding, and examining. In Edinburgh the situation was quite different. The University was the principal seat of medical education and thus an institution primarily devoted to teaching, although research became increasingly important after the Great War. Further complicating the Edinburgh story was the existence of an Extra-academical School of Medicine based at the Royal Colleges.[1] This latter approximated more to the London model.

The Royal Infirmary of Edinburgh was an autonomous institution primarily devoted to patient care. Writing in 1929, A. Logan Turner could see the history of the RIE and the Edinburgh School of Medicine as "one and indivisible."[2] This was not strictly correct. The relationship was much more one of symbiosis and occasionally mutual parasitism. The sometimes uneasy relations between the RIE and University determined much of the politics surrounding the introduction of academic medicine in this period. An important contribution to this was the status of the physicians and surgeons who served the Infirmary, a number of whom were also employed by the University as teachers and researchers. This situation created dual and occasionally conflicting allegiances and sometimes different priorities. The teachers had an allegiance to the University (and the service of intellectual endeavour) and to the Infirmary Managers, whose prime concern was sound patient care. Further, there were strains within the Infirmary itself. These resulted from the vestiges of an ancient attendance system under which two sorts of practitioner cared for patients and taught students. Although, by the 1920s, for administrative reasons, all senior doctors at the RIE were nominally University teachers, only the Professors of Medicine were University employees (that is, paid University salaries).[3] The allegiances of the so-called Ordinary Physicians, not paid to teach, were often divided between the University and the Extra-academical School. All consultants, whether professorial or not, constituted the Honorary Staff.

Writing in 1933, the Principal of the University, Sir Thomas Holland, could describe it as "the most cosmopolitan among British universities" with "19,000 graduates scattered throughout the world."[4] By this time the Edinburgh medical course lasted five years. In the 1920s thousands of students attended the school. To take the beginning and end of this period, in 1919–20 a total of 1,968 medical students matriculated, by 1929–30 the number had fallen to 1,318. The University rewarded the student with degrees in medicine and surgery (M.B., Ch.B.). The University also awarded higher degrees in these subjects (M.D., Ch.M.).[5] Other students attended the Extra-academical School, in which they studied not for the University degree but for the Triple Qualification of the three Royal Medical Incorporations in Scotland.[6] Students could take both University and Extra-academical courses (the latter of which the University was legally bound to recognize).[7] Whereas once, classes in subjects like physiology were offered as extramural courses, by the 1920s, because of the cost of equipment, laboratory courses were increasingly taken as University courses.[8] In these years about 40 to 50 students per annum qualified through the Colleges.[9] Post-graduate courses were instituted after a committee composed of representatives of the University and the Royal Colleges had been formed in 1905.[10] These courses were given at the Royal Infirmary. In all of these arrangements the entwining of autonomous Edinburgh institutions— University, Colleges, Infirmary—is visible. This unique combination was the source of Edinburgh's success, fame, intense local pride, friction, and, to outsiders, incomprehensibility.

The Medical Faculty of Edinburgh University was established in 1726. At that time a handful of professors who were practising doctors taught just about everything medical and lived off student fees and private practice. By the 1920s that world had to a great extent disappeared. Salaried basic scientists doing laboratory research had taken over the teaching of the non-clinical subjects. Compared to clinical teachers, who were almost entirely Edinburgh graduates (and most of them Scottish), professors without clinical responsibilities were recruited from far and wide. There was a variety of reasons for this: the University was an international institution, the Infirmary a parochial one (although with an international reputation); the University recruited through relatively open competition, the Infirmary by a system involving seniority that privileged Edinburgh graduates; the University authorities searched far and wide for intellectual excellence and Infirmary Managers wanted Edinburgh-trained (preferably Scottish) doctors treating their patients.

The teachers assembled to teach the basic sciences in the 1920s were of international standing. Anatomy and physiology remained the staple basic medical sciences in the Medical School. In the nineteenth century, physiology, as noted in Chapters 2 and 3, was promoted by basic scientists and a good number of clinicians as *the* discipline on which a true science of clinical medicine should be constructed. One of the prominent British proponents of this view was Edward Sharpey-Schafer who became Professor of Physiology in Edinburgh in 1899. Sharpey-Schafer, the son of a German, was born in London. He was educated at University College London, where he became Assistant Professor. He was one of the most celebrated physiologists of the day and his appointment at Edinburgh perfectly illustrates the catholic taste of the University. Yet in Edinburgh he stood aloof from clinicians as well as the basic scientists, building his own massive, autocratically-run physiological empire. When Richard Pearce from the RF visited Edinburgh in 1923 he noted: "Schafer is to hold on to Histology and has built a laboratory for this subject on the roof of the adjacent Faculty building. This is used only three months . . . of the year, while bacteriology is crying for space." After his visit Pearce recommended the "breaking up of the present department of Physiology."[11] Sharpey-Schafer outlived Pearce. In 1931 he was still in post and Gregg called him "an old and intransigent professor."[12] His militant views on the place of physiology in medicine and his account of the bankruptcy of the bedside as a source of knowledge were well known.[13] No doubt these alienated him from some of the Edinburgh clinicians (he was not popular with the basic scientists either). Sharpey-Schafer retired in 1933.

A much more important force for change in Edinburgh in the 1920s was the Chair of Chemistry in Relation to Medicine. This was founded in 1919 and the first appointee was George Barger. Barger was born in Manchester and had been a student at University College London and King's College, Cambridge. A world famous biochemist, he again illustrates how the University could look outside its walls when choosing academic scientists. Barger is important because, in him, Meakins found an intellectual and institutional ally. He and his co-workers collaborated with Barger and used his laboratories, not least because animal experimentation was forbidden on RIE property. Barger was the victim of Sharpey-Schafer's empire-building. In 1923 Pearce reported among his criticisms of the Medical School: "To crown it all one finds Barger, one of the greatest of Biochemists, teaching inorganic and organic chemistry because Schafer insists on teaching biochemistry in his department of Physiology." Pearce added that the Medical Faculty and the Principal of the University recognized this, "but fearing Schafer are waiting for his retirement."[14] Equally as important as Barger was Arthur Robertson Cushny, who succeeded to the reconstituted Chair of Materia Medica in 1918. Once a clinical chair, the Professorship of Materia Medica effectively became one of experimental pharmacology. Cushny was an accomplished, widely-respected scientist. A Scot (an Aberdeen graduate), Cushny had studied at Strasbourg, and been Professor of Pharmacology at the University of Michigan for twelve years, and for thirteen years at University College London. Cushny, like Barger, saw eye to eye with Meakins on the role of the laboratory sciences in medicine. After Cushny's death in 1926, Alfred Joseph Clark, who had also held the Chair of Pharmacology at University College London, succeeded him. Clark was English, educated at Cambridge University. He followed in Cushny's intellectual shoes, aligning himself with Barger and Thomas Mackie (see below). He had little time for clinical individualism and was in favour of bedside medicine being firmly grounded in laboratory knowledge.

At about the time that the Medical School was originally founded, various proposals were floated to gather contributions to establish a hospital in the city. An important moving force behind these proposals was the Royal College of Physicians. In December 1728 the contributors met and elected a committee of twenty-one members. That committee constituted the basis on which future Boards of Management were founded. The Town Council, the legal profession, physicians and surgeons, and the general body of contributors were all represented and continued to be so into the 1920s. In 1920 the number of Managers was twenty-six.

The six-bedded hospital opened in a small house in 1729. Licentiates and Fellows of the College of Physicians attended patients on a rotational basis. After January 1, 1738, attendance was restricted to Fellows. In the 1920s Fellowship of the College remained a necessary qualification for appointment as an honorary physician to the Infirmary.[15] Patients were also attended by a small number of surgeons from the Incorporation of Surgeons. Later, as with the physicians, only Fellows of the Royal College of Surgeons (incorporated by Royal Charter in 1778) could become honorary surgeons to the RIE. At this period the physicians and surgeons decided among themselves who was to attend. Later all appointments to the staff were made by the Board of Management. This was to remain the case in the 1920s. From the start students attended the hospital, but the physicians and surgeons they followed were not necessarily teachers at the University.

In 1736 the hospital received a Royal Charter. The following year the Managers purchased a site for a purpose-built infirmary. The first patients were admitted to the new building in 1741. While the physicians and surgeons continued to give their services gratis and in rotation, newly-qualified medical men and students began to be employed as clerks. They lived in and were paid regularly or received a gratuity on leaving. They carried out the more menial medical, administrative, and accounting work. In 1854 these men were designated Resident House Physicians and House Surgeons. Gradually the Managers changed the system of attendance in the new hospital. Two physicians, called Physicians-in-Ordinary, were appointed to attend daily. After considerable controversy, Surgeons-in-Ordinary were also appointed. In 1818 the first Assistant Surgeon was appointed and in 1869 Assistant Physicians appeared.

As noted, at first, students attended the hospital for clinical teaching but this was not University based. Students paid the Infirmary Managers a fee for this privilege. In 1748, however, the Professor of Medicine, John Rutherford, proposed to give a course of clinical lectures to illustrate the principles taught in his systematic lecture class in the University. The Managers agreed to give Rutherford a room for that purpose. This privilege was extended to all the professors at the Medical School. Special wards devoted to these professorial clinical courses were then established. This system of clinical instruction was later extended to include surgery. Gradually more chairs were established at the University, in materia medica, clinical surgery, and general pathology for example. If the incumbents were Fellows of the Colleges they were privileged with the consent of the Managers to take part in clinical teaching. The legacy of these decisions was not addressed until just before the 1920s.

In 1829 Physicians-in-Ordinary who were not University professors were given permission to give clinical lectures. Thus a dual system of staffing and teaching grew up. One comprised the University professors to whom were assigned the duties of clinical lecturing with wards allocated to them for that purpose. The second group, the Ordinary Physicians and Surgeons, were appointed primarily for conducting the daily work of the infirmary. They also acted, however, as an, extra-academical body of teachers. In 1895 they formed the Extra-academical School of Medicine of the Royal Colleges. It was not until 1927 that the physicians obtained the sanction of the Managers for instruction on the wards to be given jointly to male and female students. Only after nine more years was mixed instruction in clinical surgery given.

In the mid-1860s it was decided to erect a new infirmary. After much controversy an eleven-acre site, south of the Royal Mile, was chosen. It was south facing and sloped down from Lauriston Place to the

Meadows. The foundation stone was laid in 1870. Shortly afterwards, nearby properties in Park Place and Teviot Row were purchased to allow for the construction of a new medical school. These buildings were in full occupation by 1884. The hospital was built in Scottish Baronial style, the medical and surgical houses constituting two distinct groups of buildings. The medical house comprised four pavilions and the surgical house six. Each pavilion consisted of a basement and three main floors containing wards and an attic. The administrative departments, nurses' home, and Pathology Department were separate from the pavilions. The new hospital was opened in 1879. It had 555 beds, 279 of which were in the surgical hospital and 276 of which were in the medical hospital. The twelve medical wards had twenty-three beds in each, the surgical wards mainly had sixteen beds. Beds for special subjects, such as diseases of the eye, were accommodated in the surgical house. In 1879–80, 5,315 patients were treated.

Gradually over the next forty years the Infirmary showed all the changes associated with a modern hospital. New speciality departments, such as an Ear and Throat Department and a Medical Electrical Department (holding X-ray equipment), were created. Staff increased. More beds were added. A Diamond Jubilee Pavilion was constructed, mainly devoted to diseases of women. A small isolation and observation hospital was built in the grounds. This building will appear again as the first Biochemical Laboratory. All these changes necessitated or were accompanied by other modernizing innovations. In 1897 electric lighting began to replace the old gas lamps. Telephones were installed. A new boiler-house and a modern heating system were added. The kitchen was reconstructed and a new laundry built.

A snapshot of the Infirmary in the year after Meakins's arrival in 1919 would include the following. There were twenty-six Managers including the Lord Provost of Edinburgh and James Doonan from the Coal and Shale Miners' Associations of West Lothian. There were sixteen officials ranging from the Superintendent (a knighted, medically-qualified Lieutenant-Colonel) to the Chief Porter. The Medical Department had four professors and four Ordinary Physicians, the latter designated Senior Lecturers.[16] There were eight Assistant Physicians designated Lecturers. There were two Professors of Surgery. There were eight specialist departments including one for gynaecological disorders and another for venereal diseases. There were 799 patients in the Infirmary on October 1, 1919, and over the next twelve months 12,521 were admitted. During the same period 48,117 out-patients were treated. Of the patients admitted labourers, domestic servants, and workers in mines, oil works, and "Trades" made up nearly half. Sixty "Professional Men" were recorded as having been admitted.[17]

The dual senior staffing system of the Infirmary and the method of appointment of consultants was a source of intense amazement (and irritation) to the Americans (and to some locals). The Honorary Staff comprised University professors who had their own wards and Ordinary Physicians and Surgeons who had theirs. Financial arrangements were complicated and frequently changed. In the 1920s, as far as one can tell, the Infirmary paid none of the doctors on the medical or surgical wards. The professors of medicine and surgery were paid a salary by the University to be teachers.[18] The University paid Assistant Physicians and Surgeons honoraria to be Teaching Assistants. Residents served for six months and were qualified practitioners. They were unpaid but received a laundry allowance.[19] Ordinary Physicians were unpaid but got the bulk of the students' clinical lecture fees. These arrangements were changed in 1929.[20] All senior staff, of course, did private practice.

The first step on the ladder leading to a senior hospital appointment was to gain a post as a Clinical Tutor. These posts provided teaching experience, further clinical training, opportunities for research, and time to prepare for higher medical qualifications. A modest honorarium from the University was usually supplemented by other sources of income, including fees for acting as a demonstrator in pre-clinical University departments, private tuition, and payments from senior colleagues for assistance in private practice. After several years in post it was not unusual for a Clinical Tutor to begin a single-handed, part-time private practice. If a hospital post was an ambition, waiting for a vacancy in the ranks of Assistant Physician or Surgeon was the almost invariable custom. The next step was to become a Senior Assistant. There was much competition for all these positions. By a rule of 1904, Ordinary Physicians and Surgeons were appointed for five years "with eligibility for re-appointment at the discretion of the Managers for a second and third period of similar duration."[21] University professors, however, could stay for the duration of their tenure. But even in the case of professors, the Managers retained the privilege of re-electing them as honorary physicians at five year periods. All had to retire at sixty-five.

The Edinburgh system of staffing was extremely inbred so, inevitably, the staff perpetuated particular clinical and pedagogical traditions. Indeed it did so with great pride. Residents were almost invariably Edinburgh graduates. In 1919, when an attempt was made to appoint an American graduate to a residency, the Residents wrote to the Infirmary Managers that they felt "very strongly that the House appointments should be given to Edinburgh graduates according to time honoured custom."[22] Since the only route to becoming an Ordinary Physician or Surgeon was by way of an Assistantship so, inevitably, Edinburgh graduates filled the top positions. Assistants were generally, but not always, promoted on the basis of years of service and a wait of twelve or even fifteen years (in one medical case twenty-five) before becoming an Ordinary Physician or Surgeon was not unusual. This was a source of aggravation. It was not simply the Ordinary Physicians and Surgeons who were inbred, the professors too had been through the system. In the 1920s, apart from Meakins, who is a special case, the five medical professors with clinical duties in post at some time in the decade had all been Assistants and Ordinary Physicians. The Ordinary staff regarded appointment to chairs as properly coming from their ranks. Many of them, of course, had gained reputations as distinguished teachers in the Extra-academical School.

To understand Meakins's appointment it is necessary to return to 1913. Perhaps in the light of the report of the Haldane Commission and the potential academic turn in London medicine, the Edinburgh medical colleges and the University embarked on some real and potential reforms. The year 1913 saw a major restructuring of clinical teaching, the appointment system at the Infirmary, the creation of a new clinical chair, the establishment of a bacteriology chair, and the promotion of ambitious plans for medical research. At this time the University professors taught the University students clinical medicine and Ordinary Physicians taught Extra-academical students. However, Ordinary Physicians also taught any University students who elected to attend their clinics. They were popular teachers but disadvantaged in that, not being University staff, they were not allowed to examine University students nor were their patients to be used for such examinations. The University students, therefore, were also disadvantaged, for they might attend the clinics and wards of the Ordinary Physicians but had to be examined by other teachers and on other wards.

Early in the twentieth century steps were taken to rectify this by appointing two Ordinary Surgeons as nominal, unpaid University Lecturers. This made more beds available to the University and more patients for clinical instruction and final examination. In 1908 the government appointed a Departmental Committee with Lord Elgin as Chairman to consider the claims of the Scottish Universities to receive increased grants from the Treasury. Reporting in 1910 the Committee noted the difficulty of providing sufficient patients for clinical instruction in Edinburgh. It recommended an extension to medicine of the system recently applied to surgery and that Assistant Physicians and Surgeons be designated University clinical teachers.

A memorandum prepared by Professor German Sims Woodhead and appended to the Elgin Report became the basis of the Clinical Teaching Agreement signed on June 20 and 23, 1913, by the Managers of the Infirmary and the University Court.[23] By this Agreement, the University gave Ordinary Physicians and Surgeons and Assistants academic titles (Senior Lecturer or Lecturer). These were nominal titles that served an administrative end. In practice it provided for a more even distribution of students and a greater patient population for teaching. Ordinary Physicians and Surgeons still had the right to teach students in the School of the Royal Colleges. By the same Agreement the basement rooms of the medical pavilions (the "duck ponds," as they were known) were fitted up and used for instruction.

The Agreement also changed the appointment system. Prior to 1913 appointments to the Honorary Staff had been made by candidates applying to the whole Board of Management of the RIE. Now, nominations for appointment were placed in the hands of a Selection Committee composed of seven members chosen from the Board. Only two of the seven were clinicians. Even then the Selection Committee had to nominate two candidates who went before the whole Board for final election. Thus the power of appointment remained in the hands of the Infirmary Managers and, by definition, lay people. Americans found this astonishing.

So did some Edinburgh doctors who, by the turn of the nineteenth and twentieth centuries, were keen for reform. Edinburgh practitioners were extremely proud of the School's scientific tradition and were ever ready to reel off the names of such figures as Joseph Lister, John Goodsir and John Hughes Bennett, who were but three in a cluster of stars whose pictures adorn the walls of the city's medical institutions. Pride in that tradition goes a long way towards explaining why Edinburgh doctors were often puzzled by transatlantic ideas of reform. None the less Edinburgh teachers were beginning to share a sentiment that the School, if not in crisis, needed serious overhaul. This can be seen in a debate, at the end of the war, over the medical curriculum. In this debate expressions such as the School being "too conservative" were bandied about. Systematic lecturing came under attack.[24] This was the venerated pedagogic method that had been established in the eighteenth century and remained central to medical instruction ever since. In the systematic course (given in a lecture theatre), the Professor of Medicine (who held the most prestigious chair) gave a detailed account of virtually every disease from a clinical point of view. This form of teaching was now criticized in the light of the need for more practical instruction and the availability of good textbooks. Many participants in the debate also raised the question of whether full-time chairs should be established in medicine and surgery.

Reform of the medical chairs was central to change in the 1920s. In addition two institutions, one real and one that never materialized, figure marginally in Edinburgh's self-generated attempts at reform. Both need brief mention since they were the source of intense local support in some quarters, yet the RF and the MRC held both of little account. These institutions were the Laboratory of the Royal College of Physicians and a Lister Institute. As noticed, it is necessary to recognize the power and influence of the Royal Colleges in Edinburgh for nothing quite like them existed in America.[25] Pearce, with his determination to deal only with universities, seemed to have found them a source of irritation, a sort of superfluous layer of bureaucracy that had to be dealt with but not taken seriously. Fletcher, who had poor relations with the London Colleges and considered their ideas about research to be unscientific, no doubt nourished this sentiment.[26]

In 1885 the Edinburgh College of Physicians had recommended that a laboratory be founded "for Physiological and Pathological Investigation."[27] The proposal was approved in 1887 and in 1889 the laboratory began operating in Lauriston Lane, near the Infirmary, under the superintendence of German Sims Woodhead. In 1896, the laboratory was moved to Forrest Road, also near the Infirmary, by which time Woodhead had resigned and D. Noel Paton was Superintendent. During the 1920s the Superintendent was Anderson Gray McKendrick, an epidemiologist. He seems to have had no contact with the University. The laboratory was both a seat of research and a site of diagnostic testing. Most of the research was done by College Fellows in their spare time and had a marked clinical orientation. A great deal of published work was produced, the majority of it, certainly until 1930, being single-authored (all McKendrick's work was single-authored). Dual authorship occasionally featured before 1930. It was more common after that, when multiple-authorship began to appear. The significance of this is the evidence it provides for, first, how seriously those associated with the College adopted laboratory medicine and, second, how that adoption was accommodated into the tradition of clinical individualism. Equally interesting is that, as the laboratory's historian records, after the Great War "The Laboratory Committee . . . recognized . . . that developments in biochemistry had been so important during recent years as to make it essential that this part of the Laboratory's work should be under the charge of a fully qualified specialist."[28] A chemist, W. O. Kermack, was chosen for the post in 1920. This matter merits mention in so far as there seems to be no evidence of any communication between Kermack and Meakins, Barger, or Cushny. The College of Physicians' laboratory staff seems to have had little contact with the University advocates of academic medicine.[29]

A further, and ultimately fruitless, plan for modernizing medicine in Edinburgh merits attention. The commitment of the Royal Colleges to medical research was manifested in a scheme that failed to interest the RF primarily because of its policy to deal only with universities. In 1912 the College of Surgeons proposed an institution for pathological and clinical research as a memorial to Lord Lister. On March 19, 1913, representatives of the University, the two Royal Colleges and the Carnegie Trustees for the Universities of Scotland prepared a draft scheme for what was to be called The Edinburgh Lister Institute of Pathology.[30] The building was to be vested in the University and the work of the Pathology and Bacteriology Departments of the University would be done there.

In addition, the laboratory of the College of Physicians was to be absorbed into it and the Fellows of the Colleges were to have rights to work there. It was to be, therefore, an institution not fully under the University's control.[31] In July 1914 a site was secured for over £50,000.[32]

The war put an end to the plan, as it did to plans for London units. The scheme was soon revived after 1918. A printed letter of December 1919 signed by the Principal of the University and the Presidents of the Royal Colleges stated £250,000 was required to make the Institute functional and that the Colleges and the University "in 1913 had agreed to contribute sums amounting to £25,000."[33] In 1921 a "Scheme of Extension and Development" of the University was produced. This seems to have been sent to Pearce in advance of his visit in 1923. In this document the Lister Memorial Institute was seen as an integral part of University growth. The collaboration of the Colleges and University was described as "an epoch in the history of medical science in Edinburgh."This is much as one would expect in a city proud of its medical traditions but it was not Pearce's view. A public appeal for money for the Institute which had been planned had to be temporarily shelved because the Royal Infirmary itself had had to launch a public appeal for its own needs.The money ultimately required was now described as "£1, 779, 800" [sic!].[34] The significance of the Lister scheme and RF hostility to it is discussed in the next chapter.

The most productive step in making Edinburgh medicine more academic was the reform of its chairs. This initiative came from the University (on the recommendation the Medical Faculty). In 1913 the University, recognizing a new subject, created the Robert Irvine Chair of Bacteriology. James Ritchie, an Edinburgh graduate, was appointed. Ritchie first held a Lectureship in Bacteriology at Oxford and in 1907 became Superintendent of the College of Physicians' Laboratory. Bacteriology in Edinburgh at this time was institutionally in the shade of pathology. In 1913 Ritchie had only a small amount of space in the University Pathology Department and any bacteriological research he did was carried out at the College. Ritchie seems to have had no specified relation with the Infirmary.[35] Bacteriological work in the Infirmary was carried out in its own Pathology Department and in 1914 the RIE recognized this by appointing William Robertson Logan as its first named Clinical Pathologist with special responsibility for bacteriology.[36]

In 1924 his title was changed to Clinical Bacteriologist and in 1925 the subject was finally given independence in the Infirmary when a separate Department of Bacteriology was established. Just before this, in 1923, Thomas Jones Mackie succeeded Ritchie in the Bacteriology Chair at the University and in 1924 he was listed as Honorary Bacteriologist to the hospital although apparently his role "was never precisely defined."[37] Mackie is an important player in this story. He formed good relations with Barger and Cushny and strongly identified with the cause of the laboratory sciences in medicine. He was on excellent terms with Fletcher.

The most consequential reforms carried out before the war were centred on chairs with clinical responsibilities at the RIE. When preparing to implement the scheme based on the Elgin Report of 1910, the University Court radically reorganized these chairs. Although, since the eighteenth century, all Edinburgh medical professors had the right to act as clinical professors in the Infirmary, in fact, by 1912, only three did so: the Professor of Medicine, the Professor of Materia Medica, and the Professor of Pathology. There was no separate chair of clinical medicine. In 1912 William Smith Greenfield resigned from the Chair of Pathology. The Pathology Department of the hospital had long had close links with the Medical School and these were tightened after 1912 when James Lorrain Smith was appointed Professor of Pathology. Smith, while remaining Professor, became Pathologist to the Infirmary.[38] The Pathology Department of the University had other employees and its Assistant Pathologists also served in the Infirmary.[39] This was, as observed in Chapter 2, an important apprenticeship, a road to a position as a full physician or surgeon. David Murray Lyon, Meakins's successor, had been an Assistant Pathologist in 1912–1919. Lorrain Smith was an Edinburgh graduate who had worked at Oxford with the physiologist J. S. Haldane on respiratory function. At Edinburgh, Smith developed a method of teaching morbid anatomy based on "a study of individual cases of disease rather in that of individual organs."[40] His research was based more on physiology and pathophysiology than morbid anatomy. He studied the determination of blood volume and the metabolism of fat. At first sight Smith would seem to be a representative of modern medicine to whom the RF would be sympathetic. Yet he was also deeply steeped in Edinburgh ways of thinking and Pearce, whenever he could, bypassed him. This was no easy task, since Smith was Dean of the Medical School, 1919–1931.

Smith's appointment offered the opportunity for reform in the Medical Faculty and the implementation of a plan by which the new incumbent of the Chair of Pathology should give his whole time to that subject and a separate Professorship of Clinical Medicine could be created. This was an important development for it divorced pathology from direct involvement with clinical practice and was, therefore, part of the move to specialization in the medical sciences that characterizes this period. This possibility of separating the chairs was being debated as early as 1911. It was not until 1913 that the bureaucratic engines of the University had been negotiated and agreement with the Infirmary Managers on this matter was reached (again the sort of bargaining with the RIE that puzzled the Americans). Besides this new chair in clinical medicine the Medical Faculty also decided in 1912 to recommend to the University Court that a *second* special Professorship of Clinical Medicine be eventually instituted "to meet possible future requirements."[41]

In October 1913 William Russell, one of the Ordinary Physicians to the Infirmary, was appointed to the new Professorship of Clinical Medicine, now named the Moncrieff Arnott Chair. In an innovative move, and perhaps with the Haldane Commission in mind, the Medical Faculty recommended the appointment be more or less full time. It decreed that:

> the new Professor should devote his time and energies chiefly to the duties of the Chair and he shall be required to take care that consulting practice or professional work shall not be allowed to interfere with his duties as Professor or with the time required for the performance of these duties; his remuneration should be not less that £800 per annum; and he should be provided with a salaried assistant or assistants, and with appropriate laboratory accommodation, much of which is already available in the Royal Infirmary.[42]

To create the second clinical chair the Court cast its eye on the long-standing Chair of Materia Medica (also a chair with clinical responsibilities) and agreed to divide it into two professorships. This was done on the retirement of Sir Thomas Richard Fraser in 1918. Of the two new chairs, the first remained the Chair of Materia Medica but no longer had clinical duties. In fact the new professor, Arthur Cushny, as described above, was a pure scientist. The second chair created was in therapeutics and this had clinical responsibilities. By arrangement with the Infirmary Managers, the beds formerly in the charge of the Professor of Materia Medica were allocated to it. This division of an old chair is significant because it was recognition by the Faculty that the ancient subject of materia medica should be dismantled and two modern disciplines promoted: experimental pharmacology and clinical therapeutics. The Christison Chair of Therapeutics was to have Meakins as its first incumbent. As with the Moncrieff Arnott Chair of Clinical Medicine, the question whether the Professor of Therapeutics should be full time was raised. This matter was perhaps made more pressing by the fact that the incumbent of the Moncrieff Arnott Chair, William Russell, does not seem to have acted in a full-time capacity.

By 1917, when Fraser's retirement from the Chair of Materia Medica was imminent, the Medical Faculty was asked by the University Court's Finance Committee: "(1) how far the holder of the proposed Chair of Therapeutics should be permitted to carry on private practice; (2) what income should, in the opinion of the Faculty, be allotted to the above Chair." In the ensuing discussion it was reported that "the feeling of the Faculty appeared to be that the holder of the proposed Chair of Therapeutics should not engage in private practice but might be allowed to hold an appointment such as that of a medical officer to . . . an Insurance Company: that the salary should be not less than £800 with an addition for clinical teaching."[43]

In the event, at its next meeting the Faculty recommended a salary of £1,000 that would include clinical teaching (in addition to obligatory systematic lectures on therapeutics). It also considered a Memorandum circulated by Sir Thomas Fraser that stated:

> In addition to routine bedside instruction it is highly desirable that the Professor of Therapeutics should engage in original investigation. This would occupy much time and he should be . . . provided not only with patients but with laboratory accommodation and the newer instruments required in the modern methods of advancing knowledge of the abnormal conditions of patients and the effects of treatment.[44]

The Chair was created in 1918 but in December of that year, for whatever reason (perhaps no suitable candidate had been found), "The

Faculty decided that they were not able, in the meantime, to recommend that the Chair be filled up."[45] By February of 1919, however, it was "decided to intimate to the University Court that the Faculty are of opinion that the time has come for steps to be taken in regard to the appointment of a Professor who should commence his duties in October next."[46] The minutes record nothing about Meakins.

Jonathan Meakins was born in Hamilton, Canada, in 1882. His mother was of Scottish descent and in view of Edinburgh "clannishness" (see especially Chapter 6) this may have been a factor in his appointment.[47] He entered McGill University, Montreal, as a medical student in 1900 and graduated in 1904. Following an internship at the Royal Victoria Hospital, Montreal, he became an Assistant in Medicine to Rufus Cole at the Johns Hopkins Hospital. Cole was one of the most distinguished experimentally-minded physicians of the day. In the summer of 1907 Meakins worked at a children's hospital in the Blue Ridge Mountains where he studied intestinal disease, an interest that was to re-emerge in Edinburgh.[48] He then became Resident Pathologist at the Presbyterian Hospital, New York. Meakins was obviously gaining something of a name for himself in academic medicine. In 1909 the Rockefeller Hospital, an adjunct to the Rockefeller Institute, was nearing completion and Rufus Cole was appointed Medical Director. He offered Meakins the job of Senior Resident. In fact Meakins returned to Montreal where he entered private practice. He was also a Clinical Assistant at the Royal Victoria Hospital as well as Demonstrator in Clinical Medicine.

Meakins advanced rapidly up the McGill academic ladder. Dissatisfied, as he and a number of colleagues were, with "purely anatomical cases, both normal and pathological," they induced the Medical Faculty to establish a Department of Experimental Medicine in 1912.[49] Meakins was made Director. He was, however, unhappy at McGill and his chief wrote to London to Sir James Mackenzie and Thomas Lewis asking if Meakins might study under them. James Mackenzie, the older of these two men and Lewis's mentor, had been a general practitioner in Lancashire and had then gained an appointment at the London Hospital. Lewis was a friend of Fletcher's (they went fly-fishing together) and a physician at University College Hospital, London. Between them, Mackenzie and Lewis had been largely instrumental in creating the "new cardiology." Until the early twentieth century the study of the heart was largely based on normal and morbid anatomy. The clinical correlate of this was that the heart was investigated by percussion and by auscultation through the stethoscope in order to discover abnormalities in structure. The new cardiologists emphasized cardiac function and the investigation of the properties of the heart's muscle (such as irritability) and conducting tissues that had been described by laboratory-based physiologists. The new tool for investigating these properties at the bedside, both in everyday practice and for research purposes, was the electrocardiograph. Lewis was the acknowledged master of this instrument. The new cardiology was seen as a major example of what the new scientific medicine could offer. Meakins left for London in September 1913. Having presented his letters of introduction to Lewis and Mackenzie, Meakins started on what he later remembered as "a wonderful year."[50] No doubt it was intellectually, but he wrote at the time that his meeting Mackenzie was a "great disappointment." He explained: "Without doubt he is a great man but as far as the clinic is concerned he seems to absolutely neglect any attempt to create one. He gives no encouragement to any men but general practitioners of the most general kind." Paradoxically Mackenzie, whose work was a building block of academic medicine, was quite hostile to many of the changes associated with it. Most of Meakins's time was spent with Lewis, whom he found "very encouraging and helpful," studying electrocardiography and doing animal experimental work. Meakins also worked with the physiologist Leonard Hill on blood pressure and met the famous respiratory physiologist Joseph Barcroft.[51]

After a brief return to Montreal, the war having broken out, Meakins enlisted, serving initially at the No. 3 General Hospital (McGill) in France.[52] In 1916, however, his cardiological expertise was recognized and he was posted to Mount Vernon Hospital at Hampstead Heath in London, which had been specially designated by the War Office as a centre for the study of so-called "soldier's heart." Lewis was in charge. In the winter of 1917 Meakins was posted to a hospital in Brighton, followed by an appointment at the Red Cross General Hospital at Taplow, Berkshire, in the grounds of Cliveden, the residence of Lord Astor. During the war Meakins had grown interested in respiratory physiology. While at Brighton, by way of introduction from William Osler, Meakins met the doyen of respiratory physiologists, J. S. Haldane, who worked at Oxford.

At Taplow Meakins organized a laboratory and was fortunate to have working with him another distinguished respiratory physiologist, John Gillies Priestly. Osler, living in Oxford (which is very near Taplow), visited once a week, as did Haldane. Meakins was made a member of the Chemical Warfare Committee of the War Office. Also on the committee were Walter Morley Fletcher, Arthur Cushny, Haldane, and Barcroft and two other leading physiologists, Henry Dale and Claude Gordon Douglas. Meakins by now was well integrated into elite British medical and scientific circles and after the war became a sought-after candidate for medical chairs.

On June 2, 1919, Haldane wrote to Meakins telling him that he had met Lorrain Smith (Haldane's former co-worker), who had told him of developments in Edinburgh. Haldane explained to Meakins that there was a new therapeutics chair to be filled. The appointment would be full time and at a salary of £1,000 per annum. Private practice was excluded but, added Haldane, "this does not include Insurance Company appointments which are pretty important at Edinburgh." Haldane reported that he had written to Principal Ewing mentioning Meakins's name.[53] According to Meakins (who had not recollected the dates correctly): "It was about the middle of June [1919] when I received a long letter from Dr. Haldane informing me that my name had been proposed—I think by him, Osler and Mackenzie—as a candidate [for the Chair of Therapeutics in Edinburgh]."[54] Since a chair in clinical medicine would customarily be given to an Ordinary Physician of the Infirmary, Edinburgh had obviously been prompted into looking for an outside candidate. Haldane, Meakins remembered, had "warned the University and the Infirmary, that with any offer to me, they should state that suitable laboratory accommodation would be provided in the Infirmary grounds."[55] Other supporters of Meakins had clearly been recruited in the drive to enlist him. Cushny (newly established in the Materia Medica Chair), writing on June 13, 1919, stated how pleased he would be to have Meakins as a colleague, remarking: "As you have no doubt observed the clinical work in this country needs a good deal of burnishing up." He thought, "the greatest attraction of the Therapeutics chair is the opportunity of resuscitating clinical medicine in Edinburgh." Encouraging Meakins to come, and using the same carrot as Haldane, Cushny noted, "may I say I am told that good appointments to Insurance business and that sort of thing are to be had."[56] Things moved quickly. On June 14 Haldane reported that the Edinburgh Election Committee had decided to offer Meakins the Chair (even though Meakins had not yet applied).[57] Two days later Ewing asked Meakins to submit his name with a view to appointment.[58] Exciting the Edinburgh bureaucratic machinery into action paid dividends. About the time the Principal's letter arrived, Meakins would have received one from C. F. Martin of McGill Medical School, stating: "I do not know whether you know by this time or not that you are to be asked for on this side of the water."[59] It is not exactly clear where and what this position was, but it was certainly in Montreal. Meakins was hot property. In August, 1919 the University of Michigan wrote to him with the offer of a full-time chair of medicine at a salary of $7,500 and the promise of beds in a new building, "which we hope to make the latest and best thing in a teaching hospital."[60]

During early July 1919 negotiations over Meakins's terms were still taking place. On July 11 Lorrain Smith wrote to Meakins saying, "It is perhaps unfortunate that the Faculty a year ago decided that the Professor should be debarred from private practice." He felt that the salary of £1,200 now offered was "small" and he hoped it could be raised by £200.[61] Haldane had suggested Meakins stick out for £1,500.[62] Smith, like Cushny, noted: "Edinburgh is a great Insurance centre" and medical officers could pick up £400 to £800 a year, "while the work and time entailed are by no means excessive." Meakins had suggested to Haldane he might be permitted to see private patients in the Infirmary but Smith pointed out that this was "quite contrary to the custom of this country."[63] Meakins, however, did see private patients in a nursing home in or around Edinburgh, certainly in 1923 and probably earlier.[64] By 1924 he seems to have changed his mind and saw no space at all, in theory at least, for private practice for a professor. In a report to the Infirmary Managers that was also copied to Abraham Flexner he made his position clear. Possibly the Infirmary was considering taking in private patients to boost its income as had happened at the London hospitals. Private patients in a public hospital, Meakins wrote, might mean the professor "could build up an enormous private practice, which would, if he allowed it, soon occupy the major part of his time." It would then be "quite obvious . . . that he is not a full-time university teacher either in spirit or in fact." He also thought full-time appointments with certain hours for seeing private patients outside hospital "a hybrid arrangement." This was "neither good for the department or for the man's practice." This "hybrid position" was, in fact, the one favored by Osler on the grounds of the experience it brought. "[W]ith this contention," wrote Meakins, "I have no sympathy whatever." He had not "yet been able to find any essential difference between the illnesses of the pauper and those of the millionaire."[65]

Meakins accepted the nomination and he cabled Ewing on July 12 to that effect.[66] Ewing wrote to him on July 15 that the University Court had elected him Professor.[67] Meakins records that he was to take up his duties on October 1.[68] He received a letter of congratulation from Haldane who wrote that there was "no mistake that a new and far more scientific standard in medicine is badly wanted over here and I have no doubt that you'll take a lead in establishing it, and find plenty of keen support at Edinburgh."[69] He received other letters welcoming his move and confirming the sense that Edinbugh need revitalizing. Thomas Muir, writing from Hampstead in August, congratulated him, hoping that "we shall soon see Edinburgh begin to recover her old prestige in the description of new ideas."[70] Meakins, now married, planned to set out for Edinburgh on his own and "find rooms for myself and scout about for a furnished house with maids etc on a temporary basis."[71] His wife, Dorothy, and children would follow in spring 1920, by which time he hoped to have found an unfurnished property. On arriving in Britain he went first to London where he spent time with the elite of British physiology and physiologically-minded physicians: Fletcher, Lewis, Hill, Haldane, Barcroft, and two "new cardiologists", Thomas Cotton and John Parkinson.[72] On arrival in Edinburgh he stayed with Henry Harvey Littlejohn, Professor of Forensic Medicine, whom he had met at Taplow. His stay overlapped with that of Osler.[73] The next day he met Ewing, Lorrain Smith, and Murray Lyon, "who had been appointed a clinical assistant and detailed to my service."[74] This implies that neither he nor Murray Lyon had any choice in the matter, but in July Lyon had written to Meakins applying to be his clinical tutor.[75] Meakins was given charge of a ward and a half with thirty-four beds for men and seventeen for women.[76]

By the beginning of the twentieth century, biochemistry had gradually been introduced in a minimal way into both undergraduate medical teaching and clinical practice although with rather less flag waving than surrounded the introduction of bacteriology. By the 1920s it was also being institutionalized in hospitals where laboratories carried out diagnostic and other tests for clinicians on the wards. By this time, firmly established in the undergraduate curriculum as a discipline, biochemistry in the hospital began to be used as a locus for medical specialization and clinical discipline building. The relatively undefined place of biochemistry in clinical medicine is well illustrated in the various proposals made in Edinburgh to introduce routine biochemical testing and research work into the RIE in 1918–20. A distinction between these two sorts of biochemical work, research and routine, was by no means definitive during this period. The introduction of biochemistry into the Infirmary did not begin as an academic initiative at all. Agitation for a chemical dimension to the pathological services of the Infirmary began early in 1918. In May of that year the Infirmary Managers considered a letter from the Honorary Staff, who had unanimously agreed that the appointment of a "Chemical pathologist" to the hospital was desirable. This person they considered should be a paid officer of the Infirmary, work in the Pathology Department, and engage in research.[77] How far "need" played a role in this request and how far it was driven by a sense of Edinburgh's tardiness in modernizing is impossible to gauge. St. Thomas's, London, had had a chemical pathologist, Hugh MacLean, since 1912. It is not clear who the moving force was behind the Edinburgh proposal. The Medical Managers' Committee was asked by the Infirmary Managers to consider this request. Although not opposed in principle, the Committee did not feel it was within the realm of "practical politics" (the nation after all was still at war) and considered it would involve a "substantial addition to the annual outlay in connection with the Pathology Department."[78]

By July 1919 a quite different proposition was being discussed: a research laboratory in the Infirmary for the Professor of Therapeutics. When the Secretary of the Senate, L. J. Grant, formally notified Meakins of his duties he stated that the Professor "is to undertake research." For this purpose "laboratory facilities will be provided in the Department of Materia Medica and Pharmacology, and the Court hope to arrange for the provision of similar facilities in the Royal Infirmary."[79] Once again the RIE had to be bargained with and, in this instance, persuaded of the benefits of a biochemistry laboratory. When Grant notified the Infirmary Managers of Meakins's appointment he observed:

> The Faculty of Medicine have emphasized the importance of the new Professor undertaking research, and they are anxious that he should be provided with laboratory facilities, not only in the Department of Materia Medica and of Pharmacology, but also in the Royal Infirmary, and the University Court will be greatly obliged if the Managers will take this matter into their kind consideration.[80]

What was being appealed to here was the Infirmary Managers' sense of their being custodians of the reputation of a great teaching hospital. Research was stressed. Nothing about the value of the Professor's laboratory to patients was recorded.

At this point then, the Professor of Therapeutics' research laboratory was a separate issue from the request for a diagnostic laboratory. Pressure for an independent biochemistry diagnostic lab (as opposed to creating a post within the Pathology Department) came shortly after this. The instigator was Francis Darby Boyd, an Ordinary Physician who had succeeded William Russell as Professor of Clinical Medicine in 1919. At a meeting of Infirmary Managers on October 20, 1919, a letter from Boyd was read, "directing attention to the urgent necessity for the establishment of a properly equipped Clinical Laboratory in close association with the medical wards of the Institution."[81] In November 1919 the Medical Managers discussed a proposal (presumably Boyd's letter) for a "Central Clinical Laboratory" and the Committee decided to ask the staff whether "in their opinion there would be any disadvantage in using for it the old Observation Ward."[82] A month later the staff had "unanimously approved" the suggestion.[83] It is not clear whether this proposal and that for a research lab for the Professor of Therapeutics had been welded together by this time. They shortly became so.

The Infirmary Managers discussed these various developments at a meeting on February 2, 1920. Since Boyd's original letter, his "request had been subsequently emphasized by Dr Meakins, the Professor of Therapeutics, and it was indicated that, if provided, the Laboratory would always be available for use for all the members of the Honorary Staff." Following this, a full explanation was given from the Managers' Chair "as to the vital necessity for providing the Laboratory now asked for if the Institution was to keep its proper place as a first class hospital." The Chair informed the Managers that "The work to be done was not the teaching of students (they would not have entry to the Laboratory) but investigation of diseases of patients in the Wards under the care of the various members of the Staff from time to time." This seems to indicate that it was envisaged, at this point, that all members of the staff would use the lab and carry out their own tests, and that this activity would constitute research (to the hospital's credit) and also be of benefit to the sick. The notion of testing for patient management in one laboratory and research in another seems to have disappeared.[84] In any event, the Infirmary Managers debated the question of whether a lab was required at all and whether it should occupy the Observation Ward. The minutes record: "The subject was then discussed at some length, several members expressing the view that as it had been urged that the Laboratory was necessary to enable Drs Boyd and Meakins to adequately carry out their special work as Professors, the University Authorities might reasonably be asked to pay a proportion at least of the cost of adapting the building." It was finally agreed to report that a Clinical Laboratory should be provided and that "the Observation Ward should be allocated and altered for that purpose in accordance with the plan submitted." In addition it was minuted: "That the University Authorities shall be approached on the question of sharing the cost of converting the building chosen, it being understood however that such negotiations should not interfere with the work being proceeded with."[85] In the event the University agreed to contribute to half the conversion cost to a sum of up to £500.[86]

By June 1920, draft regulations for a "Clinical Laboratory" had been drawn up by Meakins and Boyd and sent to the medical managers for report.[87] The delicate symbiosis of University and Infirmary, of research and routine, was explicit in the final rules. The Director was to be the Christison Professor (an arrangement much the same as that governing the Infirmary Pathology Department). The concept of routine testing does appear in these rules but there was still a relative lack of distinction between routine and research. A description of the "work to be carried out in the Laboratory" referred to "organized investigations" by the Professor's Assistants and members of the Honorary Staff. The lab's second role was defined as being "the carrying out of the more complicated routine methods of physiological and pathological chemistry in relation to the diagnosis and treatment of cases of disease in the hospital which in the opinion of the advisory committee cannot be undertaken in the Ward siderooms [*sic*]."The "ordinary" apparatus of research was to be supplied from grants from the University Court and special research apparatus paid for by the workers themselves.[88] Such apparatus could be quite expensive: Meakins's own apparatus was insured for £800.[89] The Infirmary was to pay for apparatus and materials used in "routine reporting work."[90] A standing Advisory Committee was constituted.[91]

The laboratory, however, was not known as the "Clinical Laboratory" but the "Bio-chemical Laboratory."The name was proposed by James Ritchie (the bacteriologist).[92] The significance of the lab being "Biochemical" and not "Clinical" is that no morbid anatomy was carried out there, or histology, or clinical microscopy. Most of this latter was done in the side rooms and, when more specialist advice was needed, in the pathology laboratory. Neither did the lab carry out any clinical bacteriology or diagnostic serology, this too, at this time, being done in the Pathology Department. Nor did it carry out haematological investigations: blood counts, haemoglobin estimations etc. Again, these were done in the side rooms of the wards or the Pathology Department. The lab commenced carrying out routine examinations for the Infirmary in January 1921.

Notes

1. D. Guthrie, *Extramural Medical Education in Edinburgh and the School of Medicine of the Royal Colleges* (Edinburgh and London: Livingstone, 1965). Unfortunately for present purposes Guthrie mainly deals with the nineteenth century.

2. A. Logan Turner, *Story of a Great Hospital. The Royal Infirmary of Edinburgh 1729–1929* (Edinburgh: Oliver and Boyd Ltd., 1937), 1.

3. Teaching Assistants received honoraria from the University.

4. Thomas H. Holland, introduction to *The History of the University of Edinburgh 1883–1933*, ed. A. Logan Turner (Edinburgh: Oliver and Boyd, 1933), xiii–xiv.

5. John Dixon Comrie, "The Faculty of Medicine," in ibid., 100–163.

6. The two Edinburgh Colleges and the Royal Faculty of Physicians and Surgeons of Glasgow.

7. W. S. Craig, *History of the Royal College of Physicians of Edinburgh* (Oxford: Blackwell Scientific Publications, 1976), 339.

8. For classes and teachers see Royal Colleges of Edinburgh, *School of Medicine Calendar* (Edinburgh). None the less the last edition, for the session 1947–48, still included classes in experimental physiology.

9. Richard Pearce, "Notes of R.M.P. on Medical School of the University of Edinburgh," February 22–24, 1923, 5, folder 5, box 1, series 405, RG 1.1, Rockefeller Foundation Archives, RAC. See also Craig, *History of the Royal College of Physicians*, 347. Numbers increased in the 1930s as the US closed its doors to foreign graduates, see ibid. on this and also on the quality of the students.

10. Comrie, "The Faculty of Medicine," 162.

11. Pearce, "Notes of R.M.P.," 2, 9.

12. Gregg, "Edinburgh—Record System," February 13, 1931, folder 10, box 1, series 405, RG 1.1, Rockefeller Foundation Archives, RAC.

13. "The Introductory Address," *British Medical Journal* 2 (1885): 655.

14. Pearce, "Notes of R.M.P.," 2.

15. Turner, *Story of a Great Hospital*, 55.

16. The qualifier "Ordinary" had been dropped by now although in effect this category remained.

17. Royal Infirmary of Edinburgh, *Reports Regarding the Affairs of the Royal Infirmary of Edinburgh from 1st October 1919 to 1st October 1920* (Edinburgh: The Darien Press, n.d.).

18. There was also a Professor of Tuberculosis. In the 1920s this was Robert Philip.

19. Turner, *Story of a Great Hospital*, 112.

20. Comrie, "The Faculty of Medicine," 151–52.

21. Turner, *Story of a Great Hospital*, 301.

22. RIE, Board of Managers Minutes, September 22, 1919, LHSA, LHB1/1/56, EUL.

23. *Report of the Committee on Scottish Universities with a Memorandum by Professor G. Sims Woodhead, Presented to both Houses of Parliament*, 1910, cited in Turner, *Story of a Great Hospital*, 305 note.

24. Edinburgh Pathological Club, *An Inquiry into the Medical Curriculum* (Edinburgh: W. Green & Son, 1919), 236.

25. They were the American Colleges of Physicians and of Surgeons, but they had nothing like the prestige or power of their transatlantic counterparts nor did they concern themselves with undergraduate medical teaching. See Rosemary Stevens, *American Medicine and the Public Interest: A History of Specialization* (Berkeley: University of California Press, 1971).

26. For Fletcher's poor relations with the London Colleges see *Historical Perspectives on the Role of the MRC: Essays in the History of the Medical Research Council of the United Kingdom and its Predecessor, the Medical Research Committee, 1913–1953*, ed. Joan Austoker and Linda Bryder (New York: Oxford University Press, 1989).

27. John Ritchie, *History of the Laboratory of the Royal College of Physicians of Edinburgh* (Edinburgh: Royal College of Physicians, 1953), 5.

28. Ibid., 65.

29. Kermack published a short communication with a member of the staff of the Department of Therapeutics, C. G. Lambie, in 1929. C. G. Lambie, W. O. Kermack, and W. F. Harvey, "Effect of Parathyroid Hormone on the Structure of Bone," *Nature* 1234 (1929): 348. Lambie seems to have used the College's lab for animal experiments. See Chapter 8.

30. In 1901 Andrew Carnegie donated ten million dollars to the Universities of Scotland. Holland, introduction to *The History of the University*, xxiii.

31. A brief history of the scheme can be found in Ritchie, *History of the Laboratory of the Royal College of Physicians*, 58–60.

32. Printed letter of invitation to serve on the General Committee of the Lister Memorial scheme (December, 1919). A copy can be found appended to Pearce, "Notes of R.M.P."

33. Ibid.

34. "Scheme of Extension and Development," appended to Pearce "Notes of R.M.P.," 13, 20.

35. University of Edinburgh, Faculty of Medicine, Minutes of a Special Faculty Meeting, October 28, 1913. Shelf ref. DA43, EUA.

36. See Charles J. Smith, *Edinburgh's Contribution to Medical Microbiology* (Glasgow: Wellcome Unit for the History of Medicine, 1994), 134, 224. During the War a Miss Fitzgerald was Assistant Clinical Pathologist. RIE, Board of Managers Minutes, April 7, 1919, LHSA, LHB1/1/56, EUL.

37. Smith, *Edinburgh's Contribution to Medical Microbiology*, 137.

38. Comrie, "The Faculty of Medicine," 120, 123, 159.

39. For a list of the Assistant Pathologists see Turner, *Story of a Great Hospital*, 377–78.

40. Comrie, "The Faculty of Medicine."

41. The Medical Faculty Minutes of 1912 recorded: "After discussion the following motion, proposed by Professor Walker, and seconded by Professor Caird, was unanimously agreed to: 'The Faculty, adhering to the first paragraph of recommendation No. 1, page 2, of its report to the Senatus of 2nd March 1911, recommends that a special Professorship of Clinical Medicine be instituted. The Faculty further recommends that, in the Ordinance required for the purpose, the Court should take power to institute a second special Professorship of Clinical Medicine, in order to meet possible future requirements'." University of Edinburgh, Faculty of Medicine, Minutes of a Special Faculty Meeting, November 5, 1912. Shelf ref. DA43, EUA. For the approach to the Infirmary Managers, Turner, *Story of a Great Hospital*, 309, cites "Minute, Royal Infirmary, August 5, 1912."

42. University of Edinburgh, Faculty of Medicine, Minutes of a Special Faculty Meeting October 2, 1913. Shelf ref. DA43, EUA.

43. University of Edinburgh, Minutes of a Medical Faculty Meeting, December 4, 1917. Shelf ref. DA43, EUA.

44. University of Edinburgh, Minutes of a Medical Faculty Meeting, December 11, 1917. Shelf ref. DA43, EUA.

45. University of Edinburgh, Minutes of a Medical Faculty Meeting, December 3, 1918. Shelf ref. DA43, EUA.

46. University of Edinburgh, Minutes of a Medical Faculty Meeting, February 3, 1919. Shelf ref. DA43, EUA.

47. On his father's side his forebears came from Essex! On Meakins's background see Meakins, "Autobiography," 3, 867/51, OLHM.

48. Ibid., 48.

49. Ibid., 61.

50. Ibid., 70.

51. Meakins to C. F. Martin, Montreal, c.1916, 867/39/84, OLHM.

52. Meakins, "Autobiography," 76.

53. Haldane to Meakins, June 2, 1919, 867/39/39, OLHM.

54. Meakins, "Autobiography," 98.

55. Ibid., 99.

56. Cushny to Meakins, June 13, 1919, 867/39/42, OLHM.

57. Haldane to Meakins, June 14, 1919, 867/39/40, OLHM.

58. Ewing to Meakins, June 16, 1919, 867/39/43, OLHM. See also, Meakins, "Autobiography," 99. On June 13, 1919 Cushny also wrote "You will receive by the same mail as this an invitation from the Principal to enter in the new Chair of Clinical Therapeutics." Cushny to Meakins, June 13, 1919, 867/39/42, OLHM.

59. Martin to Meakins, June 11, 1919, 867/39/41, OLHM. Quite why Martin wrote is unclear, after all, they were friends and both in Montreal. Perhaps Meakins was on vacation.

60. V. C. Vaughan to Meakins, August 12, 1919, 867/35/1, OLHM.

61. Lorrain Smith to Meakins, July 11, 1919, Secretary's file, DRT 95/002, pt. 1, Faculty of Medicine, box 27, EUA.

62. Haldane to Meakins, July 10, 1919, 867/36/8, OLHM.

63. Lorrain Smith to Meakins, July 11, 1919, Secretary's file, DRT 95/002, pt. 1, Faculty of Medicine, box 27, EUA.

64. The University Court in 1922 (see Chapter 5) granted him the dispensation to see private patients. That he actually did so, see Pearce, "Notes of R.M.P.," 6.

65. Meakins to Abraham Flexner with copy of "Report for the Managers of the Infirmary," May 1, 1924, 867/35/4, OLHM.

66. Meakins to Ewing, July 12, 1919, Secretary's file, DRT 95/002, pt. 1, Faculty of Medicine, box 27, EUA. In his "Autobiography," Meakins mistakenly says July 2. Meakins, "Autobiography," 100.

67. Ewing to Meakins, July 15, 1919, 867/39/50, OLHM.

68. Meakins, "Autobiography," 100.

69. Haldane to Meakins, July 26, 1919, 867/36/9, OLHM.

70. Muir to Meakins, August 6, 1919, 867/39/54, OLHM. The only Thomas Muir in *The Medical Directory* for 1919 had a Glasgow medical degree from 1894 and

was living in East London. He seems an unlikely candidate. Muir could well have been a biochemist or physiologist.

71. Meakins, "Autobiography," 100.

72. Ibid., 101.

73. Ibid., 101. See also Harvey Littlejohn to Meakins, July 27, 1919, offering accommodation, 867/39/38, OLHM.

74. Meakins, "Autobiography," 102.

75. Murray Lyon to Meakins, July 24, 1919, 867/39/53, OLHM.

76. For some reason, which is not clear, Meakins, although clearly designated Professor of Therapeutics, appears as only a Senior Lecturer in the *Edinburgh University Calendar* until the 1922–1923 edition. See *Edinburgh University Calendar, 1920–1921* (Edinburgh: James Thin, 1920), 586.

77. RIE, Board of Managers Minutes, May 20, 1918, LHSA, LHB1/1/56, EUL.

78. RIE, Board of Managers Minutes, June 24, 1918, LHSA, LHB1/1/56, EUL. The Medical Managers who considered the request were Sir James Affleck (also an Infirmary Manager), a Consulting Physician to the Hospital (a sort of senior advisory position); George Mackay, a Consulting Ophthalmic Surgeon; McKenzie Johnston, a Consulting Ear and Throat Surgeon; and a Dr Macpherson who does not seem to have had an Infirmary appointment [not traced].

79. Grant to Meakins, July 16, 1919, 867/39/52, OLHM.

80. RIE, Board of Managers Minutes, July 21, 1919, LHSA, LHB1/1/56, EUL.

81. RIE, Board of Managers Minutes, October 20, 1919, LHSA, LHB1/1/ 56, EUL.

82. RIE, Board of Managers Minutes, November 24, 1919, LHSA, LHB1/1/ 56, EUL.

83. RIE, Board of Managers Minutes, December, 22, 1919, LHSA, LHB1/1/ 57, EUL.

84. At the Johns Hopkins Hospital the General Clinical Laboratory carried out routine tests and research, and trained students in laboratory methods. The hospital also had specialist research laboratories in biology and biochemistry. See Lewellys F. Barker, "The Organization of the Laboratories in the Medical Clinic of The Johns Hopkins Hospital," *Bulletin of The Johns Hopkins Hospital* 18 (1907): 193–98.

85. RIE, Board of Managers Minutes, February 2, 1920, LHSA, LHB1/1/ 57, EUL.

86. RIE, Board of Managers Minutes, February 23, 1920, LHSA, LHB1/1/ 57, EUL.

87. RIE, Board of Managers Minutes, June 7, 1920, LHSA, LHB1/1/57, EUL.

88. Draft Rules can be found in RIE, Medical Managers Committee, October 27, 1920, LHSA, LHB1/2/47, EUL. See also the final printed version in *Regulations for the Conduct of the Laboratory* (1921), "Scrap-Book of the RIE Biochemical Laboratory," box 1, folder 11, RCPE.

89. W. S. Caw (Treasurer and Clerk to Infirmary) to Meakins, 6 November 1920, "Scrap-Book of the RIE Biochemical Laboratory," box 2, RCPE.

90. *Regulations for the Conduct of the Laboratory.*

91. Consisting of the Director (Chairman), the Moncrieff Arnott Professor of Clinical Medicine, the Regius Professor of Clinical Surgery, a member of the Medical Staff elected by the Medical Staff, a member of the Surgical Staff elected by the Surgical Staff, a member of the Staff elected by the Staff attached to the Special Departments and a member of the Committee of the Medical Managers elected by that committee. RIE, Medical Managers Committee, October 27, 1920, LHSA, LHB1/2/47, EUL.

92. RIE, Board of Managers Minutes, November 22, 1920, LHSA, LHB1/1/57, EUL.

5

EDINBURGH, LONDON, AND NORTH AMERICA

Rockefeller attempts to transform Edinburgh medicine in the 1920s turned out to be no means as easy and as successful as Pearce had probably anticipated. In the early 1920s American visitors to the city recorded, sometimes with dismay, local opinion on what constituted sound medical practice, the most productive ways to teach, and the best means to advance medical knowledge. In London there was suspicion of American ways in doing things because of the hospital-based nature of London medical schools and the relative marginality of London University. More generally the rural ideology of the London doctors and their association of American reform with other features of modernism played a part. Things were ostensibly different in Edinburgh where there was a university-based medical school and two Royal Colleges committed to modernizing medicine through the Lister scheme. In the appointment of Meakins to a full-time chair there was an indication of a commitment of some sort to the American ideal.

Edinburgh, then, on the face of it, looked an obvious Rockefeller target. In fact, throughout the decade, there were sometimes deeply different perceptions in Edinburgh and New York of medicine and strategies for its promotion. What is noteworthy is that the features of Edinburgh medicine that the city was particularly proud of—tradition, and the collaboration of the Colleges, the Medical School, the University, and the RIE—were those that Pearce found most tiresome. Edinburgh physicians valued all the very things that frustrated their transatlantic cousins. Institutional collaboration, which was a virtue in Scotland, was seen an obstacle to progress in Manhattan. Tradition, which was a hallowed word in Edinburgh, savoured of backwardness across the Atlantic. In Edinburgh, medical institutions were seen as having been founded by wise ancestors whose foresight had been borne out by time. These institutions needed gradual change in conformity with their historical development. At a dinner in 1926, celebrating the 200th anniversary of the founding of the Faculty of Medicine, it was observed by Lorrain Smith that, "The Colleges, the Faculty, and the Hospitals were three measures of medical service devised and set up for the healing of the nation. Subsequent developments proved the wisdom of the founders and the soundness of the principles on which they acted."[1]

RF officers slowly came to terms with the fact that tradition was hallowed throughout the whole of Europe, not just Scotland. Gregg on his first visit to Europe saw "the significance of tradition" for "the first time." He compared "tradition in the United States [which] didn't amount to a damn in point of recognition of real power," with Europe, where "it was the guide line to find out how things happened to be."[2] It is notable how often the term "tradition" (or antiquated and like terms) were used as terms of criticism by RF visitors to Edinburgh. Edsall observed Edinburgh medicine late in 1922 and in that October Pearce received a letter that cannot have pleased him. Edsall wrote: "There is not much that I should want to transfer to America . . . I certainly do not think [Edinburgh students] are superior to ours at the same stage." He found "a strangely fixed tradition as to lectures and their number." He thought there was "a great deal [i.e. too much] of teaching of the student in the Clinical work (he is taught almost more than he works by himself)." Edsall complained there were a "multiplicity of teaching units" and considered there were "strange and rather difficult administrative relations between the University and the extra-mural schools." Not surprisingly, perhaps, he thought, "Cushny is good of course, as is Barger," adding, "Schafer I only saw casually. The good men seem to be out of sympathy with his course." Apart from "Meakins' Laboratory," he noted, "Research in medicine . . . in any modern sense seems almost non-existent."[3] A month later, in November, Edsall again wrote to Pearce. Beginning on a positive note, he observed, "Methods differ very greatly in Scotland as compared with England (London) and the Scotch have the sounder methods." He then immediately qualified this, noting that the Scots "are antiquated in their view point in some ways, and are so over-whelmed with students that they can't do a good job." He thought there was "a utilitarian dogmatic element in the teaching and in the atmosphere that leads them to teach the craft and the lingo of practice but not the understanding of disease." Virtually the only good thing he had to say was that, "Meakins is the most advanced man I have met."[4] In his final report, although he thought, "the Scotch product is on average, superior to the English," he concluded, "The Scotch method is now almost exactly like that by which I was trained in clinical medicine thirty years ago."[5] Whereas many of the Scots would have defended a method of clinical teaching *because* it bore a genealogical relationship to a form in use thirty or indeed a hundred years earlier, the idea of thirty years previously to a progressive American conjured up the dark ages of medical education.

Graham, in his report, was less critical than Edsall. This is not surprising: Graham was a surgeon and the RF made much better head-way reforming surgery than medicine. Although endorsing Edsall's observations, Graham simply noted that in Scotland "much more empha-sis is placed on didactic instruction and on more formal courses than is the case in the London schools." He did observe, however, that "The con-ventional criticism made in London of the Scottish schools is that the clinical material is inadequate in the latter." He considered, "This criti-cism would seem to be well-founded as regards the system of 'clinical clerks' and 'surgical dressers'." "At Edinburgh," he added, "only one hos-pital case per month is allotted to each 'dresser'; and during his period of three months he has only three cases under his care."[6] Student testi-mony bears this out. Christopher Clayson, who walked the wards in the 1920s, recalled, "I attended a class by the impressive Professor Edwin Bramwell. So did about fifty others. This meant that many of us could not hear all that was said, and for most the opportunities actually to palpate an abdomen, or to demonstrate tendon reflexes were remote."[7]

The difference between American and Edinburgh perceptions of medicine is neatly illustrated in a letter from Lorrain Smith to Pearce in March 1923. Extolling Edinburgh's virtues, Smith observed that the "wide field of Clinical Teaching in hospitals is extended by the Courses of Dispensary practice." The system he thought was "worthy of special note." He explained that: "In these Courses the students, working under the general superintendence of a Dispensary Physician must all attend patients in their own homes." He considered "the benefit of this kind of training lies in the fact that, while still an undergraduate, the student is compelled to exercise independent observation and take real responsibility for care and treatment of patients. It is recognized by all that this experience is one of the most valuable parts of Clinical training in Edinburgh."[8] Smith was careful to point out that the system had been introduced by Professor Andrew Duncan in the early nineteenth century and thus by implication had the imprimatur of time firmly upon it.

On his visit to Edinburgh in 1922 Edsall had noted cryptically to Pearce: "The most extraordinary thing about this school is the dispensary system."[9] In his final report he was more expansive and, were Smith to have seen it, he might not have described the virtues of dispensary practice as glowingly as he did. Edsall wrote that, "Those of the poor classes of citizens who do not come under the health insurance system apply to the dispensary when they need medical care." After this, "the students are assigned to them and actually take charge of them in their homes, make their diagnoses, and prescribe for them." The students could send a very sick patient to hospital but, "If he dies at home they sign the death certificate." Further: "The student keeps no record except the names and addresses and his diagnoses of his patients." Students could also prescribe and "dangerous prescriptions are expected to be held up by the pharmacist." He concluded, "it seemed to me positively bad training, and also extremely bad medical service to the poor." He thought that most of the students "who were on this work exhibited wholly inadequate training to be at all safe in such responsible activities, or really to profit by it." This was obviously not the view in Edinburgh, for Edsall recorded, "I was repeatedly urged by instructors to see it, and it was described to me as the best part of the practical training."[10]

Without making too radical a distinction, for views were subtle and varied, it can be said that there were clinicians in Edinburgh, as in

London, who put greater weight on individual clinical experience in medicine than they did on collaborative and laboratory work. They stressed such experience as essential for everyday diagnosis and, although none of them discounted the role of laboratory research in advancing medical knowledge, they claimed that the role of individual bedside work in promoting medical progress was insufficiently recognized. Like their London counterparts Edinburgh doctors often invoked Thomas Sydenham as the model bedside practitioner. They also, of course, frequently appealed to Edinburgh traditions. It is noticeable that addresses given by such physicians often began with high praise of laboratory science and this was then followed by something close to a lament for the neglect of bedside medicine. I have called such London practitioners patricians: the term will suffice for Edinburgh so long as it is not taken to imply total uniformity of opinion either within Edinburgh or with London. There were, of course, some in Edinburgh who distrusted the claim that the individual had privileged access to medical knowledge. They held that teamwork with reliance on laboratory data was the best means of practising and achieving progress in medicine. Such would also have been the view of Pearce and Fletcher. Those holding such views can conveniently be termed academic physicians but (as with the patricians) this does not imply they agreed on all points.

Edwin Bramwell was a physician who can be placed in the patrician camp, and his clinical practice is examined in Chapter 9. Bramwell came from a distinguished medical family. His father, Sir Byrom Bramwell, a native of north-east England, was successively pathologist and a physician at the RIE. He retired in 1912. He published widely, notably on neurological and cardiological subjects. Edwin, born in 1873 in north-east England, moved to Edinburgh when his father started practice there in 1879. Like his father and grandfather, Edwin attended the Edinburgh Medical School, then, after a medical sojourn in Europe, he worked in London's prestigious centre for the study and treatment of neurological disease, the National Hospital, Queen Square. In 1901 he returned to Edinburgh and in 1908 he became Assistant Physician at the Infirmary. In 1919 he was appointed Ordinary Physician and University Lecturer in Neurology. In 1922 he was elected to the relatively new Moncrieff Arnott Chair of Clinical Medicine. By this time he had a very large private practice. In 1920 he saw 750 patients.[11] Distinguished and industrious,

Bramwell seems to have been well liked as a teacher and in demand as a colleague for reform and committee work.

Bramwell's medical orientation was to the ward and to pathological anatomy. His extensive publications, almost all single-authored, were devoted largely to neurology and dominated by clinical and pathological descriptions. His view of medicine was expounded in various addresses given in the 1920s. In one he pondered how the efficacy of therapies was to be gauged. Therapeutic assessment was a key point of contest between the old and new ways of doing medicine. Bramwell observed that there was an "art of diagnosis" and that this was "being constantly facilitated by the introduction of scientific methods of precision." He had no doubt, he stated, that, "the results obtained by the laboratory worker are invaluable because of the possibilities and indications they suggest." But, he added, "the clinician is responsible for the final evidence." To support this view Bramwell turned to history and the "method of Sydenham" of whom, he reported, it had been said: "He drove home the great truth that the solution of the problem of disease . . . must be sought at the bedside by means of observation and inquiry." Whereas an English physician in this context might have then appealed to an English medical tradition to further substantiate this precept, Bramwell cited one of his eighteenth-century professorial predecessors, the "wise old physician" John Gregory. He also quoted another Scot, Sir James Mackenzie (who was to die a little over two weeks after the address was given), on the dangers of following authorities (also a favorite trope, of course, of laboratory workers). Mackenzie has been mentioned as having been at the forefront of a transformation of the study of the heart, and as a teacher of Meakins. As mentioned too, Mackenzie was an oddity in some ways and far from sympathetic to the ideals of academic medicine. He was widely known, notorious even, for his hostility to specialization and his distrust of laboratory science as a model for making clinical judgements. Bramwell also cited William Osler, who was probably perceived by most doctors in the first two decades of the twentieth century as the living embodiment of the wise clinician. Wisdom as opposed to knowledge (the product of science) was an important constituent of the clinician's vocabulary for describing the art of medicine. Bramwell warned that arriving at conclusions at the bedside was much more difficult than in the laboratory, noting, "Sir Berkeley Moynihan [a surgeon] perhaps exaggerates the position, no doubt wittingly, when he asserts that the difficulties of laboratory research are mere 'bumble puppy' as compared with those of clinical deduction."[12] Indeed, Bramwell observed, "the very prevalent and unfortunate use of the word research as the equivalent of laboratory methods and laboratory results tends to belittle the importance of clinical observation." The pitfalls the clinician might face included attributing a cure to medicaments, "when it is often the *vis medicatrix naturæ* which deserves the credit." Similarly, reasoning from laboratory results could be quite fallacious on the ward because "We have here to remember that evidence to the effect that a therapeutic agent has been proved in the laboratory to have a certain action is apt to appeal much more forcibly to the mind of the tyro, who comes to the clinical teacher fresh from his physiological studies, than a statement to the effect that a remedy does good although we know not why." "This" he said, "is an attitude of mind which we are constantly called upon to combat."[13]

In another address given two years later Bramwell made a number of similar points. First he noted that physiology was the "essential basal science" of medicine and he praised Sharpey-Schafer and the "distinguished" Edinburgh school. Then he observed that, "the mental outlook of the physician is necessarily quite different to that of the physiologist" and he deplored "the progressive tendency to assume that the student should acquire his experience of medicine as a graft so to speak, upon a mental framework of physiological knowledge."[14] Bramwell would have known, no doubt, that his speech was part of a debate that went back to the late nineteenth century. In this long-standing controversy Schafer (as he then was), in 1885, eulogized physiology and upset not a few clinicians by apparently deprecating clinical experience.[15] On another occasion Bramwell had remarked that he thought there was "a general feeling among physicians in this school that physiology occupied too much time in proportion to the rest of the course."[16] What was needed to resolve the tension between physiology and clinical medicine, said Bramwell, was a supplementary course in "applied physiology" given by a clinician. At the bedside the student would need "to cultivate an entirely different attitude of mind to that which he has been accustomed by his previous physiological training; he must concentrate on observation and study the natural history of disease." On the ward, he continued, the student would learn that "true diagnosis does not consist in naming the disease from which the patient suffers but in eliciting *all* the facts." He warned that "the cultivation of an attitude of mind which underestimates clinical observation and attaches undue importance to the results of the laboratory and to methods of precision, constitutes a grave menace to the undergraduate training at the present time."[17] It was, he wrote elsewhere, the memories of the "indelible impression" left by cases on the mind that were "an essential part of clinical experience."[18]

In a diary written in the 1930s Bramwell reflected on a range of subjects including the place of the laboratory in clinical life. He cautioned the clinician against "failure to apply the methods of the laboratory or of precision when these might be expected to afford additional information." But he also condemned the "type" of clinician who was a "scientist or ultra-scientist who over-emphasises laboratory and instrumental aids." Listing the main failings of students, he noted that they were: "Apt to attach too much importance to X-rays, bacteriological methods, instruments of precision." The conflation of the dangers of clinical instruments with laboratory facilities was common among London patricians and suggests a position with regard to technology arising from wider factors than concern about their unnecessary use. Bramwell also expressed a worry about the consultant "who fails to grasp or understand the patient's outlook."[19] This again was a concern about technology and a move in clinical medicine away from using patients' reports of their well-being as one of the guides to the value of therapy and to assessing sickness solely in biochemical terms.

Another Edinburgh patrician was William Ritchie. Born in 1873 and an Edinburgh graduate he practised for nearly the whole of his professional life in the city. He was a physician to the Infirmary and was appointed to the Chair of Medicine in 1928. His inaugural address of that year began with a detailed history of medicine and the establishment of the Edinburgh school. He had high praise for the basic sciences and applauded the role of laboratory research in furthering medical knowledge. But parts of his address revealed a distinctly older and at times particularly Scottish view that would not have been well received at Rockefeller headquarters. First he remained loyal to the epistemology of clinical individualism: "The true physician has always been a clinician, applying at the bedside his knowledge of the ancillary sciences. Sydenham, the Father of Clinical Medicine in England, took no part in the doctrines and systems of his time, but deliberately made bedside observation a scientific study." He valued the multiplicity of Edinburgh medical institutions: "When occasion arises for reviewing our organization of medical education, we have to bear in mind that it is a product of native growth and like our forms of Church government and legal procedure, an expression of our history and social life." He had high regard for the ways they were bound together: "The association of the University, the Royal Colleges and the Royal Infirmary is not based on self-interest or profit; they are linked by ties comparable to those between brothers and sisters." He set store by home-grown products grounded, as he saw them, in Scottish life, not imported from alien German or American cultures. "The system of unified control of medicine and clinical medicine indigenous to Germany, which has found favour across the Atlantic, would be alien to this country. Democratic, rather than autocratic, principles and healthy rivalry between professorial and extra-mural teachers have been most important factors in the welfare of our medical school."[20] "Unified control" and "autocratic principles" were of course exactly what Rockefeller wanted. I return to the question of "democratic" below.

In contrast to the views of the patricians were those of the advocates of academic medicine. The most important of these was Meakins. Unfortunately he left little in the way of general pronouncements about how medicine was to be practised and advanced. I demonstrate his views in concrete form, however, in Chapter 9, where I scrutinize his accounts of insulin therapy and the diagnosis of thyroid disease. There are, though, fragments that indicate his general point of view, and hardly surprisingly his opinions conform to those the RF and the MRC found congenial. Meakins was suspicious of the empirical or natural historical approach approved of by patrician physicians. In 1923 he gave an address on insulin that began with an historical section discussing "reasons for giving remedies." He observed: "There is nothing so open to fallacy as empirical observation in disease." Only scientific reasoning and knowledge, scientific presumably meaning laboratory-based, could compensate for this.[21] Meakins did not decry empirical knowledge but said it only constituted sound knowledge when explained by laboratory work. He made this clear in a memorandum of 1924, written for the Infirmary Managers, on the benefits for patients of a biochemical laboratory. He began with a claim that was distinctly prominent in American medical educational literature and with which the patricians would also have agreed: that excellence in everyday hospital practice was associated with teaching and research. He said that the reputation of the great hospitals of Britain and the rest of the world "for the diagnosis and treatment of disease is based, and rightly so, upon the accomplishments and endeavours of a professional staff who have contributed to the elucidation of the causes and cure of disease, or have excelled in expounding and teaching Medical Science." It is noteworthy that he wrote of medical science (a term recurrently used in the document), not the art of medicine. He then explained that empirical knowledge "is really the result of patient and close investigation" but, in short, laboratory studies were necessary both to elucidate the facts of an individual case and to explain empirical data more generally. He explicated this historically. Thirty years previously "the greater part of medical investigation was confined to the recording and correlation of different signs and symptoms." After this it was the "introduction of the true experimental spirit" that led to "the elucidation and cure of disease in the human subject."[22] Meakins, however, did not consider cloistered laboratory work by clinicians with no contact with patients a good thing. "The man who works in the laboratory and not in the wards," he wrote in a letter in 1923, "is even worse than the clinician who says that the laboratory cannot help him and that clinical sense is the only thing."[23]

Another proponent of academic medicine was T. J. Mackie, a Glasgow graduate who had been Professor of Bacteriology at the University of Cape Town. In 1923 after the death of James Ritchie he was appointed Professor of the same subject in Edinburgh (bacteriology was not a clinical chair so it is not surprising to find a non-Edinburgh graduate in post). He was the author of an extremely successful textbook of bacteriology. Mackie's view of the much-revered clinical art would not have endeared him to Bramwell or Ritchie. In an address given in 1929 he declared:

> Art is now being subordinated to science, and the original art of healing is being replaced by scientific method. One often hears the decadence of the medical art deplored by medical men of an older school, but the true mastery of an art is the privilege of few, and it is perhaps for the common

good that medicine is sharing in the general mechanisation that science has introduced into nearly all human affairs.

Mechanization of human affairs was of course the thing that so many deplored in these years. Mackie had little-disguised contempt for individual clinical experience. He wrote: "The data on which our practice is based must be as incontestable as those obtained by the methods of precision of the science laboratory. The vague impressions of so-called experience too often accepted as authoritative and yet so fallacious and dependent on personal equations must give way to a scientific technique of controlled observation." And again, promoting the laboratory in a manner that would have shocked clinicians, he averred: "It must also be remembered that scientific applications and laboratory methods have in modern times proved their value in medicine to such an extent that the clinic is no longer the centre of gravity of medical enterprise."[24]

The newly-appointed Professor William Ritchie had claimed that, "Democratic, rather than autocratic, principles" were the basis of the welfare of the Medical School, and that Scottish medicine was a "native growth," like Church government, and the law. This assertion provides an insight into the wider context of the doubts that elite Edinburgh doctors had about the comprehensive adoption of American academic medicine. Just as London doctors had suspicions of the new order that were grounded in a wider vision of England, so too was the Edinburgh doctors' sense of some incommensurablility between American and Scottish medicine rooted in deeper experiences of national identity. Whereas the doubts of London doctors were associated with a rural myth, in Edinburgh, suspicion of the RF programme lay in an ideology that prized Scottish civic values, especially education and civilized debate, as the bonds that held traditional society together and promoted "native growth." These goals and practices were perceived as properly stemming from the Scottish universities.

It is widely recognized that the Scots had to define their identity after the parliamentary Union of 1707 as citizens of a "stateless nation."[25] Cultural nationalism in others countries, notably nineteenth-century Latin America, grew up with political nationalism directed through calls for self-government.[26] Broadly speaking the loss of the parliament and thus independent statehood was not a major issue for many Scots until well into the twentieth century. After 1707, however, the Scots gave many and various answers to the question of what their cultural identity was as Scots (a long-standing reflection) *and as Britons.*[27] The answer to the former question, the constitution of Scottish identity, was often but not exclusively focused on the tripod of church, law, and education. Ritchie was far from alone in distinguishing these three institutions as central to Scotland's perceived uniqueness. Many Scots saw them as the basis of civil society.

After the seventeenth century, civil society was portrayed as coterminous with political society but as a counterbalance to the state. On the individual level, its roots were perceived to lie in so-called civic virtue. Discussing the Scots, and their use of the concept of civil society as a counterweight to the British state and Scottish administration, Graeme Morton observes, "civil society is the social structure which exists between the household and the state and it is an arena where extensive and intricate association can take place without personal obligation."[28] Obligation came from a sense of civic virtue. Nicholas Phillipson has argued that civic virtue was a central concern of the eighteenth-century Edinburgh literati: lawyers, clergymen, landowners, doctors, university professors and independent men of letters such as David Hume. They famously developed it as an instrument of historical and sociological understanding but they also saw it as a source of practical morality which they pursued by their active involvement in the cultural and educational life of the city—in its clubs, societies, University and churches.[29] This commitment remained central to Edinburgh affairs into the twentieth century. It should be noted, however that by no means everyone in Scotland agreed with the assumption implicit in this philosophy that Edinburgh stood for the nation as a whole.

With respect to learning, by the nineteenth century the leaders of Scottish society represented themselves as custodians of what was termed a "democratic" educational system: one open to all talents both in schools and in universities. The word "democratic" (and also "egalitarian"), it is frequently claimed, had particular resonances in Scottish society and these were inherently different to those conjured up in England. This is undoubtedly the case, although as historians have shown, different Scottish communities (and classes) gave different meanings to the term. Nowhere did egalitarianism mean actual social, economic, or political equality, rather it meant equality of opportunity. It was a concept of democracy coupled far more strongly with education than with politics. David McCrone concludes that it was an elitist and conservative ideology.[30] It was, and still is, a deep-seated assumption among many Scots that Scottish society has long been more open, democratic, and egalitarian than "what is judged to be a less mobile, status-conscious and more powerful society—England." McCrone designates this a "myth," not because he is challenging any veracity it might have, rather he is drawing attention to its use in defining social identity and interpreting social reality, particularly in a country stripped of its parliament.[31] Viewed through the prism of medicine this is a useful distinction between the two countries.

The embodiment of the democratic myth (totem even) in education was the "lad o' pairts," who was deemed to have "equality of access to an educational ladder from the parish or burgh school to a Scottish university and all that was necessary for the young, ambitious, working-class Scot was talent and intellect."[32] There is evidence that the "lad o' pairts" was not simply a myth in the sense of a complete figment of the imagination. Christopher Harvie writes: "At the time of the 1872 Education Act 14 per cent more Scots children than English children were at school."[33] In the nineteenth century many youths of peasant and working-class origin attended the universities although gradually children of the professional and commercial classes increased in proportion.[34]

With regard to university education, the research of George Elder Davie has been particularly fruitful and provocative.[35] Davie has stressed the emphasis the Scots laid on a general philosophical education and its necessity as a pre-condition to advancement in Scottish society. Identifying post-union cultural differences he pointed to "the egalitarianism of the Presbyterians" and "an educational system . . . combining the democracy of the Kirk-elders with the intellectualism of the advocates [that] . . . made expertise in metaphysics the condition of the open door of social advancement."[36] Before the late nineteenth century, Scottish universities in various ways, including their relatively high intake of those from non-elite families, were different to Oxford and Cambridge (although not University College London). Davie, who described the Scottish universities as "genuinely democratic" (an opinion not without its critics), further argued that various economic, political, and religious upheavals in early nineteenth-century Scotland led to the hope that "the universities would assume responsibility for the nation's spiritual leadership in the room of the divided church."[37] Scottish university teachers invested themselves with a central role as guardians of civil society.

Davie also describes how, in the late nineteenth century, Scottish state schools increasingly turned to early specialization of study. Universities were pressured to do the same, following the model of the new English universities. Philosophy as the foundation of all further knowledge began to fall out of favour. In the 1920s, however, for reasons detailed by Davie, philosophy regained its place at the head of the university curriculum and debate raged over the virtues of specialism and generalism. By and large the generalists were in the universities. The proponents of specialism were in the Scottish Education Department that controlled the schools and took an English point of view.[38]

The 1920s saw a continuation of the perception in Scotland that universities were meant to provide a rounded education, that they were to produce good citizens, and that their teachers were custodians of cultural values. Something of the stress on the general and suspicion of the narrowing possibilities of science is revealed in Edinburgh attitudes to medical laboratory work. Bramwell's defence of his view of clinical medicine was coupled with the sentiment that the Americans were in the vanguard of the movement to overwhelm it with specialized laboratory studies. Bramwell had obviously seen Edsall's report on British medicine, for when Edsall wrote: "Nor do I think they [the British] get . . . the fact that we are teaching [American students] . . . science, not in order to make scientists of them, but to make better clinicians of them," he added, "Bramwell, for example, "discusses [my report] . . . as if good scientific training were valuable to those men who were going to make good scientists, only."[39]

Writing of the twentieth century, Harvie has observed: "A provincial culture, distinct from that of England for various reasons, rather than superior to it. An acute awareness of Scottish intellectuals of the power of parochialism and the mediocrity of its cultural values: a sense of attraction to and revulsion against the metropolis. These factors appear to be constant throughout our period."[40] The Edinburgh medical elite of the 1920s demonstrated the same ambivalence to their own (in some cases adopted) country and to England that marked the thought of Scottish intellectuals in general. Edinburgh was dominated by the old professions that were dependent on the gentry (and increasingly on business) for their incomes.[41] Edinburgh professionals were largely apolitical although probably Liberals in a formal sense. The ferocity of Irish political nationalism of this period scarcely touched them and it is likely that the radical, literary Scottish Renaissance spearheaded by the communist (and fiercely anti-parochial), Hugh MacDiarmid passed them by or else was a source of anxiety.[42] The British gentry and aristocracy, although the latter were well in decline, were still a powerful force in London and, like Scotland, in the countryside.[43] None the less there were important differences between the two nations. The Scottish professional bourgeoisie were more distanced from the aristocracy and gentry than their English counterpart. Many from the upper reaches of Scottish society went to English public schools and Oxbridge, but "the bourgeoisie and the professions remained culturally Scottish in speech, education and temperament. They were Presbyterian by religion and individualistic by inclination." They were Scottish-educated at fee-paying schools and at the Universities of Glasgow and Edinburgh. Although they married into the gentry and land, Scotland's professional classes "while socially conservative, embody the survival of a distinctive Scottish 'civil society', and can be considered as keepers of native institutions, and hence incipient 'nationalists', resistant to further anglicisation."[44] Edwin Bramwell on one occasion drew all of the threads together. "Love of your School, of University, and of Country are sentiments which are largely determined by tradition." Tradition was "a force for good" and "whereby an emotional factor provides a stimulus which serves to translate our actions into terms of practical utility."[45]

In the case of the London elite, suspicions about academic medicine were shaped within an ideology or myth centred on hierarchy and rural life. It is harder to give such definite form to the ideology of Scottish patricians in the inter-war years. They wrote fewer general reflective essays on their society than their southern counterparts, although this itself may be symptomatic of an intensification of Scotland's long-standing identity crisis. In England spirited, middle class, amateur social analysis and criticism flourished, often promoted by Scotsmen.[46] Scottish intellectuals at home, however, who had a distinguished tradition of social inquiry, seem to have relatively neglected such studies, save for the writers of the Scottish Renaissance.[47] Evidence for this is the apparent and rather curious lack of interest shown by Scottish intellectuals in eugenics. Eugenic worries were present in Scottish legal and administrative action to curb promiscuity, illegitimacy, and venereal disease.[48] But whereas eugenic concerns permeate English and American social theory of the period they seem absent from Scottish debates.

It is noteworthy that one of Scotland's most influential global political and social theorists of this period, Patrick Geddes, had only a relatively short connection with Edinburgh and for a great deal of his working life was involved in projects outside his native country. More remarkable is that one of his most redoubtable medical disciples, the distinguished psychiatrist and classical scholar Arthur Brock, remained intellectually and geographically marginal to the capital, pursuing his lonely Scottish nationalist furrow and studies of Galen outside Edinburgh in the hinterland of North Queensferry.[49]

Scottish patrician inter-war ideology is also difficult to pin down for historiographical reasons. Modern cultural studies of inter-war Scotland are few compared with those of England. For reasons to do with the question of the centrality attached to Scotland's identity, the bulk of historians have found the country's cultural history less interesting after 1900 and to become more appealing the further back it is traced. This factor is rendered less important here, however, since the ideologies or myths of elite Edinburgh doctors in the 1920s look not so very different from those espoused in the nineteenth century. There is a strong sense in which, like their eighteenth-century forebears, twentieth-century doctors and university professors saw participation in Edinburgh life, *as men of letters*, as the highest social good. William Cullen, medical professor, writer, philosopher, social improver, and friend of David Hume and Adam Smith was the presiding deity of Edinburgh medicine. It is striking how many of the men who embraced Rockefeller initiatives were not Scots and if they were, were not Edinburgh educated. It is striking too, how many of them were basic scientists and had frequently held positions in other countries besides Scotland. In Edinburgh at least science looks like an international pursuit and medicine a local one. Ironically, it should be noted that Cullen, Hume, and Smith were three of the great Scottish innovators of their day well as being international figures.

In any case, there were important institutional differences between London and Edinburgh medicine. In London, the university was marginal to many hospital consultants in the 1920s. Indeed for many of the leaders of London medicine in these years, if they felt allegiance to a university at all, it was often to Oxford or Cambridge where a good number of them had spent their pre-clinical days. They often showed loyalty to a particular London hospital, but St. Bartholomew's did not stand for or symbolize London and its University in the way that the RIE did Edinburgh. London was not regarded by southern patricians as a sort of special society and place in the way that northern doctors saw Edinburgh. London was too large for a start, and nowhere near as close knit. For Scottish medical teachers the university was the source of all sorts of values about Scottish society.

Praise of the value of tradition was not filigree on more important substance. Scottish medical teachers saw themselves as the bearers of tradition that was among the sources of stability in a civil (and potentially explosive) society.[50] It is notable that when invoking tradition in detail Scottish teachers almost always summoned up the names of Scottish *university* teachers (with the exception of Thomas Sydenham). The heroes of the English were almost invariably general practitioners or private teachers. Ironically they were frequently self-made men and sometimes Scottish, notably John Hunter (who lived and worked in London). The English, of course, frequently regarded the Scots as honorary members of the southern nation.

The myth of the "lad o' pairts" celebrated thrift, getting on, hard work, and moral duty. These virtues were seen by the Scots as exceedingly well developed in their country, and were often traced far into the nation's history. In this regard Scottish educational ideologies were by and large conservative, or perhaps better still, preservative. Ritchie's praise of tradition, democracy, and healthy rivalry would seem to fit this account perfectly. Meakins's observation that "reactionary spirits" blocked change in Edinburgh was the response of a transatlantic modernist in a culture clash. In London and Edinburgh the, at times, slow progress of Rockefeller medicine was on the surface owing to entrenched clinical individualism. However there was a wider context in which clinical individualism was promoted and allowed to flourish. In broad brush strokes, London and Edinburgh responses to Rockefeller initiatives were similar. American medicine exemplified a threat to national identity, to English and Scottish ways of doing things, to the doctors' sense of themselves, their medicine, their culture, and their past. But the responses were nuanced. In London genteel aspirations were coupled with an idealization of rural practice, in Edinburgh a rather more independent bourgeois culture took pride in its civic traditions, especially as embodied in its university.

How then did Scottish assumptions affect RF's attempts to transform Edinburgh medicine, in particular the financing of the Department of Therapeutics and its funding of a wholly new biochemical laboratory? The Foundation's involvement with Edinburgh probably started in 1921 when Sir Harold Stiles, Professor of Clinical Surgery, visited New York with plans for the creation of the Lister Institute. The men at the RF were not impressed. In November of that year Vincent wrote to Principal Ewing that the Foundation was confining its aid to "public health and medical education, and is not making direct contributions to research work, except in so far as such work is incidental to the development of medical teaching." He did not think it "wise for this Foundation to set aside its established policy for the purpose of this co-operation."[51] How far this statement was strictly true and how far it was evasion is impossible to know, for the Lister scheme did include provision for teaching. Indeed only four years later, Pearce was telling Lord Knutsford of the London Hospital that "Our program . . . has been developed . . . with the thought of the necessity of development of certain types of effort combining both teaching and research."[52] The RF did not care for the Lister scheme because it did not like supporting anything other than a university department and it was hostile to the collaboration with the Royal Colleges. The RF's antipathy was possibly the background to Vincent's letter. Perhaps not getting the message, at some point the RF received a glowing report from Ewing of the state of the University and its still solid commitment to the Lister scheme.[53] Vincent, visiting Britain, probably in July 1922, went to Edinburgh and discussed the Lister plan with Ewing.[54] During the trip, Pearce recorded, Vincent made no promises of aid but said that Pearce would visit the city "in due course" and look into the matter.[55]

From mid-1922 onwards the RF launched a major initiative regarding British medical education. In July 1922 Pearce wrote to Walter Fletcher: "During the coming winter I plan to make a survey of all the medical schools of the British Isles."[56] Pearce and Fletcher had no doubt previously met, most obviously when Fletcher, with Wilmot Herringham representing the University Grants Committee, "enjoyed" the hospitality of the Foundation when visiting medical schools in America in 1921. They had probably met before this.[57] To facilitate his visit, Pearce had prepared an outline of the information he wished to collect and hoped Fletcher would send it out to the schools in advance. Fletcher said he was "most ready to give you any assistance in our power."[58] Pearce went first to continental Europe basing himself in Paris and hoping to be in Britain in January 1923. Writing to Fletcher from Warsaw in October 1922 he remarked on their "common interest in medical education in England [*sic*]."[59] Pearce was in England by January 1923, visiting St Thomas' Hospital and enjoying the success of MacLean's professorial unit.[60]

In Edinburgh in early 1923 hopes for the Lister scheme were still alive in some quarters when, in mid-February, Pearce took the train north. He visited a large number of medical institutions in Edinburgh, including the Royal Colleges and the proposed Lister site. He had official interviews with Ewing and the Dean of the Medical Faculty, Lorrain Smith. He also had a number of "Special interviews" with departmental heads and directors. He had various formal dinners, and most significantly, had informal "dinners or lunches" with Meakins, Barger, Cushny and "Watson."[61] The latter was Benjamin Philip Watson who was appointed Professor of Midwifery and Gynaecology in 1922. The significance of Pearce meeting informally with him is that Watson was a University employee, he had an interest in laboratory medicine (indeed he had his own lab in the Medical School), and he was clearly sympathetic to a full-time professorate.[62] However he does not appear often in correspondence and he left Edinburgh for a post at Columbia University, New York, in 1926. The paper trail suggests that Pearce's most important alliance was with Meakins, Barger, and Cushny. Only Cushny was a Scottish graduate (from Aberdeen) and he had spent most of his professional life outside Scotland.

In his notes from his visit, which were probably intended for internal consumption at the RF, Pearce recorded, architecturally speaking, that the Medical School was "excellently adapted to its purpose." Inevitably he wanted to see it transformed for "modern laboratory work." However, he thought large classes and "reverence for a traditional curriculum" made the situation with regard to space "almost intolerable."

The Anatomy Department, he considered, sacrificed valuable room to a "useless Zoological–Historical Museum." Museum-knowledge, as it might be called, was natural historical knowledge of the sort prized by devout bedside men. Not surprisingly it found little favour as a research tool with modern academic clinicians. Pearce's criticisms of Schafer and the Physiology Department have been noted. Redistribution of space in the Faculty, Pearce felt, was a priority. What was essential was "doing away with useless lecture rooms and Museums." The "doing away" with lecture rooms no doubt had as much to do with the Americans' dislike of the Edinburgh emphasis on didacticism as it did with any redundancy of space. Pearce held that with careful redistribution "many of the arguments for the Lister Memorial would disappear."[63]

In his notes Pearce devoted a section to the Lister scheme, in much of which he showed his suspicion of the Royal Colleges' involvement in University affairs. He observed without comment that "it must be remembered that the Colleges have always guarded jealously their prerogatives not only as examining bodies but as bodies controlling teaching and research." The word "jealously" here hardly signifies approval, rather it conjures the sense of vested interests encrusted in tradition which is, of course, exactly how the Rockefeller people thought of Edinburgh medical life. Pearce made this plain later in the document. He wrote that the Foundation "would hesitate to aid a project not controlled entirely by the University" and it "certainly would not aid in any project which gave anybody except the University the control of research." (In the original plan the Superintendent of the College of Physicians' Laboratory was to be put in charge of the research department of the projected Lister Institute.) The Foundation, he added, "would hesitate to aid a project including the Royal Colleges and thus aiding the perpetuation of errors due directly to the traditions of these bodies." Pearce thought the scheme "too cumbersome and all inclusive." From an American point of view, in which the doctrine of managerial efficiency prevailed, he was dismayed at "several controlling bodies but with no co-ordination." He wanted to develop "unity" in the Medical School and the Lister scheme had the "opposite effect."[64]

At the close of the discussions in Edinburgh, Lorrain Smith (a big supporter of the Lister scheme) had obviously seen that the plan was going nowhere with Rockefeller and "offered the opinion that the Lister scheme was dead." He would not let it lie down however and neither had he quite got the message about the Colleges. Lorrain Smith wondered about building a pathology and bacteriology department on the Lister site "with the co-operation of the Royal Colleges." Peace recorded, "I disclaimed any interest in the Colleges," but agreed to discuss the general problems of the Medical School with a faculty group. He did so with Meakins, Cushny, Barger, Watson, Stiles (who was sympathetic to Rockefeller ideals), and Lorrain Smith (by no means an ally but who had to be present in his role as Dean).[65] Pearce remained consistently hostile to the idea of new pathology and bacteriology labs and was convinced that the pathology lab of the Infirmary was not used to full advantage.[66]

During his trip Pearce also visited the RIE. This symbol of civic pride was not, however, immune from transatlantic incomprehension and criticism. "The real problem of this hospital," he recorded, "is not that of space or arrangement, or even of facilities, but is dependent on the method of appointing staff." To explain this he had once again to refer to the role of the Colleges, the "very ancient bodies, who pride themselves on having established the earliest course of systematic education in Medicine in Scotland." One of the functions of the Colleges, he noted (perhaps with incredulity), was to license teachers of medicine. That is, clinical and laboratory-related clinical courses on the wards of the Edinburgh hospitals, in College lecture theatres, and indeed, anywhere else in the city had to be given by teachers, whether of the University or Extra-academical School, licensed by the Royal Colleges. This role of the Colleges, Pearce observed, was "a traditional one." He then explained, perhaps with amazement, that when Meakins was called from McGill, "he could not begin his duties as an actual teacher in the Infirmary until acknowledged by the College of Physicians."[67] It was as though Meakins had undergone some humiliating ancient ritual.

Licensing of teachers, coupled with the fact that the Infirmary was not "controlled by the University" (something else he obviously deplored), led to an "anomalous situation." This was that only a minority of the clinical positions was controlled by the University (three of eight positions in medicine, two of seven in surgery). Coupled with this was the fact that the University teachers did not have enough beds to teach all their students. The upshot was that the majority of students did not receive instruction from University teachers. Thus, although "a man of

Meakins' training and point of view should have an influence on the entire student body," he did not do so.[68] The professors sympathetic to RF ideals saw it that way too. Watson made a similar point in a statement in which he described his department to Pearce. Watson observed "whilst the Professor has direct control over didactic or theoretical teaching he has only indirect control over the clinical instruction of the majority of students."[69] As noted, by this time all the Ordinary Physicians and Assistant Physicians had been given University titles but the University did not employ them. Pearce obviously saw this as a fudge and did not regard them as proper University lecturers.

The consequence of this situation, Pearce said, made it "impossible to develop a school of clinical medicine or surgery in the modern sense." He wondered, "what can be done to change this?" Having a better sense of the conservatives in Edinburgh than some of them had of him, he rejected "Revolution" (a position on which he was, in a more optimistic moment, to change his mind). The answer was "nothing but slow and gradual evolution based on the unit principle, with training during a long period of years of men with modern points of view of science in relation to clinical medicine." The three clinicians that he considered were laying the basis for gradual evolution were Stiles, Meakins, and Watson. Each gave over his "principle effort to teaching and research in the hospital." They had a desire, he recorded, shared by Cushny and Barger, to develop an honours course in clinical medicine. This was to be combined with the "developing of the Unit system of the London schools." Pearce hoped "to further the aims and ideals of the[se] men in order to change the character of clinical teaching, stimulate clinical research, train a new breed of clinician and get the most out of the world wide reputation of the Edinburgh Medical School."[70]

Pearce finished his document with some general conclusions. First was that a "progressive programme" should include "improvement in facilities for teaching laboratory subjects." Second was the establishment of "true University clinics" in close association with the former goal. Finally these things required the "abandonment of Lister project as a University plan." After various suggestions as to redistribution of space he considered that the development of "true University clinics" could be done by "giving more facilities to Stiles, Watson and Meakins." There should be, he thought, clearly with an American model in mind, the gradual "elimination of all non-university teachers" and "the integration of [the] entire service under a full time head." He iterated how important Meakins was to his thinking. He communicated this plan to the Edinburgh Faculty and hinted that if a detailed programme on these lines could be produced, Rockefeller assistance might be forthcoming. His own "Programme" was "to wait for the next [strategic] move of the Edinburgh faculty," which he assumed would be the drawing up of a plan that he expected to see when Stiles visited America in April. Whether the RF gave money to Edinburgh, however, depended on the "complicated situation . . . in regard to University and Infirmary relations, traditional policies, and vested interests" all of which had to be considered, "in the hope of altering them."[71]

After his visit Pearce wrote to Embree, Secretary of the Foundation, on February 25, 1923, apprising, perhaps warning, him of Stiles's embarkation for New York on the *Aquitania* on March 31 prior to his spending two weeks at Harvard Medical School as visiting Professor. Pearce, who was leaving Britain on April 14, did not anticipate he would see Stiles in New York and he told Embree that he thought the Edinburgh situation "so difficult" and "our interest in the Lister Memorial Institution so dubious that I could give the local authorities . . . no hope of any outstanding aid from us."[72] After outlining his hopes for Edinburgh, Pearce explained he wanted Stiles to "spend a day or two at Hopkins in order that he may get some definite idea of real University clinics."[73] Three days later he wrote to Embree that he recommended Meakins "without reserve as teacher, investigator, administrator." Fletcher, he added, "has a high opinion of him" as did Barger and Cushny. Pearce concluded, investing all his hopes in the Professor of Therapeutics, "If Meakins stays at E. I have a modest plan to help develop medicine there; if he leaves I will be in doubt. That is what *I* think of him."[74]

At this point a further complication enters the story. Meakins was never completely happy in Edinburgh and always had a longing to return to McGill. He had held for twenty years, he wrote in December 1923, the "ideal" of returning to Montreal and building up the school.[75] He had been quite frank about the matter to Pearce during the latter's visit in February 1923. Meakins wrote, "I made no bones about the matter [to Pearce] that it was my ideal to return to McGill at some future date *if* I felt that I could see any way of building up the school."[76] Pearce had told him he could do more in Edinburgh and thought Meakins should stay where he could do most. Pearce had taken a great interest in McGill and in November 1920 the RF pledged $1,000,000 to the School.[77] However, by the time of Pearce's visit to Edinburgh, Montreal's two major hospitals—The Montreal General and the Royal Victoria—and the University were locked in various conflicts over surgical appointments and teaching. Meakins recalled that Pearce had spoken of what might have been an "intolerant spirit" between the hospitals. However, if McGill put its house in order, Pearce told Meakins, he might consider helping its Medical Department "in a substantial manner." None the less there was certainly no immediate possibility of a full-time professorship and directorship of a medical department that would have been necessary to tempt Meakins back home.[78] Montreal's bad news was good news for Pearce, who was intent on building the Edinburgh School around Meakins.

Out of the blue another player emerged. At some point in the spring of 1923 Meakins received an offer from Chicago to be appointed as Dean of the Medical School. In early March 1923 Pearce, in a handwritten and seemingly rushed memo to Embree, wrote that if Meakins accepted this position, Rockefeller "plans for Edinburgh . . . would be a washout." If Meakins stayed and got the Chair of Medicine, "The future development of medicine at Edinburgh will be assured." Indeed, Pearce continued buoyantly, "all England [sic!] will feel the influence. The unit system will live, and the British schools all over the world will be affected." However, were Meakins to leave, "there will be nothing to build on." The situation was "critical" and "of much more importance to the general development of medicine in the world than is the selection of a Dean for Chicago." Supporting medicine in Edinburgh "would further our world progress." Panicking, perhaps, Pearce said he was "prepared to recommend support for Meakins for five years (annual grants) in development of true university clinic." The meaning here is not quite clear but the sense of the memorandum is that Pearce was assuming that Meakins would transfer to the prestigious Chair of Medicine after the retirement of George Gulland. With Rockefeller aid, the Chair would then be made full-time for five years. After that, "If right course is taken we could eventually endow it [the Chair of Medicine]; if not, we could drop out."[79]

The Edinburgh people had still obviously not quite caught on to Pearce's single-mindedness. In mid-March he sent Embree a letter from

Stiles (who was to leave for New York in two weeks). The letter (untraced) to Pearce had clearly been a red rag to a bull and its contents might be guessed from his comment. Pearce wrote, "I do not know what he [Stiles] means by this reference to the College of Physicians and general University scheme." Pearce was afraid that in suggesting Stiles talk with Embree in New York, "I have balled things up unnecessarily," presumably meaning that even Stiles had not yet fully comprehended Pearce's vision. Pearce explained, "if Stiles' reference means that Lorrain Smith, the Dean, is pushing his scheme for even a small building as a Lister Memorial, Stiles' statement or memoranda should be received without the slightest encouragement." "I am only interested," he wrote "in the development of a true university clinic."[80]

Stiles travelled to New York carrying with him a statement signed by Lorrain Smith. Before he departed, however, Barger wrote to Pearce describing the background to the document and setting out what he and others close to Pearce felt most important in the statement. He realized this action might be "indiscreet." After Pearce's departure a "self-constituted" committee had been formed composed of Barger, Lorrain Smith, Meakins, Cushny, Stiles, Watson, and Robert Wilson Philip. The latter had been appointed to the newly-established Chair of Tuberculosis in 1917. He is marginal to this account although he was enthusiastic about the honours school favoured by the main protagonists, and as President of the College of Physicians had a good deal of clout. Barger thought him "extremely reasonable and quite keen." Cushny was absent from the last committee meeting and was replaced by Harvey Littlejohn, Professor of Forensic Medicine. Barger described him as "one of the most powerful people of the old school, a typical product of Edinburgh." Barger's prejudices were coming into play here for although Littlejohn's credentials were those of the "old school" (his father had been the previous holder of the Chair) he was a firm supporter of Meakins and, indeed, had been the latter's host when he first arrived from Canada. Barger, in fact, reported that Littlejohn was "keen on the honours degree and thought it would regenerate Edinburgh." This was an admission, of course, that the School was going through a bad patch.[81]

Barger regretted that the final statement, drawn up by Lorrain Smith, was "not . . . as clear as it might have been." He politely put this down to the fact that Smith "seemed to be suffering from the effects of term." Indeed "Littlejohn, fresh from a holiday, told him [so]." Barger summarized the statement's main proposals. These were: £175,000 for a new maternity hospital (obviously backed by Watson), £175,000 for new pathology and bacteriology labs on the Lister site (obviously backed by Smith even though Pearce during his visit had recommended that more efficient use of current space would solve any problems), £25,000 for clinical laboratories in the Infirmary (which Barger thought "the most important item" and was no doubt backed by Meakins), and a £125,000 endowment for additional teachers (presumably backed by everyone).[82] Pearce replied that he did not think Barger's letter indiscreet although he considered the proposals "more comprehensive" and reaching "a much larger sum than anything I had in mind." He agreed the most important thing was the support of Meakins under the proposal for new laboratories in the Infirmary.[83]

The document Stiles took with him to New York contained the proposals described to Pearce by Barger (although in the final version £25,000 was taken from the Lister site labs and added to the endowment for teachers). The document, written by Smith, contained a great deal of self-advertisement of Edinburgh's achievements and may have looked to Pearce like a failure to face up to problems. It included the conclusion that "the Faculty approximates to some extent to the unit system."[84] This observation might have made Pearce either laugh or cry. The document also contained the eulogy to the course of dispensary practice that had filled Edsall with horror. In May, by which time the Edinburgh statement had been received and Pearce had returned, the Foundation Trustees met and the minutes of their meeting record that support for Edinburgh "will aid in stabilizing the entire 'unit system' in England." "Progress in Great Britain," it was noted, "will affect medical development throughout the entire British Empire and the world." It was agreed Pearce would revisit Edinburgh in the autumn to arrive at "definite recommendations."[85] Pearce told Meakins he was coming and was "especially interested in the details of the clinical laboratory, anything that might be done towards the establishment of the full-time chairs of medicine and surgery, and the remodeling of the old medical school buildings."[86] He told Stiles, formally, the same, adding, "I do not think it will be possible for me to go into the more pretentious proposals," presumably meaning Smith's plans for new pathology and bacteriology labs on the Lister site and possibly the plan for a new maternity hospital.[87] Pearce was clearly committed to new clinical labs, for he wrote to Meakins in early June 1923 asking him to get to work on the details.[88]

Pearce wrote to Stiles again in late June saying, "I trust Dean Lorrain Smith understands that my communication has been with you as chairman of the committee which presented a request to this Board." Pearce, in other words, in classic Rockefeller fashion, had picked his man, Stiles, and was having nothing to do with Smith, to whose projects he was unsympathetic. Pearce warily began to commit himself. He thought the Foundation might find £25,000 for new clinical laboratories for Meakins if a site could be found, that there was an understanding as to "the types of work to be carried on," and that ongoing expenses would be borne by the Infirmary and School. He also thought Rockefeller might find £20,000 for remodelling the School. The establishing of "clinics in the true university sense," he said, he preferred to discuss during his coming visit.[89] The next day he wrote to Meakins informally, but in similar vein, recounting the same details but also telling him what he knew of affairs at McGill and that he had heard no more about the Chicago position. Pearce was clearly sensitive about Meakins's desire to move. He also felt it best not to stay with Meakins while in Edinburgh in the autumn so that he could "avoid the appearance of being too much in touch with any one member of the faculty."[90]

Pearce's Edinburgh visit began early on Monday, October 1, 1923, and lasted until the Friday evening. His initial report to Alan Gregg and Vincent was entitled "Edinburgh problems." He spent the whole of his first day with Meakins and Stiles. The next day he made visits and had formal meetings. The Wednesday he passed with Barger and Meakins. Thursday was a mixture of formal and informal meetings. On the Friday he met the Professor of Zoology, Sheriff Crole of the Infirmary Managers, and Principal Ewing whom Pearce thought "knows nothing about medical school." Overall Pearce was optimistic and noted, "we can completely revolutionize the teaching of medicine and surgery at very little cost." The addition of £600 per annum to Meakins's salary (making it £2,000, the salary of a London unit professor) would enable him to become totally full time. £25,000 would establish a new lab. A special Faculty meeting approved all the agreed proposals including those for medical and surgical reform (annual grants and endowing one of the

Chairs of Surgery), which are dealt with in the next Chapter. Pearce, while waiting in his hotel for the result of the Faculty meeting, recorded that if the motions were carried we "will have won a great victory for medical education in Scotland—the United Kingdom—the Empire—so great a victory that R. F. will have to foot the bills on basis of revolutionary principle involved."[91]

Pearce had scarcely left Edinburgh when McGill began to revive Meakins's hopes of a return home. Martin wrote to him that among many reforms, "we want to make a full-time Professor of Medicine, and I do not need to tell you whom we want to have." He was "extremely interested to get the RF materially interested in these things" and was going to New York to see Vincent.[92] A month later, in November 1923, when McGill's plans were known at Rockefeller, Pearce got the jitters. Martin wrote to Meakins, "Pearce intends asking the Rockefeller Foundation to do something for Edinburgh that will make Medicine there so attractive for you that he does not think you will be easily dislocated from that place." Martin persisted, however, and said he wished Meakins to tell the Rockefeller people that he would prefer Montreal ("and I still have a firm belief you do") "were they willing to arrange matters here at McGill so that you could come." He added, curiously, "I do not know if I have made myself clear," for nothing seemed clearer. "You will almost certainly be called to Montreal to fill the position at McGill and the Royal Victoria Hospital on a full-time basis, and we expect that if the Rockefeller Foundation find us willing to carry out the full-time plan, they will come to our support."[93] Meakins, replying to Martin's earlier letter, said he had delayed his response "in the hopes that matters [in Montreal] would take a more concrete aspect." He reported with regard to Edinburgh that Pearce had returned to New York with definite ideas to recommend to his Board.[94]

Things moved ahead rapidly on the Edinburgh front. After the Faculty and University Court had agreed to the new clinical laboratory proposals, negotiations began with the Infirmary Managers with regard to a site.[95] These negotiations were causing friction within the Faculty. There were, said Stiles, "prominent members of the College of Physicians" who were "strongly advocating" the use of the Lister Memorial site for the new laboratory.[96] There were others who favoured the Infirmary grounds. Meakins, one of the latter party, wired Pearce for his "confidential opinion and moral support."[97] Pearce was with Meakins and thought "A laboratory on the Lister site would nullify all the good results we hope to obtain."[98] In fact, even before he wrote this, Pearce had already had his preference for a building in the Infirmary grounds incorporated into the conditions of the grant for a new laboratory.

On December 5 at a meeting of the Rockefeller Foundation's Trustees it was agreed that "to aid in the development of a true university clinic" the Foundation would provide £35,000 "for the erection and equipment of a new laboratory building on Infirmary ground."[99] Pearce cabled Fletcher the news and the latter, when he knew Meakins was apprised of the decision, wrote to congratulate him.[100] Pearce wrote to Ewing telling him of the grant on December 6, 1923, and asked for confirmation that the University and Infirmary would undertake to maintain the lab. The grant, he insisted, was to the University, not the Infirmary, and "It is to be understood that this building is for the purpose of higher teaching and research in the clinical subjects, with especial reference to the development of a true university clinic under the direction of Professor Meakins." Meakins was to get £1,000 per annum for five years from the Foundation (on top of his University salary) to release him from private practice.[101] A memorandum of 1929 records that he never received any of this.[102] Pearce invested a great deal of his expectations for Edinburgh in the lab, which he obviously saw as the dynamo driving clinical research in the city. The next few years were to see these hopes chipped away and a regretful tone enter his letters on the laboratory's use.

Pearce copied his letter to Meakins, who was now assured of the sort of arrangements both he and the Rockefeller wanted. Not surprisingly Pearce considered, "you should now decide definitely whether you or Mrs. Meakins have any desire to return to Montreal." He added, "if you have no desire . . . I think you should put an end to his [Martin's] agony."[103] It was not only Martin who was in agony but Meakins himself. Meakins reminded Pearce of their springtime conversation and felt "willing to abide by [the] . . . decision" to go where he could do most good. But that did not mean, "I have lost the ideal about McGill." He did, however, feel some obligation to stay in Edinburgh now the Foundation had provided support for his Chair and department.[104] He wrote on the same day to Martin, saying, "I am in a very difficult position and to tell you perfectly frankly, I do not know exactly what to do." It would take "many searches of mind and heart" to reach a decision.[105]

It was at this time that Meakins's doubts about the possibility of medical harmony in Edinburgh began to surface. In his letter to Pearce in which he expressed his views about Montreal he also noted that now that they had the grant for the laboratory "we start on a stage which will probably be hardest and also the least pleasant." He thought that there was "going to be a considerable altercation about the site" of the new laboratory. Worse still, perhaps, was that the "question of management and control from the professional side is going to be fraught with many difficulties." He thought that the University and the Infirmary would support him, "but amongst my own colleagues there will be a consider-able amount of criticism and obstruction." He hoped he was wrong, "but can only judge from past performances." It made him "very discouraged as to whether I will ever succeed in getting" all the clinical professors "to work together." Meakins contrasted his perception of Edinburgh reality with his own ideal, one that had a distinctly transatlantic flavour: "The lack of co-operation and co-ordination turns the place into a large number of retail departments, instead of having one organised busi-ness."[106] No doubt some of his colleagues would have been horrified to think of medicine as an "organised business." Besides belittling individu-alism, the stigma of trade (whether organized or not) was one that the British medical profession, courting gentility, had long sought to keep at a distance.

In a "Private and Confidential" letter to Pearce, Stiles identified "prominent members of the College of Physicians," including Robert Philip and George Gulland (Professor of Medicine and by then the President of the College of Physicians), as advocating the use of the Lister site for the new laboratory. They also wanted the College of Physicians' lab to be built there. The shades of the Lister memorial lingered and it is not surprising that Meakins and Pearce were hostile. Stiles thought diplo-macy would win the opponents round, especially since Sheriff Crole was in favour of the Infirmary site.[107] Pearce was delighted with Stiles's efforts, not least in his placing the Rockefeller plan in the newspapers.[108] Early in January 1924 Ewing threw his weight behind the Infirmary site too.[109] Negotiations between the University and the Infirmary Managers ensured the siting of the laboratory in the Infirmary's grounds. The one drawback of this for researchers was that animal experiments were forbidden on Infirmary property.

In the midst of all this Meakins's longing to return to Montreal would not go away. Pearce fanned the flames by stating that nothing he had said was "to be interpreted by you as indicating that I feel you are bound to stand by Edinburgh."[110] In mid-February 1924 Martin wrote two letters to Meakins. In one of them he said that a policy of a full-time medical clinic in Montreal had been decided on if funds were available from Rockefeller. They had been in conference with Pearce about this. It was hoped to amalgamate the administration of the two formerly warring Montreal hospitals. Martin wanted Meakins's opinion on staff, salaries, equipment and budget.[111] In his other letter Martin asked Meakins if he would consider himself a candidate for the position of Professor of Medicine and Director of the Department at McGill. He would have fifty beds, be in charge of all the clinical laboratory services of the Royal Victoria Hospital, and have the latitude to see as many private patients in the hospital as he cared to, although the fees would be given over to the University. Martin copied his letter to Pearce, who, Martin said, was "very sympathetic with the plan."[112] In early March 1924 Meakins replied that he would consider himself such a candidate.[113] Martin was delighted but could not issue a "definite call" until after the meeting of the Rockefeller Board in late May.[114]

In mid-May, A. W. Currie, Principal of McGill, wrote to Pearce setting out his plans. He was happy to report that the Royal Victoria Hospital would "cordially co-operate" with the University to establish a university clinic. The Director of the clinic would also be Head of Department at the Montreal General Hospital.[115] The hospitals, it seemed, had patched up their differences. On May 21 the Rockefeller Trustees approved in principle co-operation with McGill in forming a medical clinic of the sort they favoured. Currie, in advance of any formal offer of a Chair to Meakins, told him of the Rockefeller decision, assuring him that should he come to Montreal a "warm welcome will await you and Mrs. Meakins in your old home."[116] It is impossible to conceive that the Rockefeller Trustees endorsed McGill's proposal without Pearce's full backing. Clearly his whole programme ranked higher than a gamble on ensuring the success of Edinburgh by backing Meakins, whom Pearce must have known by now would return to Canada. A formal invitation did come to Meakins and he did of course accept. The decision was announced in the *Scotsman* newspaper on June 4, 1924.[117]

In spite of the difficulties that Meakins had with some of his colleagues his departure seems to have produced genuine regret all round. Outside of Edinburgh, among those who had seen in Meakins hope for the reform of the school on American lines, there was dismay. J. S. Haldane wrote that the Dean of McGill had written to him to persuade Meakins to go to Canada. Haldane told Meakins, "I wasn't going to do anything of the sort."[118] Fletcher professed himself "perturbed" and "greatly depressed."[119] Letters of congratulation and sadness at Meakins's departure poured in from Edinburgh. All expressed the view that he had done much to reinvigorate the School. A. W. Alexander thought the resignation was "calamitous from the point of view of the school."[120] From the College of Surgeons, the conservator, David Greig, wrote that Meakins's leaving was a "terrible loss" and that he had been like "a pheasant among a lot of hens" and that "it was too much to expect you could be satisfied with the pabulum on which they thrive."[121] An A. C. Baycott was "shocked" and thought Meakins "one of the two or three who are showing in this country how medicine may be done." He was worried that "the new way is not so well established that there is a chance of slipping back again."[122] Sir James Mackenzie, writing from St. Andrews, selecting the word perhaps most wounding to Edinburgh pride, thought that before Meakins's appointment, the Medical School "had fallen from being a leading school to a somewhat *parochial* state." Meakins's appointment was "like a refreshing breeze into a stuffy room."[123] Edwin Bramwell hoped the report in the *Scotsman* "will not materialise."[124] Pearce did not admit any regret but he did tell Meakins: "I think you are giving up a bigger for a smaller task."[125]

Meakins left not simply because of his longing to be back in Montreal. There were features of Edinburgh medicine that made his reforming, North American mind unhappy. Usually discreet, he revealed his misgivings to Sir Norman Walker in 1927 when he, Meakins, was being prevailed upon to return to Edinburgh by applying for the now vacant Chair of Medicine in which so much hope for change was invested. Walker was a physician in the Skin Department and was knighted in 1923 when he became President of the General Medical Council. He was a significant supporter of Meakins. In Montreal,

Meakins wrote, he had had a promise from the Royal Victoria Hospital and University authorities "that they would do practically all that I asked." "This," he said, "they have carried out and the future looks increasingly bright that they will even do more than I ask." A "powerful Medical Department" had been created. Walker was surely being told to read here that none of these things was true in Edinburgh. Meakins thought, "Edinburgh at this moment is at the parting of the ways as far as the Medical Department is concerned." "For too long," he wrote, the department has been "dominated by certain turbulent and reactionary spirits in the Extra-mural school." A fact of no benefit "so far as the professional standing of Edinburgh as a centre of medical education is concerned." As he saw it, "three separate Departments of Medicine were allowed to go their own way." "The co-ordination between them," he added, "was practically nil." Appointment to a Chair of Medicine meant the incumbent "ceased, to all intents and purposes, to do productive work." It simply allowed the professor "to make more money."[126]

Meakins was suggesting his problems had been with the Medical Department but in a letter to Pearce, unfortunately rather cryptic, Stiles implicated the Infirmary too. He wrote that, "knowing what you and I do, we cannot be surprised at his [Meakins's] acceptance of the appointment." He went on: "I sincerely hope that his acceptance will be a lesson to the Infirmary authorities, and that it will show them what is liable to happen if they continue to adopt the policy of granting no privileges to the Clinical Professors beyond those granted to the non-professorial staff." Since this sentiment was followed by a tirade against the system of re-appointment of professors and the right to appoint assistants, it was possibly this that Stiles had in mind.[127] It was not only the Infirmary and the Medical Department that came in for criticism for failure to pull together. In his inaugural address at Aberdeen in 1930 Stanley Davidson referred to the "insulation and remarkable lack of co-ordination between the scientific departments of the University [of Edinburgh] and the clinical work in the hospital wards." When he was in Edinburgh, he stated, "It was a frequent remark of mine . . . that although the medical buildings were separated from the Royal Infirmary by a space little broader than the water of Leith, from its apparent impassability it might have been the Dead Sea." "The study of the nature of disease," he noted, "demands, not the individualistic, but the collective outlook."[128]

Casting the net for a wider explanation of Meakins's departure reveals Jonathan and Dorothy Meakins as relatively young, vibrant North Americans, perhaps not quite at home in Edinburgh society and not all of Edinburgh society quite at home with them. There is more than a hint of fascination with the couple's transatlantic manner and something of a suggestion of suspicion among a few. According to two of the most promising men who worked with him, the chain-smoking Jonathan Meakins was highly regarded, a skilled clinician, charming and attractive to women. Hard-working, he was a man of regular habits who always played a rubber of bridge at the New Club on his walk home to Oxford Terrace. His wife, Dorothy (who probably had private money), was beautiful, unconventional and forthright. Edinburgh society was intrigued and horrified by her. To many they seemed a breath of fresh air. Both she and Jonathan danced well and were much sought after at social functions. Sir John Finlay in particular, owner of *The Scotsman* and leader of Edinburgh society, enjoyed dancing with Dorothy.[129]

With Meakins's departure, Edinburgh did indeed revert to its old ways, and rapidly appointed the homegrown product, Meakins's assistant David Murray Lyon, to the Therapeutics Chair. This was a decision a few were to regret. Meakins's departure provoked some panic in the Edinburgh camp that Rockefeller might withdraw its support from the School. Meakins told Pearce that Ewing was "distressed."[130] Ewing wrote to Pearce that he hoped Meakins' departure would not "make any difference with regard to the policy of a whole-time Professorship."[131] Pearce cabled reassurance: "OUR OFFER CHAIR CLINICAL MEDICINE AND LABORATORY NOT AFFECTED BY MEAKINS RESIGNATION PROVIDED MAN MEAKINS TYPE APPOINTED."[132] Pearce told Meakins the same thing. Rockefeller plans would not be altered "if the right type of man is appointed."[133]

Pearce, however, was not happy. Around this time he learned something from Stiles which shocked him. He had received from Stiles an apoplectic letter which even the latter admitted was "rather . . . grousing." In it, as noted above, Stiles denounced the Infirmary Managers and hinted at the darker reasons for Meakins' departure. He also reported that "About a fortnight ago I received an official letter from the Clerk and Treasurer of the Royal Infirmary, intimating that my first period of appointment as a Full Surgeon (five years) expired on August 3rd of this year." The letter went on that "if I wished a further term of appointment . . . I was to let him know so that he might bring the matter before the Managers." Stiles made his apparent indignation clear and told the Clerk that the Crown appointed the Regius Professor until he was 65. Stiles was informed, however, "that *all* members of the full staff had to be re-appointed every five years, that this was the rule of the Infirmary, and that like other members of the staff, *I came under the same rule.*" Stiles felt "it was rubbing it in to me that in the eyes of the Managers I was appointed on the same footing as the non-professorial staff." Nothing could make clearer the autonomy of the Infirmary because, of course, although Stiles had been appointed Regius Professor at the University he had his hospital beds as a courtesy, not a right. It is hard to imagine, however, that such a shrewd individual as Stiles did not know his conditions of service when he was appointed; the show of indignation was surely for Pearce's benefit.

There was a second matter that Stiles said was irksome: he had no say in the appointment of his assistants. This he felt was egregious given that, say, the Professors of Anatomy and Physiology had complete control in this area. He had written to the Managers on the matter and "If I get a reply . . . saying that they cannot alter the rule whereby the Full Surgeons and Assistant Surgeons pair off in order of seniority, I am determined to ask the Lord Advocate to bring the matter before the Secretary for Scotland, who recommended the Crown to appoint me." He would also bring the matter before the Earl of Balfour, the University's Chancellor. He would not "hesitate to resign over the matter."[134] Probably in response to this letter, Pearce told Stiles that he was "disturbed at some of the rumors which have reached me" and that he had heard that Meakins's departure was owing in part "to the difficulties placed in his way by the Infirmary authorities in connection with the proper organization of his teaching staff." Pearce admitted that he had wrongly assumed that Professors had the power to appoint the staff of their choice in the Infirmary. He wrote that, if the professor "has to accept men on the Infirmary staff by seniority, it is, of course impossible to develop not only proper teaching but also to insure the best care of patients and research must of necessity lag." He was astonished too, that professors had to re-apply for their Infirmary position every five years. The hospital, he said, in a typical Rockefeller contrast of old and new, "should not allow tradition to interfere with that correlation in teaching effort which insures modern care of patients." He sought assurance that departmental heads would have "absolute authority" in regard to appointments. In America, he observed, "the question never arises." It was an "unwritten law" that the departmental head "not only has the privilege but the right of choosing his own staff."[135] This was quite an issue for Pearce, as evidenced by the fact that he wrote an almost identical letter to Stiles the next day, July 11, 1924. "If," he said, "a professor of a clinical subject is to have one staff for teaching and another for the care of patients, it is not possible for either medical school or hospital to obtain the best results."[136] Perhaps inadvertently rubbing salt in the wound, Pearce sent Stiles the agreement governing appointments at McGill University and the Royal Victoria and the Montreal General Hospital.[137]

Before he left, Meakins drew up sketch plans for the new laboratory. A committee of the Infirmary recommended a site on the hospital's grounds which was adopted by the Infirmary Managers. Writing to the University Secretary, the Infirmary's Clerk stated the Managers had agreed that the costs of the laboratory should be borne by the University and that the buildings were to become the property of the Infirmary Managers. It was further agreed all members of the honorary staff would have the right to work in the laboratory and that the Director would be the Christison Professor of Therapeutics (soon to be Murray Lyon). These plans, the Clerk said, would be submitted to the honorary staff.[138]

Now, considering that the money from Rockefeller was given to the University for a laboratory that was to be under its control, the action of the Infirmary Managers looks enormously high-handed, and so it was perceived to be, at least by Harvey Littlejohn, a man with no Infirmary appointment and a fierce defender of the University. Writing in late September 1924 from the Junior Athenaeum Club in Piccadilly, London, to the secretary of the University, he stated that he considered that the "plans [for the laboratory] should be *drawn up by the University* and submitted to the Managers." He gathered that the opposite was being done and, compounding the felony, the plans were being submitted "to the *Staff* of the Infirmary for their views." "Surely," he wrote, "this is wrong, and is giving the Staff a position in regard to the Laboratory to which they are not entitled, and which may lead to difficulties in the future, as to the exact relation of the laboratory to the University." "The Infirmary," he added, "don't seem to realize that they are receiving a very valuable asset." He thought there should be some "reciprocal obligation on the part of the Infirmary to *guarantee* that the Christison Professor shall have wards allotted to him. At present these are given *ex gratia*."[139] Littlejohn had obviously been apprised that the new laboratory was to have a ten-bedded ward attached to it which was to be under the care of the Director. He was concerned that the Infirmary Managers might use this as a pretext for removing from the Professor's care the beds elsewhere in the hospital that were usually at his disposal.

Littlejohn, however, may have been on his own in this matter. Murray Lyon (now Professor) wrote to Pearce telling him of the Infirmary Managers' actions without comment. Indeed he very much approved of "how desirable it was that the non-professorial members of the [Infirmary] should be carried along in any scheme which the University wishes to bring forward."[140] None the less the Clerk's letter and that of Littlejohn were presented at a meeting of representatives of the University Court and the Managers.[141] Reporting on that meeting, Lyon told Pearce that the new laboratory buildings would become the property of the Infirmary Managers, who would maintain them. The buildings would contain twelve beds "at the service of *any* member of the Infirmary staff." This presumably was a condition imposed by the non-professorial staff when they saw the Managers' proposals. The meeting found Meakins's plans for the laboratory unacceptable, mainly because both sides professed themselves strapped for cash. Lyon sketched out some new plans. The laboratory was to be on two floors with rooms on either side of a central passage. There were to be two small wards (one male, one female, presumably). Lyon reported that the "attitude of the Infirmary Board towards the scheme is somewhat divided." The majority supported it but "some still require education as to the benefits which the institution and the patients will derive from the existence of such a laboratory." There was active opposition from only one man, "who appears to represent an interest antagonistic to the University" and who thought the "work proposed in the laboratory is amply provided for in the College of Physicians Laboratory."[142]

Matters moved slowly. In February 1925 someone, probably Murray Lyon, at a meeting of an Infirmary Managers' committee recorded that the Managers "are exceedingly jealous of the possibility of any outside control and would like to have whole management of the building in their own hands."[143] At this time the University was receiving Rockefeller aid for the Department of Surgery and Ewing wrote to Pearce for yet more help in this direction. Pearce was possibly getting a bit fed up. He told Ewing that he thought "it would be unwise to bring any new project in connection with Edinburgh to the attention of the Trustees of the Rockefeller Foundation until all problems are settled." He said "it might be as well to have the University and Infirmary settle the problem of the clinical laboratory before any new projects are seriously considered."[144]

By late March 1925 the Regulations for the "Rockefeller Laboratory" had been agreed. Littlejohn seems to have got his way for the University had the plans prepared (albeit by the Infirmary's Master of Works) and they had been submitted for the Infirmary Managers' approval. No mention was made of the approval of the honorary staff of the Infirmary. The buildings were to belong to the Infirmary Managers, who were to be responsible for their upkeep as well as for the cost of routine testing. The expense of staffing for teaching and research was to be borne by the University.[145] On the basis of this document Ewing reported to Pearce that the matter of the laboratory had been "satisfactorily settled" and "the building of the laboratory will now proceed at once."[146] In late March 1925 Ewing told Pearce that work had started and early in May the Foundation appropriated £35,000 towards the building of the laboratory.[147] Ewing had been misinformed. Late in November 1925 Murray Lyon reported to Pearce that "it was not yet possible to start on the building" since contractors building the new X-ray Department were occupying the ground. Unfortunately, the contractor employed on this job was "also employed in erecting a large building in Princes Street for Woolworth's, who apparently make a more powerful call on the contractor than the Royal Infirmary."[148] Building did commence but there is apparently no further correspondence extant until January 1928 when Murray Lyon reported that the "structure of the new Clinical Laboratory is approaching completion."[149] The next few months were taken up with discussions of the equipment required.[150] In early May Murray Lyon reported that "Part of the new Clinical Laboratory will be ready for occupying in a short time" and he sent out a questionnaire to the senior staff asking what facilities, if any, were required.[151] The lab seems to have been occupied gradually. In October Murray Lyon, at a meeting with Sir Norman Walker, reported "that people have taken space in the laboratory already." He then admitted, "Criticism of the class of work done by these people was made."[152] By November 1928 the lab was "sufficiently advanced" for the allocation of places to any member of the honorary staff who wanted one.[153] Detailed discussions were also held on the criteria by which patients were to be admitted to Ward 21, the laboratory's ward. The most important of these was that the ward was for patients requiring special investigations that could not be carried out on the ordinary wards.[154] I deal with the work of the lab in Chapters 7 and 8, but before this I turn to attempts to reform the Medical and Surgical Departments.

Notes

1. *Bicentenary of the Faculty of Medicine 1726–1926. Records of the Celebrations* (Edinburgh: James Thin, 1926), 17.

2. William H. Schneider, "The Men who Followed Flexner: Richard Pearce, Alan Gregg, and the Rockefeller Foundation Medical Divisions, 1919–1951," in *Rockefeller Philanthropy and Modern Biomedicine: International Initiatives from World War I to the Cold War*, ed. William H. Schneider (Indiana: Indiana University Press, 2002), 7–60, 22.

3. Edsall to Pearce, October 18 [1922], folder 217, box 16, series 401, RG 1.1, Rockefeller Foundation Archives, RAC.

4. Edsall to Pearce, November 13, 1922, folder 217, box 16, series 401, RG 1.1, Rockefeller Foundation Archives, RAC.

5. David Edsall, "Comparative Observations of Methods of Education in Clinical Medicine in Great Britain and the United States 1922–3," 64, 57, folder 217, box 16, series 401, RG 1.1, Rockefeller Foundation Archives, RAC.

6. Evarts A. Graham, "A Report of an Investigation of the Teaching of Surgery in Representative British Medical Schools, Based on a Visit to Great Britain under the Auspices of the Division of Medical Education, Rockefeller Foundation," 2, 5, folder 217, box 16, series 401, RG 1.1, Rockefeller Foundation Archives, RAC.

7. Christopher Clayson, "Some Glimpses of Medicine Seventy Years Ago," *University of Edinburgh Journal* 39 (1999): 92–95.

8. Lorrain Smith to Pearce, March 1923, folder 5, box 1, series 405, RG1.1, Rockefeller Foundation Archives, RAC.

9. Edsall to Pearce, October 18 [1922], folder 217, box 16, series 401, RG 1.1, Rockefeller Foundation Archives, RAC.

10. Edsall, "Comparative Observations," 58–59. Clearly Edsall considered students were over-supervised on the wards and under-supervised in dispensary work. In the former case he may have been referring to a surplus of lectures taking the place of practical work.

11. Bryan Ashworth, *The Bramwells of Edinburgh: A Medical Dynasty* (Edinburgh: The Royal College of Physicians of Edinburgh, 1986), 24–37, for patient numbers see 28.

12. Edwin Bramwell, "A Plea for Accuracy in Therapeutic Deduction," *The Lancet* 1 (1925): 265–68. Bumble puppy is also known as 1. Nine-holes (a game in which either on the ground or on a board a player endeavours to roll balls into nine holes); 2. "Whist played unscientifically." *The Shorter Oxford English Dictionary*. Moynihan probably had the former in mind.

13. Bramwell, "A Plea for Accuracy in Therapeutic Deduction."

14. Edwin Bramwell, "The Undergraduate Training in Medicine," *Edinburgh Medical Journal* 34 (1927): 746–53.

15. See the unsympathetic account of Schafer's address to the British Medical Association reported as "The Introductory Address," *British Medical Journal* 2 (1885): 655.

16. Edinburgh Pathological Club, *An Inquiry into the Medical Curriculum* (Edinburgh: W. Green & Son, 1919), 93.

17. Bramwell, "The Undergraduate Training in Medicine."

18. Edwin Bramwell, "Remarks on some Clinical Pictures Attributable to Lead Poisoning," *British Medical Journal* 2 (1931): 87–92.

19. Edwin Bramwell, private papers, courtesy of Hilda McKendrick.

20. W. T. Ritchie, "Medicine in Edinburgh," *Edinburgh Medical Journal* 35 (1928): 665–73.

21. Jonathan Campbell Meakins, "Insulin in the Treatment of Diabetes: Science, Empiricism and Superstition. Inaugural Sessional Address Delivered at the Scientific Evening Meeting of the North British Branch of the Pharmaceutical Society in Edinburgh on November 23 1923," *Pharmaceutical Journal* 57 (1923): 567–70.

22. Jonathan Campbell Meakins, "Memorandum as to the Benefits to be Derived by the Patients of the Royal Infirmary from the Proposed Clinical Laboratory," February 1924. It forms part of Meakins's "Autobiography," 867/51, OLHM.

23. Meakins to Martin, December 19, 1923, 867/39/29, OLHM.

24. T. J. Mackie, *Medical Education: An Evaluation*, Promoter's Address (Edinburgh: University of Edinburgh, 1929). There is a copy at FD1/1842, 49252, PRO.

25. David McCrone, *Understanding Scotland: The Sociology of a Stateless Nation* (London and New York: Routledge, 1992).

26. See Benedict Anderson, *Imagined Communities: Reflections on the Origin and Spread of Nationalism* (London: Verso, 1983).

27. On the latter point see Linda Colley, *Britons: Forging the Nation 1707–1737* (Yale: Yale University Press, 1992).

28. Graeme Morton, "What if? The Significance of Scotland's Missing Nationalism in the Nineteenth Century" in *Image and Identity: The Making and Re-making of Scotland Through the Ages*, ed. Dauvit Broun, R. J. Finlay, and Michael Lynch (Edinburgh: John Donald, 1998), 157–76, quote at 160. Unfortunately Morton does not explore in detail the concrete form the exercise of civic virtue took.

29. See for example Nicholas Phillipson, "Towards a Definition of the Scottish Enlightenment," in *City and Society in the Eighteenth Century*, ed. P. Fritz and D. Williams (Toronto: Hakkert, 1973), 125–47; "Culture and Society in the Eighteenth-Century Province: The Case of Edinburgh and the Scottish Enlightenment," in *The University in Society*, ed. Lawrence Stone, 2 vols. (Princeton, NJ: Princeton University Press, 1975), vol. 2, 407–48.

30. David McCrone, "Towards a Principled Elite: Scottish Elites in the Twentieth Century," in *People and Society in Scotland. III 1914–1990*, ed. Tony Dickson and James H. Treble, 3 vols. (Edinburgh: John Donald, 1992), vol. 3, 174–200.

31. McCrone, *Understanding Scotland*, 12. On his ideas of myth see David McCrone, "We're A' Jock Tamson's Bairns: Social Class in Twentieth-Century Scotland," in *Scotland in the Twentieth Century*, ed. T. M. Devine and R. J. Finlay (Edinburgh: Edinburgh University Press, 1996), 102–21.

32. Helen Corr, "Where is the Lass o' Pairts?: Gender, Identity and Education in Nineteenth Century Scotland," in *Image and Identity*, ed. Broun, Finlay and Lynch, 220–28, quote at 220.

33. Christopher Harvie, *No Gods and Precious Few Heroes: Twentieth-Century Scotland*, 3rd ed. (Edinburgh, Edinburgh University Press, 1998), 122.

34. See McCrone, *Understanding Scotland*, 102. For a view of Scottish school education as always having been inadequate and for the distinct decline at the end of the nineteenth century of any equality of opportunity that there ever was see T. C. Smout, *A Century of the Scottish People 1830–1950* (New Haven and London: Yale University Press, 1986), 209–30.

35. George Elder Davie, *The Democratic Intellect. Scotland and her Universities in the Nineteenth Century* (Edinburgh: Edinburgh University Press, 1961).

36. Ibid., xi–xii.

37. Ibid., xvii, xvi.

38. George Elder Davie, *The Crisis of the Democratic Intellect. The Problem of Generalism and Specialisation in Twentieth-Century Scotland* (Polygon: Edinburgh, 1986).

39. Edsall to Pearce, September 26, 1924, folder 217, box 16, series 401, RG 1.1, Rockefeller Foundation Archives, RAC.

40. Harvie, *No Gods and Precious Few Heroes*, 129.

41. Ibid., 5.

42. Ibid., 129–35.

43. David Cannadine, *The Rise and Fall of the British Aristocracy* (New Haven, Conn., London: Yale University Press, 1990).

44. McCrone, "Towards a Principled Elite," 185, 195.

45. Edwin Bramwell, "The Undergraduate Training in Medicine." The irony here is that Bramwell was English by birth. The family had long lived in Edinburgh.

46. See the "Introduction," and essays in *Regenerating England: Science, Medicine and Culture in Inter-War Britain*, ed. Christopher Lawrence and Anna-K. Mayer (Amsterdam: Rodopi, 2000) which are specifically devoted to "amateur" social theorists.

47. Harvie, *No Gods and Precious few Heroes*, 129–35.

48. Roger Davidson, *Dangerous Liaisons: A Social History of Venereal Disease in Twentieth-Century Scotland* (Amsterdam: Rodopi, 2000).

49. David Cantor, "Between Galen, Geddes, and the Gael: Arthur Brock, Modernity, and Medical Humanism in Early-Twentieth-Century Britain," *Journal of the History of Medicine and Allied Sciences* 60 (2005): 1–41.

50. Scottish society, it is argued, being relatively poor, is driven by powerful forces for fusion and division, egalitarianism, and elitism. See H. M. Paterson, "Incubus and Ideology: The Development of Secondary Schooling in Scotland," in *Scottish Culture and Scottish Education 1800–1980*, ed. Walter M. Humes and Hamish M. Paterson (Edinburgh: John Donald, 1983), 197–215, see especially 198.

51. Vincent to Ewing, November 22, 1921, folder 12, box 1, series 405, RG 1.1, Rockefeller Foundation Archives, RAC.

52. Pearce to Lord Knutsford, April 16, 1925, folder 245, box 18, series 401, RG 1.1, Rockefeller Foundation Archives, RAC.

53. Attached to Richard Pearce, "Notes of R.M.P. on Medical School of the University of Edinburgh," February 22–24, 1923 and presumably sent to him in advance of his visit, folder 5, box 1, series 405, RG 1.1, Rockefeller Foundation Archives, RAC.

54. Pearce to Edsall, May 2, 1922, folder 217, box 16, series 401, RG 1.1, Rockefeller Foundation Archives, RAC.

55. "Notes of R.M.P.," 6.

56. Pearce to Fletcher, July 22, 1922, folder 67, box 5, series 401, RG1.1, Rockefeller Foundation Archives, RAC.

57. Pearce visited Europe in 1920 after the formation of the Division of Medical Education. That may well have been his first meeting with Fletcher. Schneider, "The Men who Followed Flexner," 12.

58. Fletcher to Pearce, October 6, 1922, folder 67, box 5, series 401, RG1.1, Rockefeller Foundation Archives, RAC.

59. This is clearly one of those places where England stands for Britain. Indeed earlier in the letter Pearce talks of visiting "most of the Medical Schools in the United Kingdom." Pearce to Fletcher, October 12, 1922, folder 67, box 5, series 401, RG1.1, Rockefeller Foundation Archives, RAC.

60. MacLean to Pearce, January 26, 1923, folder 333, box 26, series 401A, RG 1.1, Rockefeller Foundation Archives, RAC.

61. "Notes of R.M.P.," 1.

62. On Watson's lab see ibid., 6. His University salary was £900 per annum.

63. Ibid., 2–3.

64. Ibid.

65. Ibid., 8–10.

66. Pearce to Meakins, June 26, 1923, folder 13, box 2, series 405, RG 1.1, Rockefeller Foundation Archives, RAC.

67. Pearce, "Notes of R.M.P.," 6.

68. Ibid., 5.

69. "Statement by B. P. Watson. University of Edinburgh." (Dated by hand March 1923, but that may have been when it was received at the RF), folder 5, box 1, series 405, RG 1.1, Rockefeller Foundation Archives, RAC.

70. Pearce, "Notes of R.M.P.," 5–6.

71. Ibid., 8–10.

72. Pearce to Embree, February 25, 1923, folder 32, box 3, series 405, RG 1.1, Rockefeller Foundation Archives, RAC. On the date of Pearce leaving Britain see Meakins to Martin, April 2, 1923, 867/39/96, OLHM. In fact Stiles was not leaving America until a few days after Pearce had returned, so there must have been some other reason why Pearce did not expect to see him.

73. Pearce to Embree, February 25, 1923, folder 32, box 3, series 405, RG 1.1, Rockefeller Foundation Archives, RAC.

74. Pearce to Embree, February 28, 1923, folder 13, box 2, series 405, RG 1.1, Rockefeller Foundation Archives, RAC. Underlining in original.

75. Meakins to Martin, December 19, 1923, 867/39/29, OLHM.

76. Ibid.

77. Marianne Pauline Fedunkiw Stevens, "Dollars and Change; The Effect of Rockefeller Foundation Funding on Canadian Medical Education at the University of Toronto, McGill University, and Dalhousie University" (Ph.D. Thesis, University of Toronto, 2000), 186; Marianne Fedunkiw, " 'German Methods,' 'Unconditional Gifts,' and the Full-Time System: The Case of the University of Toronto, 1919–23," *Canadian Bulletin of Medical History* 21 (2004): 5–39.

78. Meakins to Martin, April 2, 1923, 867/39/96, OLHM.

79. Pearce to Embree, internal memorandum, hand-written, March 8, 1923, folder 13, box 2, series 405, RG 1.1, Rockefeller Foundation Archives, RAC.

80. Pearce to Embree, March 19, 1923, internal memorandum, folder 32, box 3, series 405, RG 1.1, Rockefeller Foundation Archives, RAC. Stiles's letter not found.

81. Barger to Pearce, March 29, 1923, folder 13, box 2, series 405, RG 1.1, Rockefeller Foundation Archives, RAC.

82. Ibid.

83. Pearce to Barger, April 4, 1923 (copy), folder 13, box 2, series 405, RG1.1, Rockefeller Foundation Archives, RAC.

84. "Preliminary Statement by the Faculty of Medicine of the University of Edinburgh Submitted to the Board of the Rockefeller Foundation," March 1923, folder 5, box 1, series 405, RG 1.1, Rockefeller Foundation Archives, RAC.

85. Minutes of the Rockefeller Foundation, May 23, 1923, folder 12, box 1, series 405, RG 1.1, Rockefeller Foundation Archives, RAC.

86. Pearce to Meakins, May 29, 1923 (copy), folder 13, box 2, series 405, RG 1.1, Rockefeller Foundation Archives, RAC.

87. Pearce to Stiles, May 29, 1923 (copy), folder 13, box 2, series 405, RG 1.1, Rockefeller Foundation Archives, RAC.

88. Pearce to Meakins, June 8, 1923. This letter is attached to the hand-written part of Meakins, "Autobiography," 867/51, OLHM.

89. Pearce to Stiles, June 25, 1923 (copy), folder 13, box 2, series 405, RG1.1, Rockefeller Foundation Archives, RAC.

90. Pearce to Meakins, June 26, 1923, folder 13, box 2, series 405, RG 1.1, Rockefeller Foundation Archives, RAC.

91. Memorandum "Edinburgh Problems," Pearce to A. Gregg and Vincent, October 5, 1923, folder 13, box 2, series 405, RG 1.1, Rockefeller Foundation Archives, RAC. Seven months earlier Pearce had mocked the notion of revolutionary change, "Notes of R.M.P.," 5–6.

92. Martin to Meakins, October 11, 1923, 867/39/2, OHLM.

93. Martin to Meakins, November 26, 1923, 867/39/3, OLHM.

94. Meakins to Martin, November 27, 1923, 867/39/28, OLHM.

95. Memorandum from Pearce to A. Gregg and Vincent, October 5, 1923, "Edinburgh Problems", folder 13, box 2, series 405, RG 1.1, Rockefeller Foundation Archives, RAC.

96. Stiles to Pearce, December 19, 1923, folder 32, box 3, series 405, RG 1.1, Rockefeller Foundation Archives, RAC.

97. Meakins to Pearce, December 3, 1923, folder 13, box 2, series 405, RG 1.1, Rockefeller Foundation Archives, RAC.

98. Pearce to Ewing, December 6, 1923, folder 13, box 2, series, 405, RG 1.1, Rockefeller Foundation Archives, RAC.

99. Minutes of the Rockefeller Foundation, December 5, 1923, folder 12, box 1, series 405, RG 1.1, Rockefeller Foundation Archives, RAC.

100. Fletcher to Meakins, December 19, 1923, 867/40/45, OLHM.

101. Pearce to Ewing, December 6, 1923, folder 13, box 2, series, 405, RG 1.1, Rockefeller Foundation Archives, RAC.

102. "Memorandum regarding Chair of Therapeutics," June 21, 1929, Secretary's File, DRT 95/002, pt. 1, Faculty of Medicine, box 27, EUA. In 1922 the University Court had agreed that Meakins could accept consulting positions in private and public nursing homes, ibid.

103. Pearce to Meakins, December 6, 1923, folder 13, box 2, series 405, RG 1.1, Rockefeller Foundation Archives, RAC.

104. Meakins to Pearce, December 19, 1923, folder 13, box 2, series 405, RG 1.1, Rockefeller Foundation Archives, RAC.

105. Meakins to Martin, December 19, 1923, 867/39/29, OLHM.

106. Meakins to Pearce, December 19, 1923, folder 13, box 2, series 405, RG 1.1, Rockefeller Foundation Archives, RAC.

107. Stiles to Pearce, December 19, 1923, folder 32, box 3, series 405, RG 1.1, Rockefeller Foundation Archives, RAC.

108. Pearce to Stiles, January 8, 1924 (file copy), folder 14, box 2, series 405, RG 1.1, Rockefeller Foundation Archives, RAC.

109. Pearce to Ewing, January 4, 1924, folder 14, box 2, series 405, RG 1.1, Rockefeller Foundation Archives, RAC.

110. Pearce to Meakins, January 11, 1924 (file copy), folder 14, box 2, series 405, RG 1.1, Rockefeller Foundation Archives, RAC.

111. Martin to Meakins, February 14, 1924, 867/39/5, OLHM.

112. Martin to Meakins, February 14, 1924, 867/39/4, OLHM.

113. Meakins to Martin, [March] 4, 1923. This letter is catalogued as May but all the evidence points to March. 867/39/31, OLHM.

114. Martin to Meakins, March 20, 1924, 867/39/6, OLHM.

115. Currie to Pearce, May 12, 1924, 867/39/16, OLHM.

116. Currie to Meakins, May 27, 1924, 867/39/17, OLHM.

117. T. H. Graham to Meakins, June 4, 1924, 867/38/2 OLHM; John Thomson to Meakins, June 4, 1924, 867/38/1, OLHM.

118. J. S. Haldane to Meakins, June 17, 1924, 867/40/31, OLHM.

119. Fletcher to Meakins, June 20, 1924, 867/40/32, OLHM.

120. Alexander to Meakins, June 5, 1924, 867/38/4, OLHM. There was an Adam Alexander, M.D. Aberdeen, practising at the London Hospital, listed in *The Medical Directory*, 1924.

121. Greig to Meakins, June 5, 1924, 867/38/3, OLHM.

122. Baycott to Meakins, June 13, 1924, 876/38/10, OLHM. There was no A. C. Baycott in *The Medical Directory* for 1924.

123. Mackenzie to Meakins, July 11, 1924, 867/38/17, OLHM. Emphasis mine.

124. Bramwell to Meakins, June 6, 1924, 867/38/5, OLHM.

125. Pearce to Meakins, June 25, 1924, 867/38/14, OLHM.

126. Meakins to Walker, March 23, 1927, 867/39/56, OLHM.

127. Stiles to Pearce, June 17, 1924, folder 33, box 3 series 405, RG 1.1, Rockefeller Foundation Archives, RAC.

128. L. Stanley P. Davidson, "The Evolution of Modern Medicine, with Special Reference to Medical Research," *Edinburgh Medical Journal* 38 (1931): 113–25, quotes at 123, 121.

129. Jonathan L. Meakins, "Summary of a conversation with Sir Derrick Dunlop," September 11, 1979; "A summary of luncheon with Dr. Ray Gilcrist [*sic*] at the New Club," September 11, 1979. Originals in possession of Jonathan L. Meakins.

130. Meakins to Pearce, June 10, 1924, folder 14, box 2, series 405, RG 1.1, Rockefeller Foundation Archives, RAC.

131. Ewing to Pearce, June 9, 1924, folder 14, box 2, series 405, RG 1.1, Rockefeller Foundation Archives, RAC.

132. Pearce to Ewing, June 19, 1924, folder 14, box 2, series 405, RG 1.1, Rockefeller Foundation Archives, RAC.

133. Pearce to Meakins, June 25, 1924, 867/38/14, OLHM.

134. Stiles to Pearce, June 17, 1924, folder 33, box 3, series 405, RG 1.1, Rockefeller Foundation Archives, RAC.

135. Pearce to Stiles, July 10, 1924 (copy), folder 14, box 2, series 405, RG 1.1, Rockefeller Foundation Archives, RAC.

136. Pearce to Stiles, July 11, 1924 (initialled file copy), folder 33, box 3, series 405, RG 1.1, Rockefeller Foundation Archives, RAC.

137. Pearce to Stiles, July 12, 1924 (file copy), folder 33, box 3, series 405, RG 1.1, Rockefeller Foundation Archives, RAC.

138. W. S. Caw to [W.] Wilson, July 22, 1924, "Scrap-book of the RIE Biochemical Laboratory," box 1, folder 3, RCPE.

139. Littlejohn to Wilson, September 23, [1924], "Scrap-book of the RIE Biochemical Laboratory," box 1, folder 3, RCPE.

140. Murray Lyon to Pearce, September 29, 1924, folder 14, box 2, series 405, RG 1.1, Rockefeller Foundation Archives, RAC.

141. William Wilson, "The Rockefeller Laboratory" [circular letter], September 29, 1924, in "Scrap-book of the RIE Biochemical Laboratory," box 1, folder 3, RCPE.

142. Murray Lyon to Pearce, December 4, 1924, folder 14, box 2, series 405, RG 1.1, Rockefeller Foundation Archives, RAC.

143. "Rockefeller Meeting," February 5, 1925, in "Scrap-book of the RIE Biochemical Laboratory," box 1, folder 4, RCPE.

144. Pearce to Ewing, March 9, 1925 (copy), folder 34, box 3, series 405, RG 1.1, Rockefeller Foundation Archives, RAC.

145. Ewing to Pearce, March 28, 1925, folder 34, box 3, series 405, RG 1.1, Rockefeller Foundation Archives, RAC. That plans had been drawn up see Caw to "Sir," March 31, 1925, folder 14, box 2, series 405, RG 1.1, Rockefeller Foundation Archives, RAC.

146. Ewing to Pearce, March 28, 1925.

147. Caw to "Sir," March 31, 1925. See also Minutes of the Rockefeller Foundation, May 5, 1925 (copy), folder 12, box 1, series 405, RG 1.1, Rockefeller Foundation Archives, RAC.

148. Murray Lyon to Pearce, November 23, 1925, folder 14, box 2, series 405, RG 1.1, Rockefeller Foundation Archives, RAC.

149. Murray Lyon (circular letter), January 6, 1928, in "Scrap-book of the RIE Biochemical Laboratory," box 2, RCPE.

150. See for example, "Meeting of Advisory Committee of the Laboratory," May 8, 1928, in "Scrap-book of the RIE Biochemical Laboratory," box 2, RCPE.

151. Murray Lyon (circular letter), May 4, 1928, in "Scrap-book of the RIE Biochemical Laboratory," box 2, RCPE.

152. [Murray Lyon], "Meeting with Sir Norman Walker and Mr. [A] Miles," October 19, 1928, in "Scrap-book of the RIE Biochemical Laboratory," box 1 folder 6, RCPE.

153. [Murray Lyon], "Memorandum, Clinical Laboratory, Royal Infirmary," November 10, 1928, in "Scrap-book of the RIE Biochemical Laboratory," box 2, RCPE.

154. "Meeting of Advisory Committee of the Laboratory," November 12, 1928, in "Scrap-book of the RIE Biochemical Laboratory," box 2, RCPE.

6

THE DEPARTMENTS OF SURGERY AND MEDICINE

The RF's concentration on the Biochemistry Laboratory and the Department of Therapeutics was a product of considerable institutional history and Rockefeller strategy. As usual the RF picked out its man, in this case Meakins (that he held the therapeutics chair was coincidental). Although there were problems in London the RF had been able to support new medical and surgical units there, notably because they were unencumbered by the burden of history. In Edinburgh it tried to create units using the premier medical and surgical professorships but these were long-standing chairs with intricate relations with the Infirmary and with incumbents who had their own agendas. Nor following Meakins, in the case of medicine, was there an individual with whom the Foundation was comfortable. Because of these factors the result, certainly in the medical case, was far less satisfactory than the RF would have wanted. In this chapter I examine the support for surgery, the struggles around the Chair of Medicine, and the physical reconstruction of the Medical Faculty after 1928.

From the Rockefeller point of view, the reconstruction of surgical teaching and research was, after a great deal of bargaining, a relative success story. There were two departments of surgery in the Medical Faculty headed by a Chair of Systematic Surgery and a Chair of Clinical Surgery. Both of these chairs dated from the early nineteenth century. In many ways they were quite independent. When the Department of Surgery is referred to in the contemporary literature it sometimes means the Chair of Systematic Surgery and sometimes both chairs, either because of colloquial usage or because both were included in the Department of Surgery of the RIE. Context usually makes things clear. The Department of Systematic Surgery had a large lecture theatre in the Medical School. The Professor of Clinical Surgery gave his lectures in the Infirmary. Here, behind the operating theatre, the surgeons had their own pathological laboratory for histological and bacteriological work.[1] In the hospital, appointments to the position of Assistant and Ordinary Surgeon were governed by the same complex rules that governed the appointment of physicians. This meant that the Infirmary Managers had a major voice in these appointments and that promotion to Ordinary Surgeon was based on the position of the Assistants in the pecking order.[2] The professors (appointed by the University usually from the Ordinary Surgeons) received ward space in the hospital by courtesy of the Managers, who thus had a substantial voice in appointments to chairs. Each of the two professors had his own allotted beds. At the beginning of the 1920s the Professor of Systematic Surgery was Henry Alexis Thomson, who retired in 1923. He had a salary from the University of £1,250 per annum. The Professor of Clinical Surgery was Sir Harold Stiles, who had a salary of £900 per annum.[3] He resigned in 1925. The RF considered Stiles an ally (even though he had been so misguided as to present Pearce enthusiastically with the Lister scheme in 1921). Pearce, who dealt with him frequently, considered him a man of "great influence."[4] Along with Meakins and Watson, Pearce held him to be one of the three men to have the "modern point . . . of view of science in medicine." He had the "proper ideal."[5] As it turned out this did not mean that Stiles lacked any plans of his own.

When Pearce visited Edinburgh in February 1923 he had nothing specific to say about surgery although he considered it should have a "true University clinic."[6] In March 1923 he was more precise, talking of a "true university clinic, in surgery, for Stiles."[7] The committee formed after Pearce's visit whose "wish list" Stiles carried to New York made no particular recommendations regarding surgery,[8] although, beforehand,

Barger had said the committee proposed to "shift 'systematic' medicine and surgery to the Infirmary" in order to create more space in the Medical School.[9] On May 23, 1923, Pearce presented various proposals to the Foundation Trustees, including one "to provide additional annual sums for a five-year period to place one chair in medicine and one chair in surgery on a full-time basis (probably $7,000 a year)."[10] Writing to Meakins in June 1923, Pearce said of a proposed visit in October that "details concerning the possible development of true University clinics in medicine and surgery along the line of the London units, I prefer to discuss with you and Stiles when I arrive, and it might be well to keep these matters out of general discussion until I have a chance to talk with you."[11] Pearce seems to have been burned quite badly by the full-time business both at home and abroad and he was very cagey about it.

On September 3 Stiles wrote to Pearce that Alexis Thomson (the Professor of Systematic Surgery) was to give up his Infirmary position and would probably no longer give his lectures in the Medical School. If that was the case, Stiles said, "now will be the time for reorganising the surgical teaching in Edinburgh." Stiles reported he had been hard at work during the summer educating the Infirmary Managers on the "necessity of providing a larger University Unit." Of course, what Stiles wanted out of any reorganization was unknown to Pearce at this time. Stiles reported to Pearce that he happened to know the Managers were "even in favour of abolishing the Chairs of Systematic and Clinical Surgery and having one Professor at the head of one large unit."[12] At first sight this is extremely odd even if Stiles had "educated" them into this position. The formal appointment of a professor and abolishing chairs was not the Infirmary Managers' prerogative. What it indicates is the power the Managers could exercise over professorial conditions of service. Bringing together the beds allocated to the two chairs certainly was their province. By limiting or expanding professorial access to beds they could effectively impose part-time or full-time conditions on chairs.

By the time of Pearce's visit on Monday, October 1, 1923, Thomson had resigned. On the Tuesday Pearce recorded that he met Stiles, who proposed the now vacant Chair of Systematic Surgery be abolished and a "unified" surgery department created with control of all of the hospital's professorial beds. Stiles further proposed he would head the department and an associate professor should be appointed under him. This would not create a department with a full-time director but, said Stiles, a "school" of surgery with a single head—Stiles. In the hospital Stiles would now have sixty beds—twice the number he had before. Pearce thought this a "great advance," presumably in the light of Stiles's insistence that it was "useless" to consider a full-time plan for the Chair of Systematic Surgery. Stiles did not explain why this was "useless" but it did become clear that he did not personally wish a full-time appointment. In his proposal he would be head of the school and still do a great deal of private practice. Pearce undoubtedly had this spotted, for although he recorded Stiles's account of the full-time issue, he added: "I am, however, still working this through [with] Meakins."

The following day, Wednesday, it was clear that Pearce did have doubts about Stiles's plan and his reasons for promoting it. Pearce had his eyes on a full-time chair heading both departments and controlling all the hospital beds. Filling the vacancy in systematic surgery with a suitable candidate obviously seemed the sensible first strategic move towards achieving this. Pearce recorded, presumably that evening, that he had "put M[eakins] up to sounding out Fraser, the only local possibility for full-time chair in [Systematic] Surgery." John Fraser was an Assistant Surgeon. By Thursday, Pearce said he had started "a real campaign for a *full-time professor* in surgery instead of *Associate Professor*." However, Stiles "would not consider" full-time and if a single department were created it raised a "problem . . . as to the headship of combined groups." Pearce obviously saw that a newly-promoted younger surgeon could hardly be ranked over Stiles. The compromise would be to have Stiles as joint head until his retirement and then have the full-time professor take over. Quite what would happen to Stiles's chair is not clear. Anyhow, in spite of his earlier view that it was a "useless" to consider a full-time Professor of Systematic Surgery, Stiles (no doubt outvoted by Pearce and others) agreed to put that plan to a special faculty meeting.[13] It was at the time of this meeting, described in the previous chapter,[14] that Pearce (probably alone in his hotel room) sat fretting and hoping for the endorsement of a new lab for Meakins.

The Medical Faculty agreed that the Chair of Systematic Surgery be made full time.[15] But that was not the end of the matter, the University Court had to agree, as did the Infirmary Managers (again this must have amazed Pearce), and a suitable candidate had to be found.[16] On December

5 the Rockefeller Trustees endowed the chair by providing £15,000. This assured £750 a year in interest to top up the professor's salary to £2,000. The Foundation also agreed to provide an additional £750 per annum for five years to assist with the salaries of other workers in the department. The University was to "establish a true University Clinic" and eventually "unite under one head double the number of present beds."[17] The following day, December 6, Pearce informed Ewing of the offer and that it would materialize "When the development of the plans for unification of the two surgical services have been completed." The full-time incumbent was to have "the same attitude towards teaching, research and care of patients as characterizes Professor Meakins's work in medicine."[18] He also wrote to Stiles, who replied to Pearce on December 19 that he was "delighted," adding that Pearce's letter to Ewing "puts the whole position very clearly." Stiles reported that with regard to the full-time chair, a sub-committee had been formed which had created a "scheme" that had gone before the University Court, presumably successfully. However, further negotiations between the University and Infirmary were needed. He added: "The University's acceptance of the policy of a whole-time Professor of Surgery may cause some disappointment in quarters where vested interests are at stake, but I feel confident the Managers of the Royal Infirmary will meet the wishes of the University in the matter." He did not spell out what the "vested interests" were.[19] However, on January 16, 1924, representatives of the University and the Infirmary met to discuss the various Rockefeller offers. This meeting provided at least one indication of the "vested interests." The minutes record: "It was suggested by some members of the conference that objection might be taken in the interests of the Infirmary staff to the appointment to the Professorship of a person who was not already a member of the staff on the grounds of blocking promotion." That is, the Ordinary staff and some or all of the Managers regarded chairs as the peak of an exclusive, internal promotional ladder. Part-time service as a professor either of medicine or of surgery, with its access to extensive private practice, was built into the reward system for loyal attendance at the hospital. Indeed, except for the instance of Meakins, that was invariably the arrangement. The Ordinary staff was alarmed that an outsider would be brought in. The University pointed out, however, that there was no rule against this. The Managers said they would like to consider the matter further.[20] Again this latter

point would have astonished Pearce. It should not be forgotten in disentangling this political web that members of the Ordinary staff and the Managers probably fraternized socially (at the Kirk, on the golf course). They were, after all, members of Edinburgh's elite middle class. It should not be forgotten either how deeply divisive private practice could be in a relatively poor country with a wealth of senior practitioners. Derrick Dunlop recalled that when he took the Therapeutics Chair in 1936 the tension between the senior staff in the Medical Department of the RIE was intense, the atmosphere could be "cut with a knife." The bad feeling was largely generated by competition for private patients, particularly the poaching of patients that went on between consultants. There are no grounds for thinking that anything was different ten years earlier and this was, no doubt yet another reason for Meakins's departure.[21]

In May 1924 Lorrain Smith wrote "unofficially" to Pearce that they were making progress with the Managers over the Chair. An agreement to the appointment was reached with three conditions. These were: first, that the appointment to the Infirmary be for ten years; second, "that the professor shall be relieved of University duties on Wednesday afternoon and on Saturday of each week, and be free to engage in private practice"; and third, the professor at the end of the period of office be appointed to the first senior vacancy on the ordinary staff.[22] Thus the Managers did limit the full-time possibilities. How far they were acting autonomously and how far they were a conduit for surgical opinion is conjectural. However, before explanations are reduced to private material interests it should be borne in mind that the surgical staff and the Managers probably perceived the reputation of a surgical professor in *their* hospital to depend on the extent of his private practice. The public face of an infirmary was crucial to the extraction of charitable donations. There is evidence for the validity of this interpretation in the case of medicine (see below).

In an unofficial letter, Ewing sought Pearce's approval of the relaxation of the whole-time conditions. There was obviously concern in the Edinburgh camp that Rockefeller might pull out. Ewing, revealing nothing except perhaps his possible ignorance of how medicine ticked, said this change was made on the advice of the Medical Faculty "in order to secure the best candidates." Stiles had already been investigating suitable applicants and Ewing reported that two were prepared to accept the Chair on the currently proposed basis.[23] Meakins wrote to Pearce shortly afterwards about the change from full time. He thought, "this slight modification will have very little influence on the character of the work done." Although Meakins would have preferred the position established "*in toto*," he added tellingly, "I am rather surprised that they have been able to carry it so far."[24] Pearce replied to Ewing that he would need to take the matter to the Rockefeller Trustees, as he had no power to change conditions.[25]

In June, President Vincent sent what seems to have been an internal memorandum on this matter asking for action. Vincent believed: "The plan represents so great an advance in the teaching of surgery in Great Britain that even with the provision of a small amount of private practice it would have an excellent influence on the development of surgical clinics in the United Kingdom." He thought "To decline at this time to finance the proposed reorganization would put the Foundation in the awkward position of forcing a hard and fast plan, rather than supporting a wise and progressive change in the method of teaching."[26]

On June 17, 1924, Stiles wrote to Pearce in "a strictly private capacity." Stiles had talked to David Wilkie and John Fraser, Assistant Surgeons at the Infirmary, both of whom were ready to take the Chair with its two afternoons for private practice. Neither would take it if it were a full-time appointment. Stiles, presumably having not seen Ewing's letter, hoped Pearce could use his influence with the Trustees to fund the Chair under the modified conditions, virtually suggesting that for Edinburgh this was a radical departure: "Personally, I think it would be a very wise and diplomatic move to make this concession."[27] On July 1, 1924, the revised plan incorporating the small amount of time for private practice was approved at a meeting of the Rockefeller Trustees. At this meeting the Trustees also formally appropriated money in dollars to buy £15,000 to endow the Chair of [Systematic] Surgery.[28] Vincent explained to Simon Flexner the decision to let the incumbent do a small amount of private practice. Flexner, a Trustee, had been unable to attend the meeting but opposed the revised conditions. Vincent wrote, obviously thinking that in Edinburgh anything was better than nothing, that the "proposed change is in accordance with the general principle by which we have been guided, namely, rendering the kind of aid in a given situation which will mark an appreciable advance over the existing status." He had no doubt that the "proposed plan for Edinburgh would be a great advance over the existing regime."[29] By now Rockefeller bureaucrats were feeling vibrations that indicated the reform of British medicine needed caution. Acceptance of the academic model was not only slow but also meeting with possible reverses. Vincent explained to Flexner that it was "reported that all the surgical units in Great Britain will be abandoned except the one at University College, which will be maintained because of our gift to that center." The "Edinburgh people," he observed, "thought they could bring it [full-time] about, but when the final test came they were compelled to compromise." Vincent felt that had the decision over the Edinburgh Chair been delayed it might look as if the RF was trying to "dictate policy" (which, of course, it was, but only when it could).[30]

Having narrowed its candidates down to two, the University eventually appointed David Wilkie as Professor. Fraser was offered the Chair first but had obviously changed his mind because of the full-time business, even with the modification.[31] Wilkie, a Scot, had graduated in Edinburgh in 1904. The son of a jute manufacturer and independently wealthy, an income from private practice was probably not essential to him. By the time of his appointment he was recognized as a great teacher, researcher, administrator, and practical surgeon. Knighted in 1936, he died in 1938. Wilkie began his new position by visiting surgical clinics on the continent in the autumn of 1924. In October he expressed his "resolve" to Pearce to "develop a real Department of surgery." He then noted: "When I accepted the Chair I made the condition that the University should provide adequate accommodation and facilities for a Research Department and I am glad to say that they are doing their utmost to meet my demands in this connection." The University buildings, he said, "were [originally] constructed on the supposition that the didactic lecture was to form the essential feature of medical education for all time." Wilkie proposed to a committee of the Faculty of Medicine that the lectures on medicine and surgery be given in a single theatre and that "either the Surgery or the Medicine Lecture Theatre be reconstructed so as to provide rooms for practical teaching and museum accommodation." Wilkie also proposed that a new anatomical building, used for teaching women students, was "no longer being used to anything approaching its full capacity, [and that it] be handed over to be equipped as a Surgical Research Department." No doubt to his delight the Faculty approved both of these proposals and, he recorded, "the Professor of Anatomy has agreed to give over the new Anatomical building, provided the University purchase, renovate and equip the Anatomy rooms in an adjoining building which is well adapted to the purpose."[32]

Pearce replied that Wilkie's "plans for a research laboratory for the department appear satisfactory," adding, perhaps with a wistful look at the hopes he had harboured for Meakins's department, "I had supposed that this phase of the work might be taken care of in the proposed clinical laboratory but the plan which you outline is doubtless more satisfactory."[33] In January 1925 Stiles reported to Pearce that the alterations and extensions of the old, large surgical lecture theatre had provided an upper floor constituting a new lecture theatre and a lower floor of four rooms for tutorial classes. There was also a new museum of surgical pathology. He added that a Department of Experimental Surgical Research was not easily provided for, but the Professor of Anatomy had now agreed to hand over the women's anatomy building. Stiles also reported that the money required for making the new museum and for reconstructing the theatre had been granted by the University Court, "but this body cannot see its way to find the larger sums of money required for the Research Department." He was afraid its progress was "to be held up for the lack of the necessary funds." Stiles, who still had good relations with the RF, had no compunction in "writing to ask whether the Foundation would consider granting a capital sum for the reconstruction and equipment of this Department of Experimental Surgical Research." Stiles estimated that for reconstruction "a sum of £7,500 would be required and for equipment an equal sum." If they could obtain the money he thought "that we could look forward to having a Department of Surgery worthy of a large teaching school."

Stiles outlined the plans for the research department. On the upper floor there were to be two fully-equipped operating theatres for animal experimentation. One of the theatres was to be wired to an adjoining X-ray room. A small post-mortem room, a metabolism room and a kymograph room were also planned. Space was to be provided for two research workers, the Professor of Surgery, his first assistant, and a secretary. On the ground floor there was to be space for a laboratory for surgical pathology. There were also to be four rooms for research workers on this floor and a common room and library "where workers might meet in the afternoon and discuss the problems on which they are working." It was also proposed to construct a two-storey animal house "available for the Physiology, Pathology and Bacteriology Departments as well as that of Surgery."[34] Ewing wrote to Pearce shortly after, asking for £15,000 towards this reconstruction.[35]

The ups and downs of the Surgery Department continued for, in the following month, February 1925, Stiles resigned from the Chair of Clinical Surgery, probably on the grounds of health.[36] John Fraser, who had declined the Chair of Systematic Surgery, was appointed. No doubt there was plenty of time free for him for private practice. Quite what happened to the plan to unify surgery in one department and unite the hospital beds is unclear. With regard to support for the physical reconstruction related to surgical research, Pearce took a once bitten, twice shy approach. He told Ewing in March 1925 that "I think you will agree with me that it might be as well to have the University and Infirmary settle the problem of the clinical laboratory before any new projects are seriously considered."[37] Ewing replied that the matter was settled and perhaps Pearce could find a "fitting occasion" to bring the proposal for a surgical laboratory before the Trustees.[38] Cautiously Pearce wrote to Wilkie, with again a regretful note creeping in, that the "co-operation" of the surgical department with the new clinical laboratory "appears to have been abandoned." This suggests Pearce still did not know that animal experiments were not possible in the new clinical lab.

At any rate Pearce procrastinated, suggesting that he had heard major changes to the whole Medical School were in the offing and so the "immediate requirements" of a single department had to be considered in that light. By now Pearce had discovered that the proposed surgical laboratory was to be in the women's anatomy theatre and he professed New World astonishment at the fact that, in Edinburgh, women and men dissected separately. Dissecting together, he wrote, "is common throughout the world." Pearce, ever cautious, said he had difficulty understanding the details of how the estimated sums for the new lab would be utilized and he required more information.[39]

In June 1925 Wilkie duly obliged him. First, Wilkie said, he would have been happy to have worked in the new clinical lab but for the ban on animal experimentation. Second, he envisaged the facilities of the new surgical lab being available to other departments. He agreed with

Pearce that there was no need for women to dissect separately but, like Pearce, felt it was not his "business." Wilkie detailed the sorts of equipment, such as microscopes, his department was lacking. He had had a promise of £1,000 for reconstruction from the brother of his now deceased predecessor, Alexis Thomson. Wilkie felt that the developments in his department and the opportunities offered by the new clinical laboratory meant they could "break down the rigid departmentalism which has, here as elsewhere, done so much to hamper advance in scientific medicine."[40] In August 1925 he was able to send Pearce a more detailed estimate of reconstruction costs. A total of £13,375 was still required for building and equipment but, strangely, work was "well in hand."[41] An internal Rockefeller memo from Pearce in late August records that the surgical "laboratory is essential to success of Surgery and development of activities we have already aided." He suggested between £3,000 and £5,000 worth of aid for equipment, the University to fund the building work.[42] Pearce then wrote to Wilkie seeking further details.[43] Wilkie replied that he hoped the work would be finished by mid-October, but there was still no indication in the correspondence of who was going to pay for it.[44] In November the Rockefeller Trustees approved a grant of £5,000 for equipment for the new laboratory of experimental surgery.[45] The University had obviously agreed to fund the building works.[46] Pearce, as I have frequently noted, liked working with particular individuals and Wilkie was someone he obviously felt had what he called elsewhere the right "attitude."

The reconstruction of the old surgical lecture theatre to provide a smaller theatre, a museum, and practical rooms for teaching bandaging, surgical anatomy, and operative surgery was carried out in much the fashion predicted. The experimental department was also created much as envisaged. The new department was a success, attracting young surgeons from all over the world to do research. By 1928 it consisted of the professor, three assistants, twelve researchers, and twelve technical assistants.[47] It was churning out research papers, many of them on disorders of the gall bladder. In this year Rockefeller was due to terminate its annual support of £750 for staff salaries and research workers. Seeking to acquire capital to continue this annual subsidy the University obtained £5,000 from a "generous donor" and Ewing sought a further £10,000 from Rockefeller.[48] The Foundation did provide this money.[49]

This is hardly surprising. To Rockefeller eyes its involvement in the developments related to surgery must have looked like a relative success. There was a professor who was almost full-time and an active bunch of researchers.

Medicine was a slightly different kettle of fish. There were three departments of medicine in the Faculty: Systematic Medicine (or more simply Medicine), Clinical Medicine, and Therapeutics. As in surgery the term Department of Medicine means different things in different contexts. The Department of Medicine at the RIE embraced all three professors. The Professor of [systematic] Medicine from 1915 was George Lovell Gulland. The chair that he held was the descendant of the Chair of the Practice of Medicine founded at the establishment of the medical school in 1726 and was the most prestigious in the Faculty. Its most famous incumbent was probably the eighteenth-century physician William Cullen. It was not a full-time position and the professor was free to pursue his private practice. As I have noted, before Meakins's appointment in 1919 he was induced by various correspondents to come to Edinburgh by the suggestion he might one day transfer to the Medical Chair. Cushny wrote to him on June 13, 1919 that if the holder of the Chair of Therapeutics "makes good and after a time wants to take up consultation work, he would be the natural choice for the chair of medicine which is allowed [private] practice." Offering further encouragement, he wrote that the Chair "carries the best consultation practice in Scotland."[50] Similarly J. S. Haldane observed that if Meakins wanted "to do ordinary consulting practice" he should transfer to the Chair of Medicine.[51]

Various interests in the 1920s saw Gulland's retirement as a way of reorganizing the medical matters. From early on the RF had its eye on reforming Gulland's Chair as a means of implementing the unit system in Edinburgh. The Therapeutics Department after all was only assisted for political expediency: it was a way of supporting a modern clinical scientist, Meakins. In 1923 Pearce was expecting Gulland to retire in two years,[52] and he was hoping to manoeuvre Meakins into the forthcoming vacancy. Whether two years was a slip of the pen or a misapprehension is not clear, for by December 1923 Pearce knew the period before Gulland's retirement was to be "at least five years."[53] This estimate was still being used in June 1924.[54] Even if Meakins were to leave, the

Foundation's plan at this time was to move his successor from the Chair of Therapeutics to the Chair of Medicine. Rockefeller minutes of 1923 record: "If in five years when the chair of medicine is vacated, the professor of therapeutics is made professor of medicine, a full-time chair and true university clinic will be possible provided the increase of endowment (approximately L15,000) can be secured."[55]

Pearce wanted to transfer the full-time status to the Chair of Medicine, possibly to create a directorship of a wholly new medical department encompassing all three chairs and perhaps the department in the RIE, but certainly to make the old Systematic Medicine Department very high profile.[56] Thus the most prestigious chair would increasingly approximate to the American ideal. What would then happen to the Chair of Therapeutics was of marginal interest. Things however did not go to plan. In fact the five years to Gulland's departure talked about in 1924 was an overestimate. It was known in 1926 that Gulland was to retire in the autumn of the following year. Meakins (now in Montreal) had been in Edinburgh in the summer of that year. Two things seem to have happened. First, Meakins was asked by Ewing about how to reorganize the Medical Faculty and second, he was invited to put himself forward for nomination to the soon-to-be vacant Medical Chair. The invitation came from Sir Norman Walker, who in July 1926, in a letter written on the train between York and Newcastle-upon-Tyne, noted: "I have been thinking, at intervals, of the succession to Gulland's Chair and am convinced that the best, far the best, solution is for you to fill it." He observed that "All sensible persons are agreed that we must go outside of Edinburgh." Edinburgh was still "the potentially greatest medical school" and if Meakins could help "materially to restore it to that position, he "would be rendering a great service to the world." "All our sensible people," Walker said, are beginning to recognize that "we must be up and doing" and that "we need fresh blood."[57] Meakins, no doubt, agreed. Walker's message was polite but clear: there were reactionary forces at the University and Infirmary, composed of people not sensible enough to realize the Edinburgh tradition of inbreeding necessitated fresh blood. He confirmed most of these sentiments explicitly in December 1926 when he again wrote to Meakins and reminded him that the Electors to the Chair constituted a body, the Curators, which consisted of three representatives of the University Court and four of the Corporation of the

City. For chairs under patronage of the Curators, he observed, "local candidates are 'favourite sons'." He thought "the only local man who would get much medical support is Edwin Bramwell" (the Professor of Clinical Medicine) and it was possible he would accept the position. He reported that Wilkie had "gathered that the Rockefeller people, being much interested in Edinburgh, would be willing to do something for medicine." Once again he urged Meakins to apply for Gulland's Chair or (if Bramwell moved sideways) the Chair of Clinical Medicine. He felt, whatever Bramwell did, "we have no quite suitable man for the third chair" and, he added, stressing Edinburgh's insularity, "the bringing in of a complete stranger might not be appreciated locally." But, he went on, "you are not a stranger." He had no doubt that "in a team composed of Bramwell, yourself and Murray Lyon there is very little doubt who would be the Director."[58] The words "team" and "director" here seem to be significant acknowledgements of American thinking. There had never, in Edinburgh, been anyone called a director in the medical departments.

Gulland's incumbency of the chair, as recollected by Sir Stanley Davidson, embodied those Edinburgh traditions that the RF and others were eager to dismantle. Davidson described Gulland as "one of the most brilliant clinicians of his time." This along with "his natural shrewdness and sound clinical judgement" had led to his becoming "the leading medical consultant in Scotland." He had a large number of private patients and was "Medical Officer to one of the largest insurance companies in Great Britain." He was "frequently absent from Edinburgh for one, two or more days a week." This, said Davidson, in the thinking of the time, perfectly fitted him for his academic post. In those days "the main claim for appointment to a Chair of Medicine was the success which the applicant had achieved in the field of consultant practice." If it now appeared that Gulland had "sacrificed his academic life on the altar of private practice," wrote Davidson, this was because "it was believed at that time that the interests of the University could best be advanced by the Professor achieving the reputation of being the leading consultant in his area."[59] If a professor's reputation in private practice advanced the "interests of the University" it also enhanced the standing of the Infirmary. This was part of the thinking behind the restrictions placed on the surgery chair. Gulland defended other traditional features of an Edinburgh medical education. He advocated systematic lecturing, a didactic model criticized by Americans.[60]

It was not until March 1927 that Meakins wrote to Ewing and Walker about the Chair of Medicine and the organization of the Faculty. His letter to Ewing was brief, but he said that his letter to Walker contained his observations and that Ewing was free to see them but otherwise that letter was confidential for he had "spoken rather freely and at times perhaps roughly about certain men and affairs." He did say to Ewing that Edinburgh had "great opportunity," but only if "she sets her house in order to carry out a true University's function in the Medical School." He thought, "Edinburgh can still wield her premier place." However, he added the proviso that "this can only be done by having a Clinical Staff who really love the University as well as themselves and equally with their own pocket-books."[61] In his letter to Walker, Meakins observed: "When I saw you last summer my mind seemed completely made up in the negative," but he had had second thoughts "on account of the great honour for which you were asking me to allow my name to be considered." Meakins's criticisms of the medical departments and the organization of Infirmary teaching in this letter have been dealt with in the previous chapter.[62] His basic recommendations to Walker were that there should be "one large co-ordinated department of Medicine," that more assistants be appointed, that the professorships carry an obligation of serious University work, and that one professor control and administer the whole department.[63]

On June 9, 1927, Ewing wrote to Pearce that Gulland would retire on September 30 of that year. The Electors had already met when Ewing wrote, and he reported that he had impressed on them that the vacancy was an opportunity for bringing to the Medical School "some much-needed fresh blood." He had told them, were the Chair to be made "substantially" whole time he had reason to believe Rockefeller might provide "substantial assistance." At any rate the Electors were broadly in favour. Some of them, however, "expressed a rather strong opinion that in the special circumstances of the Edinburgh School a rigorous interpretation of the whole-time condition was to be deprecated, and that it would be better to allow the Professor some narrowly limited facilities for practice rather than forbid it altogether."[64] Ewing's preference (presumably on advice) was to encourage Francis Fraser from St. Bartholomew's Hospital to apply for the post. Fraser was Professor of Medicine and Director of the Medical Unit. He was a staunch supporter of academic medicine and a distinguished medical scientist.

David Wilkie, now Professor of Systematic Surgery, also wrote to Pearce on the same day as Ewing and on the same matter. He began by trying to jog or perhaps manipulate Pearce's memory: "You will probably recollect a very interesting and important conversation which I had with you and Dr. Vincent in New York last September, in regard to the future of internal Medicine in Edinburgh." He continued:

> I was much impressed by the views of Dr. Vincent and yourself that we had ideal conditions in Edinburgh for establishing a real Department and School of Medicine, and the generous offer which you made of financial support, if the authorities here would agree, when the Chair of Medicine fell vacant, to appoint on a whole-time basis a Professor who would be essentially a Director of a Department of Medicine with adequate assistance for organised teaching and research.

Unfortunately there is no other record of this meeting. Wilkie also expressed confidence that Fraser would be an excellent appointment and noted he would need a salary "at least equal to that which he at present has, and to provide him with several whole and part time assistants."[65]

The following day Lorrain Smith also wrote to Pearce. Smith had similar certainty about Pearce's view of these matters, and indicated that for "an effective department" that would "put the student in touch with modern medicine" various facilities would be required. This would involve physical reconstruction of the Department of Medicine. He also observed that the "facilities for research require to be greatly extended." Clearly he was hinting at funding that he obviously thought Rockefeller had as good as promised: "I need not at present enter into details, and I am sure any remarks I have made are only refreshing your memory of impressions formed when you visited us before."[66]

Ewing, Wilkie and Smith were in for a shock. Pearce wrote to Ewing that he remembered discussing the chair of medicine with Wilkie, "but beyond stating that I considered it very desirable that the chair should be put on the basis of a real university clinic, I am quite sure I said nothing that would commit the Rockefeller Foundation to 'substantial assistance'." The RF did not make such statements in advance of an official proposal he said. Anyhow he doubted the Trustees would consider the plan favourably. By now Pearce had jettisoned the idea of transferring the incumbent of the Chair of Therapeutics to the Chair of Medicine. First, for personal reasons: he was dissatisfied with Murray Lyon. Second, he was not keen on two full-time chairs (the Chair of Therapeutics would remain full time if Lyon moved). Pearce's lukewarm response to Ewing was hidden behind statements of policy. Until Murray Lyon's department was shown to be a success, he wrote, he doubted the Trustees would consider further aid. In fact, he added, "there may be some natural doubt as to whether more than one chair in medicine should be on this basis." He also expressed concern as to whether the relations between the Infirmary and the Medical School would "guarantee definitely the greatest possible success of true university chairs." "Much must be done," he wrote, "to educate the Infirmary authorities in regard to their duties and responsibilities to proper teaching."[67]

Wilkie received a similar cold douche. Pearce did not think under "the conditions as now exist," the Board "would be likely to consider favorably a proposal of aid." He was sorry if anything that was said the previous autumn was "capable of misconstruction." Pearce seemed to be hinting that he wanted the Chair of Medicine to have wide, autocratic powers perhaps including control of the new laboratory which, at this point, was nearing completion: "We could not consider your problem until the Infirmary and the University have worked out a method of clinical teaching on a true university basis." In such a system, he said, "the department or chair of medicine . . . has control over the hospital service, including appointment to staff, joint budget, etc., analogous to the best type of university clinic in this country and in Germany with a system of interns and residents so that there might be a definite succession in service."[68]

Francis Fraser, whom Edinburgh hoped to net for the Chair, was part of the charmed circle of elite clinical scientists and in August 1927 Pearce wrote to him. "Dear Fraser," he began in the familiar fashion. Pearce wanted to know what "the gossip" was about Gulland's Chair. He understood Fraser had "been mixed up in it." Pearce reported that Edinburgh "made some propositions to us some months ago, but in view of their indefinite character we did not get enthusiastic. I am curious to know what has happened."[69] Fraser replied in September 1927 ("Dear Pearce") to the effect that things were in turmoil and that Gulland had been invited to stay on for another year. He added that Wilkie had said "the point on which they [the Electors] disagreed with you [Pearce] was on the scope of the new Chair and the responsibilities of the new Professor." Fraser reported that Norman Walker and Wilkie had approached him over the Chair but no detailed proposal was made. "I would not dream of moving from here except to a Chair that offered me greater scope and responsibilities than I now have."[70]

Pearce wrote to Wilkie in late September indicating the source of his dissatisfaction: "The real problem it seems to me, aside from hospital relations, is to decide upon the organisation and inter-relation of the three clinical chairs (considering Therapeutics as one of three clinical chairs). The present attempt to consider Therapeutics as a full time clinical chair may be an embarrassment in planning full time for one of the two chairs of Medicine."[71] In other words, in America or Germany one professor filled a single chair and ran a whole department of medicine. Rockefeller was lumbered with a full-time chair of therapeutics until the subvention to Lyon's salary finished. On his appointment the RF had agreed to supplement Lyon's salary by £1,000 per annum for five years.[72] He was completely debarred from private practice.

Pearce wrote in similarly exasperated tones to Fraser, "It is true that they approached us concerning support for a full-time chair, but as they had absolutely no plan of development, no policy, and as a matter of fact their request was merely a request for funds, we could not do anything but decline to consider the request." "It seems to me," he went on, "they do not understand their own problem and are not prepared to take steps to bring about a solution of the problem which exists." Pearce considered that "they should review the situation in regard to their three chairs devoted to clinical medicine, counting therapeutics as one of these chairs and see if they cannot bring about a readjustment."[73]

Pearce, of course, was an astute politician and as Meakins had been in Edinburgh that summer, Pearce wrote to him wanting to have his "story about it." Pearce declared: "As you may know, we received a request to help them put it [the Systematic Chair] on a full-time basis, but as their request was so indefinite as to the conditions of establishing the chair, we declined to act."[74] Meakins replied that when he was in Edinburgh "things were in rather a muddle." He gathered that "practically every Physician and Assistant Physician on the Staff of the Royal Infirmary is struggling to acquire the position." He could understand this since "it carries with it about £1250 a year, an enormous prestige and comparatively little extra work." Meakins's diagnosis of Edinburgh's problems was no doubt one with which Pearce would have concurred. Meakins thought that "Their great difficulty at the present time is their pathetic poverty of local talent." He attributed this "to the fact that there are sixteen men on the Royal Infirmary Staff in Medicine practically all of whom are striving to be consultants. Edinburgh cannot support such an army." Thus "the struggle for existence is so keen that they have time for nothing else and the University suffers."[75]

In October 1927 Wilkie wrote to Pearce with a suggestion Pearce might have been waiting for all along. "In regard to the Chair of Medicine, I think that the opinion here is gradually veering round to the appointment of some one from outside Edinburgh on a whole-time or a modified whole-time basis. Would you be so kind as to let me know how you would favour a proposal to transfer the whole-time status from the Chair of Therapeutics to that of Medicine?" Wilkie acknowledged "This is purely a personal suggestion on my part," and admitted, "I have not even mentioned the matter as yet to Murray Lyon." Perhaps, however, he knew Murray Lyon would happily relinquish his full-time status in order to get into private practice (which is what he eventually did). Wilkie anticipated that this solution "might solve some of our difficulties and lead to a more intimate co-ordination of the three University Chairs in connection with the teaching of Medicine."[76] Pearce did not quite say it outright but it was obviously the sort of resolution he was looking for. He replied, at first cautiously: "Your queries concerning the chair of Medicine at Edinburgh place me in a rather difficult position, as it has always been a policy of the Rockefeller Foundation, after making a gift to an institution, to avoid anything that might appear as interference in the local problem, or, indeed, that might appear like giving advice." Pearce, however, gradually warmed to what, after all, was almost certainly one of his preferred solutions. "If, after proper consideration," he wrote rather casually, "you should decide that the best interests of medicine at Edinburgh are served by transferring the whole-time status from the Chair of Therapeutics to that of medicine, there would be and could be, no criticism on our part, and we should feel that you had solved your problem in what seemed to you the best possible way." He threw out the broadest of hints that that was what he wanted: "Personally, I believe that you are now in a position to consider the problem of these three chairs from the point of view of the best interests of teaching and research in medicine at Edinburgh on a university basis." As ever with Pearce the dead hand of Edinburgh "traditions" was invoked: "future development should be stressed rather than present conditions or past commitments and traditions. I think you are on the right track." He iterated this opinion at the end of the letter: "I believe personally, that if you approach this problem as you indicate you anticipate approaching it, you will probably reach the proper solution and one which should redound to the great benefit of teaching and research in medicine at Edinburgh."[77]

But Wilkie by no means had the power to bring these things about and Pearce remained despondent. In mid-November 1927 he wrote to Fletcher that the Edinburgh situation was "so difficult" that it seemed to him "unwise to intervene directly in any way." The thing he found "the most distressing" was "the attitude of the hospital." He went on: "It does seem that now with the opportunity to appoint a real professor of medicine on a university basis they should reconsider the situation in regard to the two chairs of medicine and therapeutics, scrap all preconceptions and decide how these three departments may be reorganized so that there may be at least one man with a true university chair of medicine." He continued, intimating once again that there was no reason why the lab should be tied to the therapeutics chair or indeed that the therapeutics chair should be the full-time one: "I hope there is no thought that our aid for the chair of therapeutics and the gift of a laboratory in any way interfere with the proper reorganization of medicine at Edinburgh." Again the burden of the past kept Edinburgh from the future: "The problem is theirs and they should decide it without regard to the past, though in Edinburgh with all its traditions this is difficult."[78]

In February 1928 Pearce, still almost without hope, noted in his diary: "Situation in medicine in Edinburgh difficult. Murray Lyon's work is going well, but he is a local man and he has not great influence."[79] The word "local" in Rockefeller dialect almost always connoted not first rate. On the same day Alan Gregg in London observed in his diary: "Murray Lyon has, it is true, been handicapped, but is not [*sic*] great success as yet."[80] Of the Chair, Pearce recorded: "The vacant chair of medicine was not offered to Fraser, but it was discussed with Fraser and he said he would consider nothing but a full-time chair." He noted another development: "Since then it has been offered to Hugh MacLean of St. Thomas's, [*sic*] who has not yet made his decision. If MacLean declines, Wilkie says there is not other solution except the appointment of a local man." Pearce faced reality: "He [Wilkie] agrees that it would be ideal to bring the three chairs under one head, but this is impossible at present."[81] MacLean, obviously, declined the appointment, and some speculated that this was the result of local sabotage.

Wilkie's forecast was borne out. A "local man," William Ritchie aged 54, was appointed to the Chair in February 1928. Born in 1873 and an Edinburgh graduate, he was a physician to the Infirmary and had practised for nearly the whole of his professional life in Edinburgh. Ritchie was not quite what Rockefeller had hoped for but he did have a distinguished record as a clinician endeavouring to apply the laboratory sciences to the bedside. In the second decade of the century he was at the forefront of the new cardiology. Ritchie distinguished himself by being one of the first investigators to describe auricular flutter. As noted in Chapter 5, however, he revealed in his inaugural address a keen commitment to tradition and clinical individualism.

In April 1928 Alan Gregg recorded in his diary that the RF still hoped to unify medicine in Edinburgh: "We can do nothing for Ritchie at present but if he can bring together the Department of Medicine, the Department of Clinical Medicine, the chair of Therapeutics, in a compact organization we might consider something a year or two from now when a decision must be made in regard to Murray Lyon's appropriation." Gregg was in Edinburgh and Ritchie had gone to him and made a proposal that the RF aid his Chair "by remodeling present laboratory space and small lecture hall." Ritchie was not referring to the hospital but to the Department of Medicine in the medical school, which obviously had its own lab. Gregg continued: "Ritchie wants to do experimental work on animals and tells me of [the] rather surprising fact that in Murray Lyon's laboratory no animal experimentation may be done since there would be opposition from the Royal Infirmary to securing a license for animal experiments on the premises. I told Ritchie that I did not know of this restriction." Gregg and Ritchie lunched "and had a long talk about conditions in Edinburgh." Gregg said that the present co-operation of Rockefeller with Wilkie and Murray Lyon was drawing to a close and that "the question of attitude of Edinburgh Faculty towards capitalization or some form of continuance would naturally be uppermost in our minds."

In other words, were Edinburgh to support full-time chairs the RF would look to help in some way. The downside for Ritchie was that Gregg "thought it was very doubtful whether another type of aid would be considered, especially on the scale indicated by Ritchie (L4,000 a year)." The RF was not about to get tangled up in a new scheme with a "local man" appointed to a part-time chair.

Gregg said he felt a responsibility to explain his "attitude towards broader aspects of the clinical organisation in Edinburgh." He began by saying he "was not at all sure that with the development of the experimental method in clinical medicine a type of Faculty organisation which had very well served the needs of the past was adequately satisfactory." Singing the Rockefeller refrain he went on: "A single Department of Medicine on a University basis with a coordination of the present separate and independent teaching services in the Infirmary would be preferable." He "asked Ritchie what his attitude towards the maintenance of the present system was." Ritchie replied that it was his belief that the present system was the best one. Although the interview was "friendly" it was possibly with a groan that Gregg recorded: "Ritchie is 54 years old, and consequently has nine years as a Professor of Medicine. I was not impressed by his grasp of the situation nor his comprehension of possible advances in teaching and clinical medicine." Ritchie, of course, had his own grasp of the situation and it was perhaps Gregg with his monocular view of medical education and change who could not fully fathom the Scottish mind. Nor did Gregg think much of Ritchie's grasp of what experimental medicine was. Ritchie, Gregg reported, was "enthusiastic about Wilkie's work, but thinks this is entirely the result of Wilkie's personality, and that the conditions of Wilkie's work have very little to do with it." In other words where the RF saw proper training in experimental medicine and the right departmental organization as central to medical progress Ritchie saw personal factors as crucial (as of course he did in ordinary clinical practice). Gregg, although he reported Ritchie "Eager to get some experimental work started," thought him "rather cloudy about it even so."[82]

Gregg was not the only one to groan. Fletcher wrote to Pearce in May 1928: "I am afraid you must be greatly disappointed, as I am, with the lack of vision being shown at Edinburgh."[83] Pearce was. He replied: "Of course I am disappointed with Edinburgh. They asked us last April to support a full-time chair, but I replied that they would have to work out many problems before we could consider that. I then hoped they might get Fraser or MacLean, after which we could come in to assist in development."To Pearce the future looked bleak: "What can be done now I do not see." "The real problem before us," he went on, "will be that of Murray Lyon a couple of years from now. Frankly I do not see how we can capitalize our present aid to his department." He added, in the by now customary fashion: "If Edinburgh would develop a unified department of medicine including the chairs of medicine, clinical medicine and therapeutics, and improve its relations to the Infirmary, it is possible we might do something. This of course is confidential for your ear only in case you have some opportunity to influence the trend of effort."[84] Quite why it was confidential is hard to figure: Edinburgh had been told it enough times.

Although Ritchie was far from being Rockefeller's choice he was by no means inactive as a professor. His most productive research days may have been behind him but he threw himself energetically into reform of the teaching. He is principally remembered for organizing co-ordinated lecture courses in pathology, bacteriology, medicine, surgery, materia medica, and therapeutics. By this method the student would be introduced to the same subject from different perspectives at the same time of the year. This innovation was made shortly after his arrival.

The medical folk in Edinburgh knew there was only one way to enlist RF support for the Department of Medicine and down that road they did not wish to go. They turned then to other possible sources of funding and other means for modernizing the school—the Lister scheme, in Pearce's words, being "perfectly dead."[85] On July 19, 1928, Stanley Davidson wrote to Fletcher. Davidson was an assistant physician at the RIE and lecturer in medicine. He had graduated at Edinburgh with first class honours in 1919. He had previously been at Trinity College, Cambridge when Fletcher was a tutor. They were now friends. He was an extremely promising clinical scientist who left Edinburgh for a professorship in Aberdeen in 1930, but returned in 1938 to the Edinburgh Chair of Medicine, where he had a most distinguished career. Davidson reported to Fletcher that, when in London recently, he had discussed with his friend Sir Robert Horne "the question of raising funds for medical research in Edinburgh.""In my opinion," he went on, "the reason why the medical side has lagged behind the surgical, both in this and in other Universities, is an economic one. Unless a person has private means it is quite impossible to do research work in medicine, as the number of research posts in this University is almost negligible. In consequence we lose much valuable talent every year." He reported on Ritchie's teaching reforms adding that Ritchie "is very anxious that a department of experimental medicine should be started in Edinburgh. This is essential because, as I told you in London, experimental work on animals cannot be performed in the new clinical laboratory in the Royal Infirmary." In optimistic vein, he noted, "there is a light beginning to shine at present in Edinburgh, and everyone is dissatisfied with the present state of affairs." "Now," he considered, "is the time to strike if we are to bring back the Edinburgh school to its former brilliance."

Davidson then got down to the point, which concerned the estate of William Dunn. This, at over a million pounds, had been left to charity and was administered by trustees. Initially the money was used in small amounts to help the needy. In 1918, however, the trustees changed direction and began to fund medical research. Fletcher was the man they turned to for advice. Davidson reported that the Dunn trustees "state they still have a sum of £40,000 which can be given for research purposes." Telling Fletcher something he already knew, Davidson went on: "Moreover, they have asked you to submit to them a plan for its use. They state that your scheme has not yet been submitted." Calling on Fletcher as friend as well as MRC Secretary, he endeavoured to enlist his aid to divert some of this money north. He told Fletcher that the trustees had asked for "a statement of the present position in Edinburgh and the necessities of the situation." Davidson had probably engineered this through Sir Robert Horne. He had told Ritchie about the trustees' request and Ritchie was "drafting a statement [about Edinburgh's requirements] which will be forwarded both to you and to them [the trustees]." Davidson then frankly admitted to Fletcher: "If I could persuade you to espouse the cause of Edinburgh I feel sure that an appreciable portion of the funds would be allotted to us."

Ritchie, Davidson reported, was asking the Dunn trustees for the endowment of four Fellowships, each of £250 a year, for research in experimental medicine. The holders of these Fellowships, Davidson said, "would be entitled to work in the clinical laboratory of the Royal Infirmary, in

Professor Ritchie's own department of medicine or in any other University department as may be considered necessary for the research in view." In addition Ritchie wanted £5,000 for reconstructing his department within the University buildings. Reconstruction, Davidson explained, meant "the adaptation of the present premises into suitable laboratories for experimental research. The premises and equipment of the department have undergone virtually no change within the past thirty years." Fletcher would receive a copy of Ritchie's letter at the end of the week.[86]

Ritchie's letter to the Secretary of the Dunn trustees began with an historically-framed description of the Edinburgh School, the Royal Colleges, and the Infirmary, stressing the School's size and its "pre-eminent position as a centre of medical learning" since the eighteenth century. Ritchie explained how there was an urgent need for the funding of experimental research in clinical medicine since it was virtually impossible without a private income. He wanted £20,000 to endow fellowships and £10,000 for reconstructing the medical department.[87] Fletcher had by this time reported on two proposals to the trustees and Sir Jeremiah Colman, a Dunn trustee, now asked him to consider Ritchie's in addition.[88] Fletcher was, of course, apprised of Ritchie's proposal and was now where he liked to be: pulling the strings that disbursed medical research money. Fletcher replied to Colman on July 27, 1928, that he had seen the proposal and indeed had had a long talk with Ritchie, who happened to be in London, that very morning.[89]

Pressure on the trustees on Edinburgh's behalf came right from the top. In September 1928, Lord Balfour, Chancellor of the University, wrote to Colman, pleading the Medical School's case.[90] Colman replied that the business was effectively in the hands of Fletcher.[91] Balfour then corresponded with Fletcher who told him, "I hope to visit Edinburgh next week in order to look into the proposals."[92] It is hard to imagine Fletcher and Balfour had not been in informal contact prior to this. Anyhow, Fletcher did visit Edinburgh and a little later wrote a letter to Ritchie that cannot have pleased him. Fletcher began: "I find myself in great difficulty when I am asked to express an opinion upon the financial scheme you proposed to the Dunn Trustees. At the same time I am most keenly desirous of doing anything I can to help the progress of the Edinburgh Medical School and of doing nothing that will impede it." Then came the warning of problems ahead: "I will tell you frankly, if

I may, the difficulties I feel about your scheme in its present shape, and I shall be grateful if you will tell me just as frankly what you think of my points." The first lay difficulty lay with the £10,000 requested for "re-modelling and equipping the set of rooms with lecture theatre that you occupy in the University buildings as professor of medicine." It was "obvious that those rooms should be modified and equipped as you suggest for the immediate purposes of your teaching by demonstration and otherwise, as well as for your own accommodation as professor and that of your immediate assistants." But Fletcher thought it was "the obvious duty of the University, who presumably have some sinking fund for necessary repairs and the reconditioning of existing buildings, and have as well an important grant from the Government through the U.G.C. [University Grants Committee] for the efficiency of medical teaching." There was a second difficulty with the plan. Ritchie had suggested "that the proposed alterations should be not only for the conduct of ordinary teaching which the University has already undertaken, but in order to gain some new laboratories for experimental research." Fletcher reminded him, "I think you agreed with me when we discussed it, that research workers under you, if they were really to get new knowledge, would have to carry their investigations either along biochemical lines, or pharmacological, or bacteriological, or physiological, and that the proper place for their work would be one or other of the well-equipped laboratories in those subjects that stand all about you a few yards away." There were problems of space but, said Fletcher, reminding Ritchie, this "ought surely to be met, as I think we agreed, by improving the accommodation in the existing special laboratories." Fletcher obviously did not think Ritchie equipped to supervise research along biochemical, pharmacological, bacteriological, or physiological lines. Fletcher had further objections to new labs in the Department of Medicine:

> If, on the other hand, research workers under you had to work in immediate relation to patients, they would have to work not at a distance in your rooms but within the Royal Infirmary itself. After leaving you on Thursday, I went all over the newly completed laboratories equipped by the Rockefeller Foundation in the Infirmary. These are most beautifully built and equipped and give ample room, on my calculation, for 37 separate workers at least. At present there are barely ten workers there.

Fletcher understood that Murray Lyon had the lab under his administrative supervision but he also understood any Infirmary physician had the right to work there. Ritchie therefore had "complete claim on any laboratory rooms or other accommodation in that building." Fletcher added, with a hint of condescension, "Perhaps I am wrong, and if so, you will tell me." He knew he was right and said: "Do you think that Edinburgh is justified in asking for money to equip new laboratories for clinical research when they have just received a beautifully-equipped building, able to accommodate at least three times as many workers as those now using it?" Fletcher wanted the Dunn money for the basic sciences.

Fletcher also noted there was a third professor of medicine, Edwin Bramwell, and that he might desire to have research workers under his guidance. "Where will he seek accommodation?" Fletcher asked. The answer seemed obvious. It would be, he replied to his own question, "either in the new clinical laboratories within the Infirmary, or within one of the University scientific departments immediately adjoining it." Fletcher then drew what was, for him, the obvious conclusion. What should be implemented was the American model of large-scale organization under a single professor: "It would seem to be undesirable from every reason of economy and efficiency to contemplate separated research laboratories for three different groups of workers under three different professors of medicine within one Medical School." Such an organization would only be a further obstacle to the sort of department he and Pearce envisaged in Edinburgh. He said nothing about Ritchie's plans for the endowment of research fellowships.[93]

On the same day Fletcher intimated his concern to Ewing. He began: "I spent some time last week at Edinburgh seeing Professor Ritchie, who was good enough to show me his present rooms, and in discussing the project generally with him and several of his colleagues. I also had the pleasure of seeing the excellent new laboratories at last completed in the Royal Infirmary under the Rockefeller benefaction." He assured Ewing he was anxious to do anything he could to encourage medical science at Edinburgh and "avoid anything that could possibly impede it." Clearly he felt Ritchie's plans were in this latter category for he went on: "I cannot help thinking, however, that the proposals now made are perhaps not along the best line of advance." He hoped to discuss the matter with Ewing later (probably at the Athenaeum, possibly at Brooks's or the United University Club). With Ewing on his side Ritchie's plans would be as dead as the Lister scheme.[94]

At this point another player entered the correspondence: T. J. Mackie the Professor of Bacteriology, whose militant views on the power of laboratory science and the comparative impotence of bedside medicine have been described. Mackie was a confidante of Fletcher, who addressed him "Dear Mackie" (Murray Lyon, in contrast, was always written to as "Dear Professor Murray Lyon"). On October 17, 1928, Fletcher wrote to Mackie about Edinburgh's problems in a manner suggesting a great deal of previous intercourse had taken place. Fletcher observed: "At present there seems to be no common agreed policy. It is easy to see how great the difficulties are, chiefly personal."The "personal" probably referred disparagingly to Ritchie and Murray Lyon. Promising nothing, Fletcher threw out the broadest of hints: "You spoke of your own shortage of rooms for research workers in bacteriology. Have you ever thought out a plan of reconstruction and its probable cost?"[95]

Ritchie in the mean time, having received Fletcher's cool response to his remodelling proposal, responded cautiously. He wrote to Fletcher that he was "glad to have your letter giving me so frank an expression of opinion regarding my appeal to the Dunn Trustees." Ritchie obviously considered that without Fletcher's support, diluting the laboratory idea was the best course of action and he observed: "The remodelling and equipping of my premises in the University Buildings is an object of secondary consideration." He still had hopes for the other part of his scheme and he observed that "the most urgent need in our medical school at present is undoubtedly the endowment of Research Fellowships in Medicine, this is the prime object of my appeal." Optimistically, he added: "I observe that you do not comment on this part of the scheme, and am therefore led to hope that it has your cordial approval and support." Not prepared to relinquish anything monetarily he ended by hoping Fletcher could feel he could "support the major part of my scheme" and that Fletcher might "be able to recommend to the Dunn Trustees that the whole of the benefaction of £30,000 for which I am appealing may be applied to the foundation of Research Fellowships in Medicine."[96] Fletcher never did comment on the fellowship scheme but it is hard to imagine him supporting research fellowships in medicine that were not under MRC control. Anyway other developments stifled this proposal.

On the same day as Ritchie wrote, Mackie also wrote to Fletcher. The letter was marked *"Private and confidential."* In it Mackie lamented that the "problem of getting the school into fighting trim for research is a most difficult one." He recounted the projected Lister Institute history, noting "You will remember the authorities of the Rockefeller Foundation refused to give any financial support to this scheme. This hypothetical institute has really hampered progress." Like Pearce, and presumably Fletcher, he clearly took the view that research was University business, observing: "The College of Physicians' Laboratory, I think, has no real life now as a research department and has no place in the scheme of things in Edinburgh except for routine examination. It represents, however, very strong vested interests!" He outlined his own University accommodation to Fletcher. Noting that there were fifteen people working in his department, it was, he said, "a tight fit." It had been suggested to him that he should "utilise some of the space in the new Clinical Laboratory in the Infirmary." This, he said, "is of little use to me because it is exceedingly difficult to divide one's attention between two separate buildings and in any case practically all my work involves animal experimentation." His main endeavour was to "push on experimental work in the University." Hinting perhaps at what he saw as Lorrain Smith's inertia, he observed, "I might say that the University Pathology Department would also require additional accommodation if it were working at full pressure," however, "probably for a few years to come there will be no urgent demand." Something had to be done "if our school is to justify its position." The Medical School was a "big pile of building," too much of which consisted of lecture theatres and a museum "which nobody ever looks at." Mackie had "thought of approaching the Rockefeller Foundation but was discouraged on hearing that they had been extremely dissatisfied with our present activities (or perhaps lack of activities.)"[97]

On October 23, 1928, Barger wrote to Fletcher that "Clark [Cushny's successor], Mackie, Wilkie and I met today in my laboratory and talked for 2 hours on 'reform'." "We have," he said, "banded ourselves together to see what we can get done." These four effectively took over all plans for modernization and Ritchie dropped out of all further correspondence with Fletcher. These were the four professors whom Fletcher obviously regarded as the force of modernization in Edinburgh. Barger told Fletcher that their main concern was to "persuade you [Fletcher]" to advise the Dunn trustees to give money for the reconstruction of the medical buildings and not for fellowships. They wanted to pool the resources of departments, utilize wasted space, and take down the large anatomy museum, "hitherto sacrosanct to the memory of the late principal Turner." Barger proposed that he and Mackie meet Fletcher in London on November 3, 1928. Barger hoped that if Fletcher approved of the scheme in a general way he could persuade Ewing to get the University Court to appoint a committee to make plans. The medical members of the Court, Barger said, were not "laboratory people," but he hoped they could get the Dean (Lorrain Smith) to serve. He thought they could persuade him to agree. This was quite likely: Smith's pet Lister scheme was dead and any reconstruction of the medical buildings was bound to benefit his Pathology Department. The anatomy museum was the biggest problem and the greatest need, besides space, was for a new library. The chief beneficiaries of more space, Barger said, would be Ritchie and Mackie. "We can't," he added, "tackle Schafer's laboratory nor his library as yet." Schafer ruled his own empire and collaborated little or not at all. Barger's last sentence was pessimistic. The plan, he wrote, "does not solve the fundamental problem of the school and infirmary which at present seems insoluble."[98] Fletcher must have replied to this but no copy of his letter seems to exist. At any rate he appears to have been sympathetic.

Shortly after this Mackie reported to Fletcher that Barger had "unfortunately met with an accident in the lift in his department" and it was doubtful he could make the London meeting.[99] He was in the Infirmary under Wilkie's care. Mackie still hoped to meet Fletcher prior to the latter's meeting with Ewing at the Athenaeum which, as outlined above, had been organized by Fletcher to scotch Ritchie's plans. Mackie clearly knew of the meeting and possibly its purpose. Mackie and Fletcher agreed to meet on Sunday morning November 4 at the Athenaeum, two days before Fletcher's meeting with Ewing. Mackie was to hand Fletcher plans for a proposed reconstruction of the Medical School.

On October 31, 1928, Barger wrote from his sick bed to Fletcher. Barger had had "a few casual words with Ewing who did not seem to think you were prepared to do anything, but I told him that I thought if the University put forward the right plan, you would be favourably impressed." Barger told Fletcher that "Mackie, Wilkie, Clark and myself have prepared a list of spaces which by reconstruction could be utilised and we are particularly keen on securing a part of the large anatomical museum." Adverting to what the modernizers saw as the old Edinburgh problem, he went on: "I think this might be made a test case. If the University is not prepared to overcome the resistance of the tradition of past generations for modern scientific needs, I for one am no longer interested in the scheme." Barger had been unable to tell Ewing much about the plans and he cautioned Fletcher that he should not appear to have more information than Ewing, for that would "put him off." Barger had only spoken to Ewing about reconstruction in "quite general terms" so he warned Fletcher "please go carefully." Ritchie had obviously been told something (perhaps not much) of the plans because Barger went on: "There is no harm in his [Ewing] knowing that Mackie, Wilkie, Clark and also Ritchie and the new Professor of Medical Jurisprudence, Sydney Smith, who is very keen on a medical library, are all of the same opinion but it would be a mistake for the principal to think that the four of us had a definite committee." The reference to the "four of us" (Barger, Mackie, Wilkie, Clark) indicated where reform was coming from—notably only Wilkie was a clinical teacher. Whether Ritchie had been told of their opposition to fellowships seems doubtful. Further, the Lister scheme may have been dead but perhaps it was not buried, for Barger continued: "We have said little to Smith about it." Barger further alerted Fletcher to Ewing's lack of knowledge of what was going on: "Ewing is so far ignorant of medical affairs that he thought the requirements of Bacteriology had now been completely met. I told him that that was very far from being the case." Barger repeated his warning: "So please do not put him off by showing too much inside information of our affairs. If you can get him to consent to a general scheme of domestic reconstruction, that would be very good and later you could see for yourself what might be done."[100]

In the midst of all this politicking Fletcher wrote to the Sir Jeremiah Colman explaining why he had not reported on the proposal that Ritchie had sent the Dunn trustees. After his visit to Edinburgh, Fletcher told Colman, "it became apparent, as indeed I had expected, that the situation was by no means a simple one and that there was by no means unanimity among the professors and others chiefly concerned at Edinburgh as to the advisability of adopting the specific proposals made by Professor Ritchie as against other ways of helping the School at Edinburgh."[101]

Mackie met Fletcher at the Athenaeum on November 4 and duly handed him some outline plans. The project involved making more space for basic science laboratories but what is interesting is that Ritchie had not abandoned his original scheme. The plans for the Medicine Department handed over by Mackie state: "The Professor proposes reconstruction and the creation of laboratories for research by converting the whole of the lecture theatre along with some other alterations in existing rooms."[102] Perhaps Ritchie had not told the gang of four of Fletcher's opposition to the idea of a lab for himself.

Fletcher and Ewing postponed their meeting of Tuesday of that week until the Thursday, 8 November. Fletcher recorded that they only had twenty-five minutes but, "I gave him all my views very frankly and some points startled him." First, "I advised him to get the younger professors together (Wilkie, Mackie, Barger, Clark, possibly with Ritchie) as soon as possible, the men who have the future in their hands, to draw up a practicable scheme." Second (the Lister scheme rearing its head again), "I said it was his job to get over the diplomatic difficulties of saving Lorrain Smith's face or any other face. I said I thought the details of the scheme for the Edinburgh Lister were bad and dangerous." Ewing had said he would look into this and asked what money might be available from the Dunn estate for reconstruction of University buildings. Fletcher replied (sounding like an RF representative): "I thought that was the wrong question to ask. The proper way to go to work was to have a good scheme worked out, the best practical ideal; when we had that ready he would be in a much better position to ask for money."[103] Fletcher wrote a brief letter to Mackie saying that he had spoken "frankly" to Ewing but gave no details.[104] Mackie replied with good news: "I might say we have been able to convert Lorrain Smith, for the time being anyway, from the Lister scheme and he agreed with me a few days ago that our best plan for some years to come is to reconstruct."[105] Fletcher also wrote arranging to meet Barger in London. By the end of the month Colman of the Dunn trust was becoming restless and he wrote to Fletcher that he felt it "rather important that I should be able to report something to the Trustees."[106] Fletcher, of course, was in no position to report anything very much of a positive nature.

Things were moving though. Just about this time Ewing told Fletcher that he had "drawn the attention of the University here to the necessity of having a comprehensive scheme prepared for improving and extending the existing accommodation for teaching and research in a number of our medical subjects." He had "reported to them [the members of the Court] a considerable part of the substance of what you said. They were duly impressed, and a committee has been appointed to go into the question fully and to consult an architect."[107] Fletcher was not yet sufficiently impressed. In December he wrote to the Secretary of the Dunn trustees relating that he had said to Ewing that he "could not possibly support any application from Edinburgh for any money either from the Dunn Trustees or any other source unless Edinburgh would enter upon a definite and coherent policy for the development of the Medical School." In his opinion, "Professor Ritchie's proposals were only patchwork, and money spent upon them might in great part be found to have been thrown away if and when a more thorough scheme is attempted." He reported that he had reminded Ewing that the RF had given a benefaction of £35,000 to Edinburgh five years ago, as a result of which fine clinical laboratories had been built after much delay. The Foundation was "dissatisfied with subsequent developments there and have withheld further support that they formerly contemplated giving." Fletcher considered "that the [Dunn] Trustees should be advised to regard the Ritchie proposals as withdrawn, at least pending the much more thorough consideration which is now being given to the whole subject by the University Committee." "Certainly," he added (no surprise here), "Lord Balfour with whom I have discussed the whole subject at Whittingehame, would desire me to say that they do not have his support."[108]

Later in the month Fletcher related the saga in the frankest of fashions to Pearce. He began: "As to Edinburgh I have much to tell you, of course in confidence." He described Ritchie's application for Dunn money, commenting: "As I had expected, the scheme was merely patchwork, having no relation to the real needs of the place for radical alteration, both structural and functional." He explained how he had stayed with Lord Balfour "and told him the truth." Fletcher related how he had seen Ewing and "said everything with the button off the foil." He told Ewing that he was "bolstering up engineering, in which Edinburgh could never compete, say, with Glasgow, and was ignoring his real asset, the

Medical School; this had gone downhill since the war, when it might have led the way." Fletcher pulled no punches: "the Medical Departments," he said, "were ridiculous in having nine vast auditoria when two at the most were needed, with pitiful research accommodation; radical internal reconstruction was needed." He had no hesitation in apportioning blame: he felt "Lorrain Smith as Dean was incompetent, and as Professor had had no research of any kind in his laboratory for twenty years." This was not all, for the "younger professors had no chance at present; the Rockefeller laboratories had been shamefully delayed." He complained that "there was still unused space in the Rockefeller building for at least 35 workers, while Ritchie, 50 yards away had been asking for new rooms." He had told Ewing that "the Lister Institute scheme was fatally misconceived, was quite moribund and yet actively dangerous because it gave excuse for delay in real reform elsewhere." Fletcher approved the efforts of Barger, Clark, Mackie, and Wilkie but the "great stumbling block of course is Lorrain Smith. Schafer, moreover, is too old to help and yet will not die."[109] Fletcher was also deeply critical of Murray Lyon.

Relying on Fletcher's advice the Dunn trustees resolved in December 1928 that Ritchie's proposal "do lie on the table."[110] Meanwhile in Edinburgh an architect had been brought in to plan the reconstruction of the School. In February of the following year, 1929, Fletcher visited Edinburgh and stayed with Wilkie. Before his arrival, Barger, probably speaking for the gang of four, told him: "We are particularly anxious that you should see the plans."[111] There is no detailed record of this visit but on March 19 Ewing told Pearce, "Sir Walter Morley Fletcher was here a few days ago. He saw the plans and went into them carefully with the Professors concerned, and expressed his warm approval."[112] In fact three days earlier Wilkie had told Pearce of the plans and that they had "been approved by the University Court." Wilkie copied this to Fletcher, and perhaps a little optimistic in the light of Rockefeller dissatisfaction, he finished on the sort of presumptuous note that characterized his persuasive style: "Should you be approached officially in the matter of giving financial support to this scheme from the Rockefeller Foundation I feel quite certain that you will consider such application with sympathy and interest."[113] Wilkie probably knew more than he let on, for Ewing, in his letter of March 19, wrote Pearce the following: "Once again I venture to invoke your support in applying for assistance from the Rockefeller Foundation to the Edinburgh University School of Medicine." He explained that plans for reconstruction had been drawn up and that the "Architect's estimate for the work of reconstruction is in round figures £60,000." Ewing appended details of the "Scheme." Besides a library and more space for the basic sciences it also recommended the "division of the medical theatre and reconstruction of other rooms for the department."[114] The proposal for the medical department had 1,600 square feet allotted for research. In spite of this concession to Ritchie, the basic scientists had won.

On the same day, March 19, that Ewing wrote to Pearce he sent the scheme of proposed reconstruction to the Dunn trustees.[115] Immediately mobilizing his allies, he later told Fletcher he had written to Lord Balfour of this development and the latter had written to Colman supporting the plan.[116] Unfortunately at the time Fletcher was kept in the dark over this development and a fortnight later he was writing to Ewing asking about the state of play so he could tell the Dunn trustees.[117] Ewing replied apologetically that he had been away from Edinburgh and explained the situation.[118] Fletcher then wrote to Colman that "I would say at once that in my opinion the proposed alterations would greatly improve the efficiency and enlarge the resources of the whole group of Departments constituting the Medical School."[119] Meanwhile, perhaps surprisingly, Pearce indicated support might be available from Rockefeller if the Dunn trustees co-operated. He handed the whole business over to Alan Gregg to deal with.[120] Privately on April 4 he told Gregg: "When I turned down in 1922 the large plan of Edinburgh for a Lister Memorial Institute, the cost of which ran to a very high figure, I told them that by reconstruction of the medical school building they could get all the space they needed without the expense of a new building." He revealed that behind the scenes, "I have unofficially intimated to Fletcher and to Barger and Wilkie that if they decided on this reconstruction we should be interested in taking a share of the cost." The Ritchie question then came up. Pearce, once again lamenting the lack of use of the clinical laboratory, noted that as:

> space is mentioned for the Department of Medicine, one important point should be brought out. Please make it clear to the Edinburgh authorities that while we have no desire to minimize the importance of Ritchie

having space, it should be distinctly understood that the laboratory of clinical medicine which we built was intended for clinical laboratory and research work in *the three departments of systematic medicine, clinical medicine and therapeutics*, and that in any rearrangement of space it should be definitely understood that from our point of view this laboratory was intended for general work in the field of medicine.[121]

This was just a way of saying that Ritchie should not have private space for research outside of the new lab which was obviously still seen as a locus that might eventually become part of a single department overseen by a director.

On April 23 Fletcher reported to Ewing that he had had a "good talk" with Colman and that the trustees wanted an assurance that in helping Edinburgh they would be doing something of permanent value. Fletcher had told him "that was certainly so." Then Fletcher passed on the good news: "The Trustees met yesterday, and Colman will be writing to you. He told me they had agreed to make you a benefaction, and he will be offering you, I understand, something between £15,000 and £20,000. I am inclined to think that that does not represent the maximum you may get if the situation develops favourably." Fletcher thought £20,000 was "quite certain." He reported that he had told all this to Gregg who thought the Foundation might come up with £30,000 if the University could find £10,000.[122]

On April 23, 1929 Gregg, in London, noted in his diary that Fletcher had "gone over the plans for reconstruction in Edinburgh and thinks the arrangements are ingenious and the proposal as sound and valuable as, for example, the Dunn Trustees' undertaking in Oxford and Cambridge." The following day he was in Edinburgh. He noted that he had met Ewing and intimated that the Foundation would put up £30,000. He had met Barger who had told him that "the unanimity in the Faculty is remarkable." Barger, he said, "told Dean and the Principal RP's [Pearce's] views regarding Murray-Lyon, and he is sure that M-L has already had an intimation that our support will not continue." On the Ritchie question Barger had told Gregg that he thought the "co-ordinated courses in pathology, bacteriology, bio-chemistry, medicine and surgery are working out very well." He considered "Ritchie's department the best place for these courses to be given." He added "this justifies some of the space being given to Ritchie."[123] Clearly Ritchie had not given in and as noted above, in the end, some of the extra space he got was probably turned into laboratories.[124]

The following day, April 25, Barger was told again about the money issues in a letter from Fletcher, who added that he had "an instinctive feeling, of course, against spending money in bricks and mortar when it is so badly wanted for wider and more liberal support of the right men." However, he felt in this instance, "reconstruction is a really urgent need, and I am sure that, if as this proceeds it becomes clear that the Edinburgh Medical School is working as a complete organism for the steady promotion of knowledge, liberal money help needed for the workers is not likely to be long lacking."[125]

After Gregg's visit to Edinburgh, Barger reported on the trip to Fletcher. Gregg was shown round the old building and lunched with Ewing. He returned for private talks with Barger and then "went on to Lorrain Smith for half an hour ('to show that he had learned his lesson')." The last phrase, presumably, meaning that Lorrain Smith was being told that Foundation would put money into the Medical School but not into anything like the Lister scheme. Barger observed that "Mackie, Clarke, [Sydney] Smith and I have remained in perfect agreement throughout and on good terms with Lorrain Smith, although we have led him rather than that he has led us." Revealing Ritchie's marginality he added: "We have also the support of Wilkie, (and of Ritchie for what it is worth)." "Ewing," said Barger, "is grasping, or wants to get as much as he can." Ewing was hoping for £25,000 from the Dunn trustees and £35,000 from Rockefeller. This of course would have made up the full £60,000 required but it is hard to imagine either of these bodies would have put up such money without any contribution from the University.[126]

Something else was afoot, however, and it was irritating Barger. The RF subvention of £1,000 per annum to Murray Lyon's salary was coming to an end. Murray Lyon was moving heaven and earth to get his debarment from private practice lifted. In November 1929 a Special Committee considered his case and eventually reported in his favour. The report demonstrates the lukewarm feeling in Edinburgh towards a full-time system. The Committee noted it restricted the choice of candidates, that full-time professors "lose touch," and the profession outside the hospital was deprived of consulting with the "highest authorities."[127] At any rate, in April 1929 Barger had already written to Fletcher that Ewing did have another fund he could apply to the reconstruction of the Medical School, "but wants to keep that for other needs. I strongly suspect," he said, "to make up the difference between £1400 and £2000 which the Rockefeller no longer wish to pay for Murray Lyon's salary." Ewing, Barger reported in a rage, "seems to think he is honour bound to continue the £2000." He observed, "Some of us are furious about this" and if "Murray Lyon is henceforth allowed to practise £1400 is all he needs." At any rate Ewing had told him they could go ahead even if they raised only £50,000 from external sources. Barger had been able to tell Ewing that Gregg had £30,000 or "in case of extreme need," £35,000. But Gregg did not see the latter to be the case and Barger agreed. "I doubt," wrote Barger, "whether Ewing fully understands the frank psychology of the Rockefeller people."

Barger then turned to related issues, revealing a great deal about local politics. He began by observing that "a curious thing happened today." He reported that "Stanley Davidson received a telegram from Horne implying that a rumour had been circulated among the Dunn Trustees (by someone in Edinburgh?) that the scheme would not be a success and was a waste of money." Obviously speaking to something Fletcher knew, he wrote that it "seems as if the tactics which resulted in MacLean not coming are being repeated." None the less he elaborated saying that, "It may be that some extra-mural lecturers wish to hamper our teaching as we are apt to cut them out." He gave a couple of examples, noting: "normally, as you know, a candidate for the Edinburgh MB may take a limited number of courses extra-murally but of late years, this has become more difficult, e.g. my teaching (and examinations!) have cut out the extra-mural analyst who ran a course formerly, and lately, improved co-ordination in the Third Year has threatened the extra-mural teachers still further." The point was obvious: any moves to academic medicine and the creation of large departments with University professors in charge threatened the extra-mural teachers. Hence the possibility that MacLean might be appointed a full time professor in 1928 was sabotaged.[128]

Fletcher replied that he had "heard no whisper here of any difficulty with the Trustees. If Horne is perturbed, it might be worth his while for him to talk to me, when I could give him powder and shot for argument with real or suborned doubters, and might also get on the track of the real source of trouble, if any."[129] Fletcher was obviously not worried and in buoyant mood for he wrote to Pearce that the developments at Edinburgh, should they come to fruition, were on "the best permanent lines." Although, he thought, we "must pray for some stroke of providence to show a way of getting the Royal Infirmary position straight."[130] In the next day or two Fletcher's optimism was justified. On April 29 Colman wrote to him: "Just a line, as I know you will be glad to hear that the full body of the Trustees voted £20,000 for Edinburgh to-day," on the understanding Rockefeller provided £30,000 and Edinburgh made up the rest.[131] Fletcher replied that he had had a "private reassurance" Rockefeller would cough up.[132]

Perhaps Barger's description of Ewing as "grasping" was not entirely inaccurate. On hearing the news of the Dunn gift, Ewing had written to Colman asking him for £25,000.[133] On May 1, 1929, he received the news that the trustees had turned him down and he wrote to Fletcher that it was a "little disappointing." Still, ever one to conserve University money, he was writing to Gregg to see if Rockefeller would up their contribution by £5000.[134] Fletcher was not sympathetic, asking Ewing: "Ought you to think it '*disappointing*'?" "A few months ago," Fletcher reminded him, "there was not a penny in sight from outside. Last October the Dunn Trustees were extremely cold about any scheme for Edinburgh, and the Rockefeller people were so disgruntled about the delays and failures connected with their large benefaction at the Royal Infirmary that it seemed impossible to hope that they would give any further help at Edinburgh." However: "In this short time the situation is so changed that you now have £50,000 practically for certain."[135] He did not think Rockefeller would increase its contribution. Pearce, however, took the "Edinburgh problem" to his Trustees and asked for £35,000.[136] This they came up with after a warm recommendation by Gregg.[137]

On May 28, 1929, *The Times* reported both gifts and announced work was scheduled to start in the summer vacation.[138] On June 21 Fletcher could report to Pearce that Edinburgh was "acting with great promptitude. Barger tells me that the welcome sound of hammers is already resounding through the building."[139] Gregg visited Edinburgh again in November 1929. He reported "lecture rooms much improved. Much space gained for laboratories. Surprising progress in the last six months. This money will have been well spent."[140] Reconstruction largely took the form of rationalizing space. The principal beneficiaries were the basic sciences: Pharmacology, Chemistry in relation to Medicine, and Bacteriology. In spite of Fletcher's objections Ritchie seems, in part, to have got his way. In the Department of Medicine the lecture theatre was divided horizontally, the upper floor becoming a demonstration room and the lower "a suite of research laboratories."[141]

Physical reconstruction of course did not suddenly make the medical school modern in the way some would have liked. Fletcher still painted a bleak picture. Writing to Sir Thomas Holland, the new Principal, in March 1931, he observed that "Edinburgh 50 years ago was one of the great medical schools of the world. To-day it has hardly any international standing, and stands not particularly high among the various provincial schools of Britain." He thought, "It has declined rather than advanced since the war. In these days of rapid progress even to stand still is to be rapidly left behind," and he considered, "If the men of enlightenment and goodwill in Edinburgh could get together now, scrap ancient lumber and go ahead on the only possible modern lines, Edinburgh might, I feel confident, suddenly leap into a leading position again." Iterating a familiar observation, he concluded, "It is of course some of her greatest potential assets that make some of the chief practical difficulties when the pace has to be rapid. If evolution could have been spread over half a century or more, things would have been easy."[142]

Notes

1. "University Clinic, Edinburgh: Surgery," [? 1923], folder 5, box 1, series 405, RG1.1, Rockefeller Foundation Archives, RAC.

2. "Agreement between the University Court and the Managers of the Royal Infirmary Regarding Clinical Arrangements and Pathology," June 20 and 23, 1913, folder 5, box 1, series 405, RG 1.1, Rockefeller Foundation Archives, RAC. There is surely also a copy of this agreement in EUA.

3. "University Clinic, Edinburgh: Surgery."

4. Memorandum from Pearce to Embree, February 25, 1923, folder 32, box 3, series 405, RG 1.1, Rockefeller Foundation Archives, RAC.

5. Richard Pearce, "Notes of R.M.P. on Medical School of the University of Edinburgh," February 1923, 6, folder 5, box 1, series 405, RG 1.1, Rockefeller Foundation Archives, RAC.

6. Ibid., 9.

7. Pearce to Embree, March 19, 1923, folder 3, box 32, series 405, RG 1.1, Rockefeller Foundation Archives, RAC.

8. "Preliminary Statement by the Faculty of Medicine of the University of Edinburgh Submitted to the Board of the Rockefeller Foundation," March 1923, folder 5, box 1, series 405, RG 1.1, Rockefeller Foundation Archives, RAC.

9. Barger to Pearce, March 29, 1923, folder 13, box 2, series 405, RG 1.1, Rockefeller Foundation Archives, RAC. Barger says this arrangement will get rid of "the boiled-down 'Oster' " [*sic*]—whatever that meant!

10. Minutes of the Rockefeller Foundation, May 23, 1923, folder 12, box 1, series 405, RG 1.1, Rockefeller Foundation Archives, RAC. This had probably been discussed with Stiles, since the written proposals he took with him said nothing to that effect.

11. Pearce to Meakins, June 26, 1923, folder 13, box 2, series 405, RG 1.1, Rockefeller Foundation Archives, RAC.

12. Stiles to Pearce, September 3, 1923, folder 32, box 3, series 405, RG 1.1, Rockefeller Foundation Archives, RAC.

13. Memorandum "Edinburgh Problems," from Pearce to A. Gregg and G. E. Vincent, October 5, 1923, folder 13, box 2, series 405, RG 1.1, Rockefeller Foundation Archives, RAC.

14. See pp. 119–120.

15. Ibid.

16. Lorrain Smith to Pearce, November 22, 1923, folder 13, box 2, series 405, RG 1.1, Rockefeller Foundation Archives, RAC.

17. Minutes of the Rockefeller Foundation, December 5, 1923, folder 12, box 1, series 405, RG 1.1, Rockefeller Foundation Archives, RAC.

18. Pearce to Ewing, December 6, 1923, folder 13, box 2, series 405, RG 1.1, Rockefeller Foundation Archives, RAC.

19. Stiles to Pearce, December 19, 1923, folder 32, box 3, series 405, RG 1.1, Rockefeller Foundation Archives, RAC.

20. UE Court and RIE Board of Managers' Representatives Minutes, January 16, 1924 in "Scrap-book of the RIE Biochemical Laboratory," box 1, folder 3, RCPE.

21. Andrew Doig, Edited transcript of interview with Helen Coyle, November 20, 1997. The expression "cut with a knife," remembered Doig, was probably Dunlop's, and if not it certainly summed up his experience.

22. Lorrain Smith to Pearce, May 22, 1924, folder 33, box 3, series 405, RG 1.1, Rockefeller Foundation Archives, RAC.

23. Ewing to Pearce, "Exhibit B," May 23, 1924, folder 14, box 2, series 405, RG 1.1, Rockefeller Foundation Archives, RAC. Presumably the Infirmary Managers had to be involved in the private practice concessions since a full-time professor would be expected either to be teaching or to be attending his hospital patients.

24. Meakins to Pearce, June 3, 1924, folder 33, box 3, series 405, RG 1.1, Rockefeller Foundation Archives, RAC.

25. Pearce to Ewing, June 4, 1924, folder 33, box 3, series 405, RG 1.1, Rockefeller Foundation Archives, RAC.

26. Vincent to [?], June 14, 1924, folder 12, box 1, series 405, RG 1.1, Rockefeller Foundation Archives, RAC.

27. Stiles to Pearce, June 17, 1924, folder 33, box 3, series 405, RG 1.1, Rockefeller Foundation Archives, RAC.

28. Minutes of the Rockefeller Foundation, July 1, 1924, folder 32, box 3, series 405, RG 1.1, Rockefeller Foundation Archives, RAC.

29. Vincent to Flexner, July 2, 1924, folder 33, box 3, series 405, RG 1.1, Rockefeller Foundation Archives, RAC.

30. Ibid.

31. Stiles to Pearce, February 24, 1925, folder 34, box 3, series 405, RG 1.1, Rockefeller Foundation Archives, RAC.

32. Wilkie to Pearce, October 16, 1924, folder 35, box 3, series 405, RG 1.1, Rockefeller Foundation Archives, RAC.

33. Pearce to Wilkie, October 27, 1924, folder 33, box 3, series 405, RG 1.1, Rockefeller Foundation Archives, RAC.

34. Stiles to Pearce, January 21, 1925, with "Plans of the New Department of Experimental Surgical Research," folder 34, box 3, series 405, RG 1.1, Rockefeller Foundation Archives, RAC.

35. Ewing to Pearce, January 28, 1925, folder 34, box 3, series 405, RG 1.1, Rockefeller Foundation Archives, RAC.

36. Stiles to Pearce, February 24, 1925, folder 34, box 3, series 405, RG 1.1, Rockefeller Foundation Archives, RAC.

37. Pearce to Ewing, March 19, 1925, folder 34, box 3, series 405, RG 1.1, Rockefeller Foundation Archives, RAC.

38. Ewing to Pearce, March 28, 1925, folder 34, box 3, series 405, RG 1.1, Rockefeller Foundation Archives, RAC.

39. Pearce to Wilkie, May 5, 1925, folder 34, box 3, series 405, RG 1.1, Rockefeller Foundation Archives, RAC.

40. Wilkie to Pearce, June 2, 1925, folder 34, box 3, series 405, RG 1.1, Rockefeller Foundation Archives, RAC.

41. Wilkie to Pearce, August 6, 1925, folder 34, box 3, series 405, RG 1.1, Rockefeller Foundation Archives, RAC. See also John Dixon Comrie, "The Faculty of Medicine," in *The History of the University of Edinburgh 1883–1933*, ed. A. Logan Turner (Edinburgh: Oliver and Boyd, 1933), 100–163, quote at 134.

42. Memorandum on "Surgical Laboratory for Edinburgh," August 27, 1925, folder 34, box 3, series 405, RG 1.1, Rockefeller Foundation Archives, RAC.

43. Pearce to Wilkie, August 31, 1925, folder 34, box 3, series 405, RG 1.1, Rockefeller Foundation Archives, RAC.

44. Wilkie to Pearce, September 18, 1925, folder 34, box 3, series 405, RG 1.1, Rockefeller Foundation Archives, RAC.

45. Minutes of the Rockefeller Foundation, November 6, 1925, folder 12, box 1, series 405, RG 1.1, Rockefeller Foundation Archives, RAC.

46. Pearce to Ewing, November 9, 1925, folder 34, box 3, series 405, RG 1.1, Rockefeller Foundation Archives, RAC.

47. Wilkie to Pearce, June 25, 1928, folder 33, box 3, series 405, RG 1.1, Rockefeller Foundation Archives, RAC.

48. Ewing to Pearce, June 22, 1928, folder 35, box 3, series 405, RG 1.1, Rockefeller Foundation Archives, RAC.

49. Comrie, "The Faculty of Medicine," 34.

50. Cushny to Meakins, June 13, 1919, 867/39/42, OLHM.

51. Haldane to Meakins, June 14, 1919, 867/39/40, OLHM.

52. Pearce, "Notes of R.M.P.," 9.

53. Minutes of the Rockefeller Foundation, December 5, 1923, folder 12, box 1, series 405, RG 1.1, Rockefeller Foundation Archives, RAC.

54. Vincent to W. Buttrick, June 14, 1924 (Exhibit A), folder 33, box 3, series 405, RG 1.1, Rockefeller Foundation Archives, RAC.

55. Minutes of the Rockefeller Foundation, December 5, 1923, folder 12, box 1, series 405, RG 1.1, Rockefeller Foundation Archives, RAC.

56. Vincent to [?], June 14, 1923, folder 12, box 1, series 405, RG 1.1, Rockefeller Foundation Archives, RAC.

57. Walker to Meakins, July 23, 1926, 867/39/62, OLHM.

58. Walker to Meakins, December 22, 1926, 867/39/63, OLHM.

59. Stanley Davidson, "The University of Edinburgh, Report on the Department of Therapeutics," LHSA, GD 1/58, EUL. Andrew Doig to whom I am most grateful for calling my attention to it deposited this invaluable document.

60. G. Lovell Gulland, "The Teaching of Medicine," in Edinburgh Pathological Club, *An Inquiry into the Medical Curriculum* (Edinburgh: W. Green & Son, 1919), 185–89.

61. Meakins to Ewing, March 23, 1927, 867/39/57, OLHM.

62. See page 125.

63. Meakins to Walker, March 23, 1927, 867/39/56, OLHM.

64. Ewing to Pearce, 9 June 1927, folder 16, box 2, series 405, RG 1.1, Rockefeller Foundation Archives, RAC.

65. Wilkie to Pearce, June 9, 1927, folder 16, box 2, series 405, RG 1.1.

66. Lorrain Smith to Pearce, June 10, 1927, folder 16, box 2, series 405, RG 1.1, Rockefeller Foundation Archives, RAC.

67. Pearce to Ewing, June 21, 1927, folder 16, box 2, series 405, RG 1.1, Rockefeller Foundation Archives, RAC.

68. Pearce to Wilkie, June 21, 1927, folder 16, box 2, series 405, RG 1.1, Rockefeller Foundation Archives, RAC.

69. Pearce to Fraser, August 24, 1927, folder 16, box 2, series 405, RG 1.1, Rockefeller Foundation Archives, RAC.

70. Fraser to Pearce, September 12, 1927, folder 16, box 2, series 405, RG 1.1, Rockefeller Foundation Archives, RAC.

71. Pearce to Wilkie, September 20, 1927, folder 16, box 2, series 405, RG 1.1, Rockefeller Foundation Archives, RAC.

72. This £1,000 per annum was originally for Meakins. He took none of it. He engaged in some private practice instead. "Memorandum regarding Chair of Therapeutics," June 26, 1929, Secretary's File, DRT 95/002, pt. 1, Faculty of Medicine, box 27, UEA.

73. Pearce to Fraser, September 27, 1927, folder 16, box 2, series 405, RG 1.1, Rockefeller Foundation Archives, RAC. In a similar vein, when, in 1925, the irascible, not to say conceited, Almroth Wright, at St Mary's, Paddington, drew up an application to the RF for a grant he virtually stated that Rockefeller should donate money and he could be trusted to use it wisely. Not surprisingly he seems to have received no reply. See E. A. Heaman, *St. Mary's: The History of a London Teaching Hospital* (Montreal & Kingston, London, Ithaca: Liverpool University Press, McGill-Queen's University Press, 2003), 215–16.

74. Pearce to Meakins, October 4, 1927, 867/36/12, OLHM.

75. Meakins to Pearce, October 6, 1927, 867/36/13, OLHM.

76. Wilkie to Pearce, October 28, 1927, folder 16, box 2, series 405, RG 1.1, Rockefeller Foundation Archives, RAC.

77. Pearce to Wilkie, November 14, 1927, folder 16, box 2, series 405, RG 1.1, Rockefeller Foundation Archives, RAC.

78. Pearce to Fletcher, November 15, 1927, folder 16, box 2, series 405, RG 1.1, Rockefeller Foundation Archives, RAC.

79. R. M. Pearce, Diary, February 6, 1928, folder 16, box 2, series 405, RG 1.1, Rockefeller Foundation Archives, RAC.

80. A. Gregg, Diary, February 6, 1928, folder 16, box 2, series 405, RG 1.1, Rockefeller Foundation Archives, RAC.

81. Pearce, Diary, February 6, 1928.

82. Gregg, Diary, April 21–26, 1928.

83. Fletcher to Pearce, May 8, 1928, FD1/1841 49222, PRO.

84. Pearce to Fletcher, May 21, 1928, FD1/1841 49222, PRO.

85. Pearce, Diary, February 6, 1928.

86. Davidson to Fletcher, July 19, 1928, FD1/1841 49222, PRO. Sir Robert Horne was Viscount Horne of Slamannan, Scottish lawyer, politician and businessman.

87. Ritchie to Secretary, Dunn Trustees, July 21, 1928, FD1/1841 49222, PRO.

88. Colman to Fletcher, July 24, 1928, FD1/1841 49222, PRO.

89. Fletcher to Colman, July 27, 1928, FD1/1841 49222, PRO.

90. Balfour to Colman, September 25, 1928, FD1/1841 49222, PRO.

91. Colman to Balfour, September 27, 1928, FD1/1841 49222, PRO.

92. Fletcher to Balfour, September 29, 1928, FD1/1841 49222, PRO.

93. Fletcher to Ritchie, October 16, 1928, FD1/1841 49222, PRO.

94. Fletcher to Ewing, October 16, 1928, FD1/1841 49222, PRO.

95. Fletcher to Mackie, October 17, 1928, FD1/1841 49222, PRO.

96. Ritchie to Fletcher, October 19, 1928, FD1/1841 49222, PRO.

97. Mackie to Fletcher, October 19, 1928, FD1/1841 49222, PRO.

98. Barger to Fletcher, October 23, 1928, FD1/1841 49222, PRO.

99. Mackie to Fletcher, October 30, 1928, FD1/1841 49222, PRO.

100. Barger to Fletcher, October 31, 1928, FD1/1841 49222, PRO.

101. Fletcher to Colman, November 2, 1928, FD1/1841 49222, PRO.

102. "Reconstruction of Medical School Buildings, Teviot Place" (with annotation "handed to Sir Walter on the 4–XI–28"), FD1/1841 49222, PRO.

103. Fletcher, untitled memorandum [?], November 6 [*sic*], 1928, FD1/1841 49222, PRO. This date is incorrect. It must be November 8 at the earliest.

104. Fletcher to Mackie, November 9, 1928, FD1/1841 49222, PRO.

105. Mackie to Fletcher, November 10, 1928, FD1/1841 49222, PRO.

106. Colman to Fletcher, November 27, 1928, FD1/1841 49222, PRO.

107. Ewing to Fletcher, November 28, 1928, FD1/1841 49222, PRO.

108. Fletcher to Secretary, Dunn Trustees, December 7, 1928, FD1/1841 49222, PRO.

109. Fletcher to Pearce, December 20, 1928, FD1/1841 49222, PRO.

110. Letter from Sir Jeremiah Colman, December 20, 1928. FD1/1841 49222, PRO.

111. Barger to Fletcher, February 20, 1929, FD1/1841 49222, PRO.

112. Ewing to Pearce, March 19, 1929 [copy], FD1/1841 49252, PRO.

113. Wilkie to Pearce, March 16, 1929 [copy], FD1/1842 49252, PRO.

114. Ewing to Pearce, March 19, 1929, with "Scheme for the Internal Reconstruction of the Medical Buildings," folder 17, box 2, series 405, RG 1.1, Rockefeller Foundation Archives, RAC. The details of the scheme were not appended in a copy to Fletcher, FD1/1842 49252, PRO.

115. Ewing to Secretary, Dunn Trustees, March 19, 1929, FD1/1842 49252, PRO.

116. Ewing to Fletcher, April 6, 1929, FD1/1842 49252, PRO.

117. Fletcher to Ewing, April 3, 1929, FD1/1842 49252, PRO.

118. Ewing to Fletcher, April 6, 1929, FD1/1842 49252, PRO.

119. Fletcher to Colman, April 15, 1929, FD1/1842 49252, PRO.

120. Pearce to Fletcher, April 4, 1929, FD1/1842 49252, PRO.

121. Pearce to Gregg, April 4, 1929, folder 17, box 2, series 405, RG 1.1, Rockefeller Foundation Archives, RAC.

122. Fletcher to Ewing, April 23, 1929, FD1/1842 49252, PRO.

123. Gregg, Diary, April 23–24, 1929.

124. Comrie, "The Faculty of Medicine," 129.

125. Fletcher to Barger, April 25, 1929, FD1/1842 49252, PRO.

126. Barger to Fletcher, April 28, 1929, FD1/1842 49252, PRO.

127. UE Court Special Committee Report, November 7, 1929, Secretary's File, DRT 95/002, pt. 1, Faculty of Medicine, box 27, UEA.

128. Barger to Fletcher, April 28, 1929.

129. Fletcher to Barger, April 29, 1929, FD1/1842 49252, PRO.

130. Fletcher to Pearce, April 29, 1929, FD1/1842, 49252, PRO.

131. Colman to Fletcher, April 29, 1929, FD1/1842, 49252, PRO.

132. Fletcher to Colman, May 1, 1929, FD1/1842, 49252, PRO.

133. Ewing to Colman, April 26, 1929, FD1/1842, 49252, PRO.

134. Ewing to Fletcher, May 1, 1929, FD1/1842, 49252, PRO.

135. Fletcher to Ewing, May 3, 1929, FD1/1842, 49252, PRO.

136. Pearce to Fletcher, May 13, 1929, FD1/1842, 49252, PRO.

137. Pearce to Fletcher, May 27, 1929, FD1/1842 49252, PRO.

138. *The Times*, May 28, 1929. Also a clipping in FD1/1842, 49252, PRO.

139. Fletcher to Pearce, June 21, 1929, FD1/1842 49252, PRO.

140. Gregg, Diary, November 25, 1929, folder 17, box 2, series 405, RG 1.1, Rockefeller Foundation Archives, RAC.

141. Comrie, "The Faculty of Medicine," 129.

142. Fletcher to Holland, 31 March 1931, FD1/3199, 49252, PRO.

7

A HOSPITAL LABORATORY

Biochemical testing in laboratories as an adjunct to patient care (clinical biochemistry) appeared in Britain chiefly in the 1920s. Before the Biochemistry Laboratory opened in Edinburgh in 1921 the Infirmary had two laboratory services: that of the Pathology Department and a so-called clinical laboratory which was mainly devoted to electrocardiography.[1] The surgeons had their own laboratory facilities and did not call much on the Pathology Department.[2] There were also ward "side rooms" for carrying out simple tests and microscopy.

During the nineteenth century, chemistry was increasingly held to be an important example of a basic science with the power to change medicine. Very early in the century, examination of the urine for chemical change was hailed as practical proof of the subject's clinical value. Richard Bright's description of his now eponymous disease that linked dropsy with the presence of albumin in the urine was soon regarded as one of the first demonstrations of the merits of chemical pathology.[3] In the early part of the century a new chemistry based on organic compounds was created and later a chemistry of life, biochemistry, was built from this. These developments mainly originated in Germany. One of the many ways in which researchers with biochemical interests sought to establish their discipline in Europe and America was by gaining access to the pre-clinical medical curriculum (as had the physiologists before them). In universities, biochemistry largely remained within physiology departments where so-called chemical physiologists unravelled animal and human biochemical processes.[4] The subject, along with experimental physiology, was proclaimed as heralding a future revolution in clinical practice. However, apart from urine testing, biochemistry had little place conceptually or practically in clinical medicine before the First World War. The close links of biochemistry to physiology are important for understanding the perceptions, approaches, and enthusiasms of those who embraced the subject and the doubts and uncertainties of those who did not.

Apart from one small case study, the history of the institutionalization in Britain of clinical biochemistry in hospitals has not been charted.[5] There seems to have been no pattern. In some instances biochemical tests began to be offered by older pathology laboratories and in other cases, as in Edinburgh, wholly new institutions were established. The relative lack of coherence of clinical biochemistry as a specialty is demonstrated by the varying terms that designated those filling new positions: biochemist, chemical physiologist, or chemical pathologist.[6] In Edinburgh in the 1920s, biochemistry instruction for medical students was split between teachers of the basic sciences and clinicians. Barger taught first-year medical students organic chemistry. Physiological chemistry for second-year students was in the hands of W. W. Taylor in the Physiology Department. Taylor, who was not medically qualified, gave a practical course of which an account was published in 1922. An annotated, interleaved copy in Edinburgh records: "30 hours allotted for this course in the term." The course included the qualitative and quantitative testing of a range of organic substances and body products. Some of the tests were purely to demonstrate theory, such as those performed on egg white. Others, however, had clinical potential, especially those done on urine.[7]

In the RIE, in side rooms attached to the wards, patients' urine had been routinely examined since the nineteenth century. For the most part the examination involved determining the urine's colour and odour, measuring its quantity and specific gravity, testing for an alkaline or acid reaction, and for the presence of albumin and sugar. Microscopy might occasionally be added to these examinations. In 1875 a patient on an Infirmary ward had a urine test detailed as: "Urine is normal in amount. Sp. Gravity 1026. Of strong acid reaction. Under the microscope the deposit shows amorphous urates and a quantity of renal epithelium. There is albumen—no sugar. Of phosphate there is abundant deposit when the urine is rendered alkaline. Chloride and urea are normal."[8] By the early twentieth century a range of quantitative and qualitative urine tests was at the clinician's disposal and students were taught them on the wards. In the patient's home, tests, if ever they were done, were often very simple.[9] Even after the lab was opened, urine testing by and large remained a side room activity in the Infirmary. Although these tests derived from and displayed the value of science, carrying them out and interpreting them were regarded as clinical skills. Urine examination remained principally directed at determining the existence and state of renal insufficiency. In 1918, a medical text noted that the "Examination of the Urine corresponds, in renal diseases, to the physical examination of other organs."[10] Testing was also regarded as a valuable asset in the diagnosis of a few non-renal disorders, most notably diabetes.

During the first three months of the course in clinical medicine, besides urine testing, clinical tutors taught students side room methods of examining blood, stomach contents, sputum, and faeces.[11] (See Figure 7.1) With regard to blood, students learned to examine it with a microscope (to count cells) and with a haemoglobinometer and to perform the Widal test for the diagnosis of typhoid fever. The much-used Wassermann reaction for syphilis was universally recognized as requiring special skills beyond those of the ordinary practitioner.[12] In Edinburgh this test was carried out in the Pathology Department until the Bacteriology Department opened in 1923.[13] Of the side room tests gastric analysis was remembered as particularly tedious as many samples required titration to determine acid content. Student help was appreciated and students discovered that being willing to assist in the side rooms as an undergraduate facilitated post graduate preferment.[14]

The key to the establishment of clinical biochemistry was not the urine but blood testing and the claim that such testing was essential to patient care and that, in many instances, it could only be properly carried out in specialized settings. Such a claim was to a great extent based on the creation of a new field of study: metabolic disease. By 1915 biochemistry

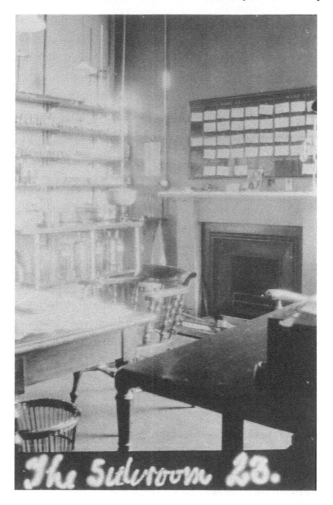

**Fig. 7.1: A side room, RIE, 1920s. LHSA copy of a photograph
taken from an album originally belonging to
Dr George Lewis Malcolm-Smith. By courtesy of LHSA.**

had become what one author called an "enormous" science.[15] The massive
Physiology and Biochemistry in Modern Medicine of 1921, by J. J. R. Macleod,
Professor of Physiology at Toronto, evidences the huge number of biochemical substances, pathways, and mechanisms that had been described
by the year the Edinburgh lab opened. Central to animal biochemistry were
metabolism and its disorders. In the middle of the nineteenth century,

physiologists and organic chemists investigating foodstuffs had concluded that the prime building materials of the body were proteins, carbohydrates, and fats. They taught that these substances were broken down and rendered absorbable by digestion and that the products were then either built into tissue, stored for future use, or employed immediately as sources of energy. Students learned that "the essential nature of the metabolic process in animals is one of oxidation," in which large unstable molecules were broken down into simple stable ones.[16] This process—catabolism—liberated energy as movement and heat.

Proteins, the body's principal building blocks, were absorbed as amino acids and those "not required" by the tissues had various fates.[17] These latter could be determined by studying one of the fundamental constituents of protein—nitrogen. Most of the nitrogen in the body and blood existed as amino acids and protein but—of clinical relevance—the nitrogenous residues of protein breakdown also appeared in the blood, constituting about one per cent of its total nitrogen. This was the non-protein nitrogen (NPN). Its principal constituents of clinical importance were urea, uric acid, creatine, creatinine, and ammonia.[18] The nitrogen of urea (urea N) constituted about fifty per cent of the NPN in blood and roughly ninety per cent of the total nitrogen of the urine.[19] By 1920, changes in the blood concentration and urinary output of these nitrogenous substances had been catalogued in a variety of conditions, notably renal failure. But pathological levels of these substances could also occur when the kidney was normal: in liver disease for instance, or in diabetic coma.[20] In acute kidney disease protein itself could appear in the urine and was, as Bright had shown, easily detected.

Carbohydrates were broken down in the gut and absorbed as the simple sugars, notably glucose. After absorption sugar was either stored as glycogen in the liver and muscles or oxidized; the glycogen of the liver was slowly released maintaining more or less constant blood sugar levels. Such *glycogenolysis* was accelerated when the organism's fuel requirements increased. The metabolic pathways by which glucose was broken down in the body were obscure but it was agreed that lactic acid, carbon dioxide, and water were three of the end products of the oxidation of this prime energy-producing substance. Sugar, not normally present in urine, could easily be detected in pathological conditions and, using more sophisticated techniques, was measurable in blood.

Fats were absorbed into the body after being broken down into fatty acids and then formed again into fat molecules more usable by the organism.[21] Blood normally contained only a small amount of fat. Developments of biochemical technique had made it possible, by 1921, to determine the fat and the cholesterol content of the blood. Fat metabolism had a complex relationship to carbohydrate metabolism in which the liver played a crucial role. Excess carbohydrates were stored as fats and in the absence of carbohydrates, fats were oxidized as an energy source. The normal end products of fat metabolism, produced by way of various acid intermediaries, were carbon dioxide and water.

In the 1920s biochemistry was gradually institutionalized in clinical settings as physiologically-minded practitioners worked to show that many disorders could be redescribed using metabolic concepts. This, they said, made blood testing a key to disease diagnosis and management. Many who promoted laboratory science in clinical medicine emphasized how the clinician should use blood levels of various substances in diagnosis and management rather than relying solely on symptoms and signs elicited at the bedside. This was true not only of biochemistry but also of the new discipline of haematology, supporters of which stressed the significance of blood counts to define disease and monitor sickness or recovery. In these various contexts academic physicians began to emphasize that the management of their patients was "controlled" (and conversely, how patient management by more traditional clinicians was not). The lab was more than simply an adjunct to the study of disease. It was the institutionalization of a new way of thinking about pathology.[22] Education in the use of the lab data by those unacquainted with ideas about metabolic disease was a way of teaching them those ideas.

Bringing blood biochemical tests into clinical medicine was a rather different matter from introducing urinalysis. The latter, after all, was an initiative of regular clinicians. Before the First World War quantitative blood chemistry scarcely had a place in patient care. Of his Montreal days, 1909–13, Meakins recalled, "a biochemical point of view . . . was almost unknown in Clinical Medicine."[23] A British text of 1913, Panton's *Clinical Pathology*, was devoted to such laboratory investigations "as have a practical bearing upon the diagnosis and treatment of disease."[24] The section on blood was overwhelmingly concerned with haematological and serological techniques. A short chapter was devoted to "The Chemical and

Physical Examination of the Blood." It covered spectroscopic examination, naked-eye inspection and microscopic procedures for detecting, but not measuring, abnormal levels of fat, glycogen, bile pigments, and uric acid. The estimation of specific gravity was described. The only quantitative chemical tests noted were those for alkalinity and oxygen content. The latter was said to be "beyond the scope of ordinary clinical pathology" and "not devoid of risk." The author observed that "no purely chemical examination of the blood has at the present time any wide application in clinical medicine."[25]

After the war things began to change, largely on the basis of American attempts to apply biochemistry, especially blood biochemistry, to the bedside. Much of this work was carried out by Donald Dexter Van Slyke, chemist at the Hospital of the Rockefeller Institute in New York, and by Otto Folin at Harvard University. Focusing on Van Slyke, Olga Amsterdamska has shown how important his work was in redefining disease in biochemical terms.[26] The technological dimensions of such transformations were crucial. Workers in chemical physiology at this time developed a host of comparatively simple methods for measuring biochemical products in blood. The move to blood biochemistry was evident in Todd's *Clinical Diagnosis* of 1918, an American manual of clinical pathology for practitioners and students. The text covered haematological, serological, and bacteriological methods, microscopy of various products, and chemical examination of urine. Blood chemistry appeared in the section "Less Frequently Used Methods," where it was noted that, until recently, the study of blood chemistry "interested the biochemist rather than the clinician." However, the author observed, "Within the past few years . . . methods have been so simplified and so many facts of clinical value have been gathered that certain chemic examinations are beginning to play an extremely important rôle in clinical medicine." Todd specifically cited as valuable the estimation of sugar, creatinine, urea, NPN, and total nitrogen.[27]

Even so, before about 1920 testing for chemicals in the blood was scarcely recognized outside of specialist publications. In the second edition of *The Newer Methods of Blood and Urine Chemistry* of 1920 the authors noted: "Chemical analyses of the blood have for years been looked upon as belonging to experimental physiological chemistry, and, in no sense of practical use such as are urinary analyses, gastric contents analyses, etc."[28]

Within three or four years of this observation, the situation had begun to change in many large hospitals. In 1923 two Americans, priding themselves on what they described as their country's pioneering work in this regard, could say: "In recent years, the chemical analysis of the blood has assumed a position of prominence in clinical medicine."[29] Still, in Edinburgh in 1922 it was a relative novelty for a clinical meeting of the British Medical Association to have demonstrated to it, in the Biochemical Laboratory, "chemical tests of renal function, including estimations of blood urea and non-protein nitrogen."[30] However, by 1924, in Britain, the London physician Walter Langdon Brown could note "a shifting of the main interest from the urine to the blood." He observed, "it is only of late that resort has been made to routine examination of the blood for any other purposes than to count its corpuscles, to estimate its haemoglobin, and to search for microbes."[31] The RIE story fits this pattern exactly. In 1920 it had no biochemical laboratory; by 1924 it had one churning out results, especially of blood examinations, on a regular basis.[32]

At Edinburgh University in 1920, Taylor, in his course on physiological chemistry, seems to have taught pre-clinical medical students how to estimate the NPN of blood. An appendix to his book noted that for "the determination of blood sugar, urea, uric acid, creatinine . . . the clinical significance of which is becoming more fully recognized" readers should consult the works of Otto Folin.[33] If biochemical testing was a mark of modernity Edinburgh seems to have lagged behind Cambridge where, since at least 1920, pre-clinical students had carried out estimations of blood glucose, chlorides, urea, and NPN.[34] Edinburgh students did not, apparently, in their clinical training, learn any side room methods of examining blood for its biochemical constituents.[35] The side rooms were scarcely ever, perhaps never, used for such a purpose. Since the Edinburgh medical curriculum was overwhelmingly directed to turning out general practitioners this is not surprising (the Americans thought it was). For the most part, GPs in Britain were not regarded as having the time, apparatus, or competencies for blood testing.[36] This seems less true of the United States and would fit with the perceptions of American visitors, described in previous chapters, who seemed to consider laboratory methods well within the competence of ordinary practitioners.[37]

A number of points about biochemical expertise around 1920 merit notice. First, in the case of many tests, when seemingly abnormal, there was by no means consensus among clinicians and chemical physiologists as to their pathological significance. Second, even within each of the two communities there could be differences of opinion as to the significance of particular tests. The value of measuring various protein metabolites, discussed below, exemplifies both of these points. Third, what clinicians might consider satisfactory tests, biochemists might not. Thus, in the 1920s, the author of a treatise on side room methods could note of the clinician's traditional means of estimating urea in urine: "It is freely condemned by chemical physiologists as being too inaccurate, but for clinical guidance it forms a good enough indication for treatment."[38] This, it might be noted, was said of a test some thought had no value at all.

The clinical chemistry of the blood figured little in general medical texts at this time. For example, the eleventh edition of Frederick Taylor's *The Practice of Medicine* of 1918 which, the author declared, "has been brought as far as possible up to date," contained a long section on "Examination of the Urine." Taylor described qualitative chemical tests (sometimes in association with microscopy) for determining the presence in urine of albumin, "other proteids," blood, lead, urea, chlorides, sulphates, phosphates, calcium oxalate, uric acid, urates, and various urinary pigments as well as sugar and other substances occurring in diabetes. He also described spectroscopic examination of the urine and how to determine acidity and alkalinity. Quantitative chemical tests for albumin, sugar, urea, and uric acid were also detailed. He noted, however, that estimation of the latter was "not suited for ordinary clinical work."[39] Taylor assumed, in other words, that, for the most part, the attending clinician would carry out all chemical testing of urine. As far as blood was concerned Taylor described standard haematological procedures using the microscope and haemoglobinometer. The only biochemical tests on blood he described were a quantitative one for ascertaining alkalinity and a qualitative one for discovering excess sugar. The latter was to be applied in "exceptional cases" when urine was unobtainable. A reaction for precipitating calcium salts from blood which were to be examined with the microscope was also described.[40]

By 1920, however, Osler and McCrae's *The Principles and Practice of Medicine* recognized the value of blood analysis in uraemia and nephritis to be respectively "of great value" and "particularly important." The text also recommended determinations of urea-nitrogen, NPN, uric acid, and "creatinin[e]." The blood picture of diabetes was described although no specific recommendations for testing were given.[41] There were at least two possible reasons for these references to blood chemistry. First, the updating of Osler's by now "classic" textbook by Thomas McCrae, a distinguished North American academic clinician. Second, the publication in 1919 of new and simpler methods for determining many of the substances commonly found in blood and urine.[42] McCrae, however, was in tune with physiological medicine in other ways. His was one of the few texts of the period to see relevance in measuring basal metabolism, specifically noting its elevation in hyperthyroidism, making it "an important aid in diagnosis."[43]

Some indication of Edinburgh sensibilities at this time is given by examination of successive editions of Hutchison and Rainy's very popular *Clinical Methods*. Harry Rainy was an Ordinary Physician at the Infirmary. The text described the skills regarded as necessary for a sound GP. Two points merit notice in the 1916 edition. First, although this was a work mainly devoted to physical examination, a great deal of space was given to clinical bacteriology. Second, urine examination also received extensive coverage. The 1920 edition was unchanged in these respects. By 1924 blood chemistry was recognized in an account of tests for the quantitative estimation of urea and glucose and in a description of the Van den Bergh reaction (a test for bile pigment). No further tests were added to the 1929 edition. The authors' perception seems to have been that knowledge of blood biochemistry might sometimes be valuable and that some tests would be within the capabilities of practitioners without access to laboratories.[44]

There was in principle, but certainly not always in practice, a division of labour in the new Biochemistry Laboratory into investigations done for the physicians and surgeons on the wards of the Infirmary and those done as research work. The distinction between routine and research was still being created at this time. Research tests were carried out at the worker's expense, paid from his or her own pocket, or by means of an outside grant or from University funds. Curiously, when the lab opened no one was employed by the Infirmary to do routine testing. Throughout most of the decade the lab had a physiologist and a biochemist. These positions were sometimes part time and the Director had a degree of flexibility in defining their roles. Technically the workers were Assistants in the Department of Therapeutics and the incumbents were paid by the University. When the lab opened Harold Whitridge Davies (a medical graduate) was the physiologist and Charles Harington the biochemist. Both spent the bulk of their time on research. They also supervised routine testing although it seems likely that during the lab's first years they (especially Harington) carried out quite a number of such tests themselves, possibly sharing the work with unpaid research workers. David Murray Lyon, for example, Meakins's successor and, at the opening of the lab, an Assistant Physician and Lecturer (but not paid to work in the lab), was involved in some routine testing, since his signature occasionally appears on test reports. In the early years Davies undertook most of the estimations of basal metabolic rate (BMR). The lab also had a non-graduate technical assistant, William Archibald, paid 15s.[45] per week by the University. In 1922 one of his duties was to collect pancreatic tissue from the city abattoir for the extraction of insulin. A "Lab boy" and a technical assistant were taken on around this time. At its opening the lab also had a part-time secretary. Probably from the beginning too, there was a charwoman for cleaning the rooms and glassware.[46] Although personnel changed, the core lab staff remained roughly this size through the decade. Davies, Harington, their successors, and the unpaid research workers who came and went are discussed in the next chapter.

The lab commenced testing in January 1921 and its Annual Reports record the number of specimens received and the number and types of examination done.[47] (See Figure 7.2) Various features of the lab's work in the 1920s evidence the ways in which, for some at least, it became important to, if not an indispensable part of, patient care. First was the gradual increase in the workload. In 1921 when the lab opened, 396 specimens were received.[48] Ten years later, in 1930, this number had risen to 2,341. Perhaps more striking is the number of examinations carried out on these specimens. In 1921 these amounted to 782, and in 1930 a total of 5,739 examinations were done (see Graph 7.1). Second, and far more impressive, is the rise in the number of tests on blood performed, compared to urine. In 1921, 429 blood examinations were carried out and, in 1930, 3,831 (see Graph 7.2). Third, although less consistent, is the increasing variety of tests. In 1921 ten different sorts of biochemical test were recorded as having been performed on blood, in 1930 nineteen different sorts of examination were carried out.

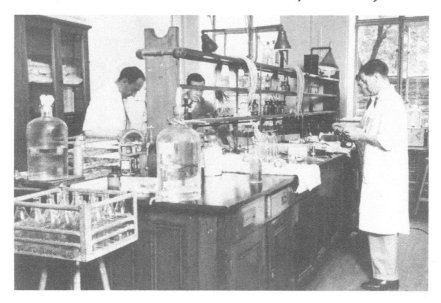

Fig. 7.2: C. P. Stewart (centre), H. Scarborough (left) and other staff
in the Clinical Laboratory, RIE, no date. The view from the window
is towards Middle Meadow Walk. (RIE, LHSA GD 14A/4/7.)
By courtesy of LHSA.

The work of the lab in 1921 very much set the pattern for the decade. The load over the ten years increased dramatically but its shape remained much the same. Major fluctuations in the lab's statistics can probably be accounted for by research interests or the introduction of new or simpler tests. In 1921, the numbers of blood specimens received and examinations carried out greatly surpassed those for urine.[49] Determinations of BMR, an estimation that made heavy demands on the lab's time and resources, were frequent from the start and climbed steadily.[50] The 101 requested in 1921 increased sixfold to 613 in 1930 (see Graph 7.3). Faecal fat analysis and small numbers of miscellaneous examinations were also done. Figures in these categories increased gradually although the numbers were never a very significant fraction of the total. The miscellaneous tests comprised a very broad church encompassing, among many other things, the analysis of body fluids, oatcakes, jam, wallpaper, plums, and gin. Increasing disproportionately to any other test, although relatively small in number, were examinations of

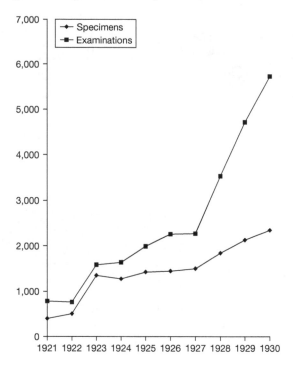

Graph 7.1: Specimens and examinations 1921–30. Graph by author.

cerebrospinal fluid (CSF), which rose by a factor of thirty, from three in 1921 to ninety-one in 1930.[51] (See Graph 7.4)

The lab's establishment had consequences that had been predicted. By the end of its first year it was clear that the lab was having more demands placed on it than it could fully handle without compromising research work. When the regulations were drawn up, Meakins had anticipated a problem of conflict between work "for the benefit of Hospital patients" and the "proper research duties for the University."[52] At this time, after all, the Infirmary was not paying anyone to do routine testing. The Infirmary's Medical Managers' Committee considered Meakins's Annual Report of 1921 and it suggested that Meakins call a meeting of the lab's Advisory Committee "to consider as to how the routine work performed by yourself and your University Assistants may be relieved."[53] On July 26, 1922, the Advisory Committee reviewed the routine biochemical examinations done in the first year and considered the question

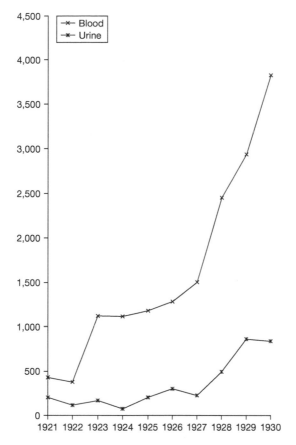

**Graph 7.2: Total examinations of blood and urine 1921–30.
Graph by author.**

of their "interfering with research work." Meakins was instructed to prepare a report for the Medical Managers although it had already been prepared and was appended to the minutes.[54] The Report noted that "a rough estimation" of the routine tests done in the first six months of 1922 revealed that they almost doubled when compared with the same period in 1921. It observed that the Advisory Committee was of the opinion that if the "volume of work increased" it would "seriously interfere with the University work of the Research Assistants and the Professor of Therapeutics." But, pressing the importance of testing, the Committee

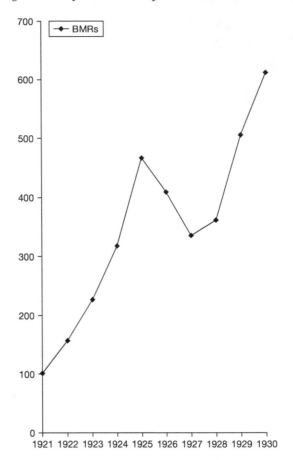

Graph 7.3: Basal Metabolic Rate estimations 1921–30. Graph by author.

was "unanimously of the opinion that the routine biochemical work, which had been done in the Biochemical Laboratory, was essentially important for the proper care of the patients in the Infirmary." The Committee was "strongly of the opinion that the laboratory should be provided with some additional assistance to carry on the routine work." Among the possibilities suggested was the employment by the Infirmary of the laboratory assistant, William Archibald, currently paid by the University, to carry out the routine work under direction.[55]

The Infirmary Managers considered the report of the Advisory Committee on August 7, 1922. They noted the increase of the work of

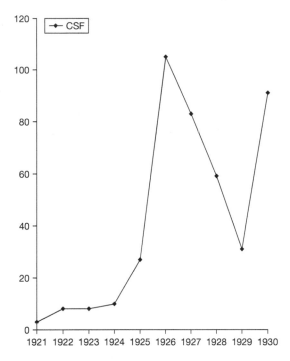

Graph 7.4: Cerebrospinal fluid examinations 1921–30. The number of specimens received cannot be quantified. Graph by author.

the lab and its "highly technical character," which prevented it being done in the side rooms. They also noted that there was "a growing sense of the importance of such examinations for the proper care and treatment of patients in the Hospital." A decision on the desirability of a surgical operation, they observed, "may, in many instances, only be determined by such means." The Managers considered that taking over Archibald was the most economical way of dealing with the problems.[56] This was done; Archibald got a wage increase and the money released from his transfer was used to pay a lab boy and technical assistant.[57] Demand for tests continued to increase, however, and in March 1925 the Advisory Committee noted the laboratory's difficulties in meeting the number of requests. For example, the lab's facilities permitted the determination of only three BMR tests each day but on some days as many as five were requested. It was suggested it be pointed out to the Infirmary Managers "that a great deal of routine work at present falls upon University-paid assistants."[58] The response of the Infirmary to this is not entirely clear. It appears that a further full-time technical assistant was not taken on until 1928.

From its opening, the lab was performing the sorts of tests on blood and urine that were to be the staple of its work over the next ten years. In the instance of urine what the lab provided were more precise quantitative estimations of substances for which side room tests were regarded (at least by chemical physiologists) as inaccurate, for instance for urea, or which required special apparatus or much time, for example the determination of ammonia nitrogen.[59] For present purposes, during the decade tests carried out in the lab on blood and urine can be usefully, if arbitrarily, grouped under four headings. First, under protein metabolism, were tests largely used for the estimation of nitrogenous substances. Consistently these comprised a significant fraction of all tests performed. By 1930, they accounted for 2,099 (1,848 of them on blood) of the total of 5,739 tests carried out in that year.[60] (See Graph 7.5) These tests were principally for NPN, urea, creatinine, and ammonia nitrogen. Renal disease must have been an important determinant of tests in this category. Second, under carbohydrate metabolism, most tests done were estimations of sugar. Diabetes, of course, was by far and away the major determinant of such investigations. By 1930 investigations related to fat metabolism had grown sufficiently large to constitute a third category. Investigations of fat, cholesterol, and bile in the blood (along with faecal fat examination) were presumably carried out in relation to malabsorption syndromes and hepatic and biliary disorders. The fourth heading, acid–base balance, is anomalous for reasons related to research and is described below. Besides these major categories the lab carried out occasional tests on blood for substances such as alcohol and carbon monoxide. The urine examination returns show sporadic reports of tests for such things as arsenic and specific amino acids. BMR estimations and CSF examinations will be considered as categories in their own right.

In the lab, tests for protein, carbohydrate, and fat metabolites were most frequently performed on blood. Urine tests were carried out mainly in the side rooms. Tests performed for protein metabolites in urine in the lab in 1921 amounted to little more than one hundred investigations, a minuscule fraction of the side room tests or of the patient population.

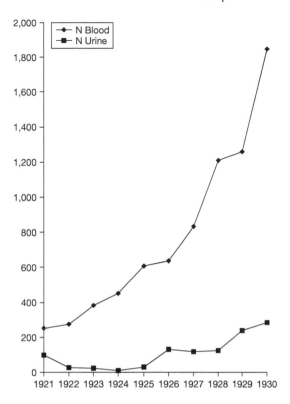

Graph 7.5: Total examinations of nitrogenous substances in blood and urine 1921–30, comprising, variously: urea nitrogen, nonprotein nitrogen, ammonia nitrogen, creatinine, total nitrogen (insignificant numbers for blood), acetone (generally insignificant), urea concentration in urine (2 tests in 1923 only) and ammonia (insignificant). Graph by author.

There is no very obvious pattern to the examination of nitrogenous substances in the urine. In fact, tests for them fell off markedly in the four years after 1921, only resuming their original levels in 1926 and increasing thereafter. Even by 1930 only 251 estimations of the principal nitrogen metabolites in urine were done. There was, in fact, little agreement in the literature as to the value of these tests. Urea, as noted above, was the main constituent of the protein metabolites. Urea was a venerated substance in the history of medicine, being the first organic compound to be synthesized in a laboratory. So many processes contributed to the excretion of urea that increases or decreases were considered diagnostic of nothing in particular and it was usually used as an indicator of general metabolism. The total nitrogen in urine (which was increasingly measured in Edinburgh) was regarded as a better marker of this.[61] An American text of 1923 noted: "In clinical work [urine] urea estimations have been practically abandoned."[62] This was not quite true in Edinburgh, but the 41 urine urea estimations of 1921, rising to 118 in 1930, were scarcely significant figures. Urea could be estimated in the side room but most methods were, in the word of one authority, "complicated," although another author wrote that there was one test that could "be carried out by anybody."[63] There was no consensus as to whether urea excretion was decreased in renal disease.[64] It was, noted one writer, increased in the acute stage of fevers and acute inflammatory diseases and diminished in "chronic cases."[65] Its estimation was regarded as particularly valuable in estimating renal efficiency when it was done as part of the "urea concentration test" in which specimens were examined one and two hours after a dose of urea.[66] Two estimations of urine urea, specified as the components of a concentration test, were done in the lab in 1923, a year in which no other urea estimations at all were carried out. There is plenty of evidence, however, of urea concentration tests being carried out on the ward and the estimations being done in the side rooms. Urine creatinine was occasionally estimated in the lab but the figures are irregular. In sum, clinicians of whatever persuasion did little to avail themselves of the *quantitative* tests for protein metabolites in urine offered by the laboratory, just as they rarely seem to have used them on the side rooms. Such tests did not figure in either research or everyday management.

Tests for nitrogenous substances in the blood were a quite different matter. The Edinburgh laboratory offered tests for all the common nitrogen-containing substances. These metabolites were known to accumulate in the blood in acute and chronic renal disease although there were wide differences of opinion as to their relative merits as monitors of these conditions.[67] Blood urea and NPN levels in particular were widely agreed to be valuable, although one British authority thought any determination other than urea "superfluous" other than for research purposes.[68] In 1919 Folin and Wu noted, "probably no other determination will be as useful and important to the clinician as the determination of the blood urea."[69] Two American authorities held NPN to be particularly useful in very early nephritis when vomiting might be the only symptom.[70] American authors in effect produced a taxonomy of the changes in the nitrogen products in blood in renal failure, describing how uric acid, urea, and creatinine accumulated differentially.[71] A blood uric acid was not estimated in the Edinburgh laboratory until 1926.[72] Creatinine was held by some to be a very sensitive indicator of the severity of chronic nephritis, one volume stating that "there is no one ingredient [of blood] that is more important to estimate than is creatinine [in this disease]."[73] Both blood urea and NPN were frequently estimated in the lab. Indeed the most frequent blood test in 1921 was for NPN, 124 examinations being done. Blood urea and NPN estimations climbed almost in tandem making it likely, as a small number of clinical records confirm, that they were usually done on the same patients. In 1930 just about 700 of each were carried out. Creatinine was less frequently estimated. The lab performed 15 determinations in 1921, a figure that gradually climbed to 443 in 1930. Again it is likely that it was estimated in the same patient at the same time as urea and the NPN.

The measurement of carbohydrate metabolites was intimately related to the introduction of insulin in 1923 and will be dealt with in Chapter 9. There is no doubt, however, of the importance of blood sugars in the lab's establishment of its authority. As already noted, in Edinburgh urine was routinely examined for sugar in the side rooms. No quantitative estimations of sugar in urine were done in the lab in 1921, but 21 quantitative estimations of blood sugar were made in that year and 50 in 1922, after which figures rocketed to 682 in 1923 and, following a small mid-decade fall, rose to 1,197 in 1930 (See Graph 7.6). It is possible many of these estimations were for Murray Lyon's diabetic out-patient clinic. Estimations of urine sugars rose too, but far less than blood. There were also means to determine acetone bodies. These appeared in blood and urine in diabetic acidosis. They were estimated rarely in Edinburgh, although thirty-four urine acetone estimations were done in 1930. The rarity is possibly based on the test being redundant in the clinical situation since the combination of clinical acidosis, sugar in the urine and raised levels of it in the blood, pointed to diabetic acidosis (rather than, say, the acidosis of renal failure). Acetone bodies were certainly tested for in patients in the MRC insulin trial in 1923, but these tests do not appear in the lab's records.

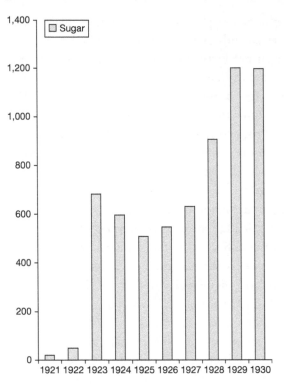

Graph 7.6: Blood sugar estimations 1921–30. Graph by author.

Measurement of substances related to bile and fat metabolism did not take off until mid-decade. One examination of blood for "bile pigment" was carried out in 1922 and one for "fat" the following year. In 1924 fat determinations jumped to twenty-eight and cholesterol appeared at twenty-nine for reasons indicated below. These later slowly and erratically rose to 199 and 65 respectively in 1930. The figures for fat and cholesterol determinations are puzzling since there was little agreement in the 1920s as to the significance of raised or lowered levels of these substances although they were known to vary with diet. Fat was recognized as being raised in diabetes, and cholesterol in certain sorts of nephritis and complete biliary obstruction. Case note evidence of their use is meagre and it is possible that they were performed in relation to research interests. Another test on blood which appeared in mid-decade was the Van den Bergh reaction, which gave what was described as either

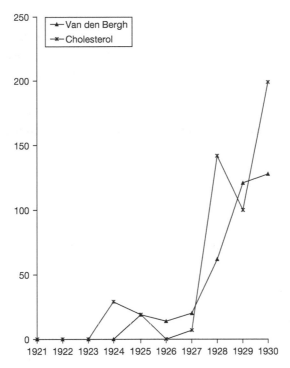

**Graph 7.7: Tests for blood cholesterol and van Den Bergh
reactions 1921–30. Graph by author.**

an *indirect* or *direct* response, allowing the clinician to distinguish between
different sorts of jaundice. Nineteen were done in 1925 and 128 in 1930,
but again case note evidence of its use is slight and the possibility arises
once again that the tests were done in association with research interests
(See Graph 7.7).

The demands placed on the lab raise the question of who its
principal users were. In the first eighteen months of the laboratory's life,
630 specimens were received: 109 from surgeons and 521 from physicians.[74] The latter breakdown is hardly surprising. Nearly all the research
worldwide on the biochemistry of disease in this period had been done
on medical conditions. It is possible too that laboratory challenges to
clinical judgement generally went against the grain of rugged surgical
individualism. As noted in Chapter 3,[75] surgeons at St Thomas's initially
preferred their clinical acumen to blood tests when these were offered

by the hospital's new laboratory. It is striking that, in the first eighteen months of the Edinburgh lab's life, nearly a half of the specimens from the Medical Department of the hospital were sent by Meakins (247 of 521). In fact, nearly two-thirds of the specimens received in the first eighteen months came from three physicians known to be engaged in research.[76] This does not mean they were exploiting the lab's resources for their own research, rather their research interests indicate that they took a biochemical view of patient management and, further, distinctions between research and routine had not been clearly formulated. Other staff, who had backed the lab's establishment, seem to have made little use of it. For example, Edwin Bramwell sent thirteen specimens in 1921.

Figures for 1925–30 tell a similar tale although they also show the increasing demand put on the lab by workers of all sorts. Surgeons contin-ued to send roughly a fifth of the total, but sometimes far less.[77] In 1930 three known researchers in the lab sent more than 1,100 specimens, nearly half the total received.[78] In this year Edwin Bramwell's figures had risen from his first year total of thirteen to nintey-one, a modest usage. The figures for William Ritchie, who became Professor of Medicine in 1928, are not much greater. Bearing in mind that reported statistics ostensibly refer to tests deemed necessary for patient management, not research, what determined the different everyday use of the lab of the two apparent communities of Infirmary physicians—laboratory researchers and non-researchers? Perhaps, more subtly, was there a distinction between those interested in dynamic and physiological problems and others more inter-ested in a case history and morbid anatomical approach to disease? The former were surely more likely to have been the greater users of the lab. There are, unfortunately, no patient records for those known to be doing research in the lab so it is difficult to know what factors determined the large numbers of tests done by them. How, if at all, were research and rou-tine management distinguished? Were laboratory researchers testing more patients than other clinicians or were they performing more tests on indi-vidual cases? That routine and research were not easily distinguished was acknowledged at the time. In 1925 someone, probably Murray Lyon, called to a meeting of the Infirmary Managers dealing with the projected new Rockefeller laboratory recorded: "The question of the separation of rou-tine from research work was touched on and it was agreed that a division between these was exceedingly difficult and perhaps impossible."[79]

One way of addressing this issue is to compare research publications with statistics compiled from routine tests carried out on patients on the wards. The answer that emerges from such an inquiry is that patient management and research were clearly distinguished in many instances. In between, however, and a very large in between it was, the laboratory-minded obviously saw good management as based on extensive biochemical testing, the results of which might well end up as a research publication. To take an obvious example, Murray Lyon requested many tests, mainly for blood sugar, which were performed on samples taken at the diabetic out-patient clinic. The results were used in his publications since Murray Lyon saw blood testing as the proper way to investigate diabetics. He was routinely researching the effects of insulin on diabetic management just as much as he was investigating his patients. Without doubt too the routine BMR determinations done by Davies in 1921 were directed to patient care. They were also the basis of the paper he published with Meakins in January 1922 (see Chapter 8).[80] In one sense, the paper was published as a research claim, in another sense it was published to show that the test was important to good management. This is clear from Davies's report to the MRC of his year's work, October 1921– October 1922. He wrote: "Routine determinations of Basal Metabolic Rate—Prof. Meakins and I have made over 200 determinations in various pathological conditions and expect shortly to publish our results."[81] Lying in a similar grey area were the four cases of familial nephritis, investigated by John Eason and George Malcolm-Smith in 1922 and reported in 1924. Three of the four were brothers and were admitted to the Infirmary with acute renal symptoms. All three had urea concentration tests, a procedure involving the measurement of urine urea before and after a dose of the substance. Between the three of them at least nine estimations of urine urea were carried out. This seems a perfectly legitimate clinical procedure in such cases. However, only three urine urea tests were reported as having been done in the lab that year. The estimations, not a difficult procedure, were probably carried out in the side rooms. The patients also had the NPN in their blood estimated. Again a legitimate examination, but technically more difficult, and these tests are probably included among the 172 NPN estimations reported that year. At any rate Eason and Malcolm-Smith got a publication out of it.[82]

In other instances, it is clear that tests were done on patients purely for research purposes and the examinations which were probably done in the lab were not reported in the annual returns. To take one example: in April 1925 Dorothy Potter published a paper based on eight months' work ending in March 1924 in which she examined the phosphate content of blood in conscious and anaesthetized patients. An Edinburgh graduate, Potter worked as a house surgeon in the Royal Maternity Hospital in 1924 where the clinical aspect of the research was probably carried out. The blood analyses were almost certainly made in the lab (the Maternity Hospital was very near the Infirmary). In November 1924 she submitted a paper to the prestigious *Quarterly Journal of Medicine* from the Department of Therapeutics. Something in the region of one hundred determinations were done as well as about thirty alkali reserve estimations. However, lab numbers reported for both of these tests were negligible or zero in this period. This is hardly surprising. Potter's work was obviously "pure" research since virtually nothing in the testing contributed to patient management.[83]

A paper in the *Edinburgh Medical Journal* of 1925 shows how difficult it is to draw the lines between routine and research, and how different types of physicians used the lab to do different sorts of research. This study was principally authored by A. Logan Turner and came jointly from the Departments of Pathology and Therapeutics. Turner was a distinguished consultant surgeon to the Ear and Throat Department. The paper described four cases of the rare condition xanthomatosis, in which fatty nodules formed just beneath the skin. One of the patients was admitted to the Infirmary for a month in 1923. He had, the paper records, at least nine blood fat estimations and four blood cholesterol tests but only one blood fat estimation was reported by the lab that year and no cholesterol tests at all. But two other patients described in the paper and who were admitted in 1924 had, between them, in excess of thirty blood tests for each of fat and cholesterol. In the same year lab estimations of these substances leaped to twenty-eight and twenty-nine respectively. The figures would certainly seem to relate to these patients, although the correlation is not perfect. One of the co-authors, A. C. White, an Edinburgh graduate with a keen interest in biochemistry, described how one of the patients "was put on a mixture containing sodium sulphate to test the claim put forward by the French school of its decholesterinising powers." The second patient was treated with various hormonal preparations. In both cases, research and management amounted to the same thing.[84] The publication makes the point that the lab could be justifiably used in bedside "care" and research on the same patient. The research itself in this instance was of two sorts although published in the same paper. One was natural historical (the case history), the other physiological (the therapeutic investigations). Possibly the natural historical approach was Turner's and the physiological White's. Physicians could be modern minded in a variety of ways.

Another example spells out the complex relations of research, routine, and varying approaches to clinical medicine. In January 1925, Murray Lyon, William Robson, and A. C. White published on "The Use of Intarvin in Diabetes Mellitus." Intarvin was a commercially synthesized product that was claimed to have an effect on the biochemistry of fatty acid oxidation. The research was, in many ways, very "modern": it was collaborative between clinicians and laboratory workers and involved the trial of a drug of which the actions were predicted on the basis of laboratory work. The Edinburgh study relied on giving the "disagreeable" drug to four diabetics and two normal subjects. The diabetics on standard diets with added Intarvin had repeated measurements made of blood sugar, fat, and acetone, and of urine acetone and sugar. There was no record in the lab reports of acetone in blood or urine being measured in 1924.[85] This then, even though patients were being treated, was perhaps seen as research, not routine work; but the waters remain muddy. It is possible economic as well as intellectual criteria entered the distinction between routine and research in this case. If a grant had been available for the work, although the report does not indicate this, the workers may have distinguished it from routine management in this way. Another feature of this report is that it straddled the old and the new in its methodology. There was an attempt to use a series of patients and "control" them with normals, yet the presentation of the results took the traditional case history form. Other similar studies make the same point about lab use. For example, the serum calcium of a number of patients was investigated in the middle of the decade in a range of patients but not as part of routine management. Hardly any serum calciums appeared in the lab reports at this time. The authors of this study, however, thanked the University for a grant from its Moray Fund and presumably this was used to defray the cost of the tests.[86]

Even when workers were scrupulous in separating routine from research, none the less research interests still entered into the way that laboratory-orientated physicians managed their patients, in the sense that good management was perceived in biochemical terms. In one area— acid–base (alkali) balance—it is quite clear that a small number of workers requested or carried out practically all of the various routine tests. Acid–base balance was central to metabolic studies and was a prime research area through which clinical biochemists promoted their subject in the 1920s. It was the key to many metabolic disorders. A central feature of all metabolic processes was known to be the production of acids and alkalis. The body's maintenance of its acid–base balance was central to physiological regulation. Research indicated that the elimination of the acids produced by metabolism was the mechanism for bringing this about. The blood was consistently alkaline in reaction and its capacity to "mop up" these excess acids was known as its alkali reserve.[87] This "buffering" capacity of the blood, it was broadly agreed, depended on its bicarbonate content.[88] Acidic products were eventually disposed of by excretion in the urine as ammonium salts and phosphates and by the exhalation of carbon dioxide from the lungs.[89]

Various pathological conditions were associated with the excessive retention of acid metabolites. This condition was known as acidosis and was regarded as the biochemical equivalent of the clinical condition called "air hunger." In renal failure, for example, normal body acids accumulated in abnormal amounts. Ketosis (characterized by the presence of ketone or acetone bodies in blood and urine) was a special case of acidosis and described the specific abnormal acids appearing in the blood in diabetic coma. Acidosis was an important concept for the clinical biochemist since it redefined clinical conditions in biochemical terms. Its definition was by no means universally agreed.[90] Rare in ordinary medical circles around 1920, by end of the decade acidosis was meriting extensive technical discussion in textbooks in which chapters on "Diseases of Metabolism" began to appear.[91]

Even though in acidosis normal or abnormal acids accumulated in the blood, the key biochemical feature of the condition was not that the blood became acid (it never did) but the depletion of the alkali reserve. Thus blood and urine tests gave a picture of acidosis but each might look considerably different depending on whether the kidney or some more general metabolic disorder was the cause. In renal disease the normal mechanisms of acid excretion might fail but in diabetic coma they might well be hyperactive. Thus, in renal acidosis, phosphate excretion could be defective and blood levels might rise and urine levels fall.[92] The ratio of ammonia nitrogen to urea nitrogen in the urine was raised in most cases of non-renal acidosis but in the acidosis of nephritis, ammonia nitrogen excretion could be impaired.[93] Tests for these various substances in urine and blood were thus considered important for distinguishing among such disturbances.[94] Carbon dioxide combining power or alkali reserve was measured using venous blood and a "blood gas" apparatus.[95] A safe although laborious way of assessing alkali reserve, however, was not by examining the blood or urine but by sampling and analyzing exhaled gases to measure the so-called alveolar air. Gas analysis of all sorts was a field in which the Department of Therapeutics excelled and many of its publications centred on it.

Acid–base balance was central to Meakins's research interests and Annual Reports of routine tests related to this area strongly correlate with his presence in the Infirmary and, later, with that of other workers with similar interests. Meakins was carrying out biochemical research on human blood, specifically on blood gases, in Edinburgh before the lab opened.[96] He continued this work after its opening and by April 1923 he could report that the department had undertaken a "systematic investigation" of the relation between respiratory symptoms and cardiovascular lesions. These investigations involved measuring the oxygen saturation of the arterial blood (often more than once) in at least twenty RIE patients between 1921 and 1923. Here a practically clear line was drawn between research and normal management, for only three measurements of arterial oxygen saturation were reported in the lab's routine statistics for these years.[97] Similarly a number of oxygen saturation tests were reported as having been done on thyrotoxic patients in 1923, but only one was reported in the statistics.[98] Nevertheless in 1921 forty-two estimations of alkali reserve were reported, the maximum done at the beginning of the decade.[99] Numbers fell to four in 1924, the year Meakins left, and none were done in 1925.[100]

That alkali reserve was usually considered a research investigation was indicated in a lab report of 1925: "Blood gas analysis and determination of the blood alkali reserve come more properly in the category of research, but requests are occasionally received by this department for the routine carrying out of these procedures. The necessary apparatus is installed in the laboratory and principally used by the staff in their own research work."[101] It seems highly likely that it was members of the Therapeutics Department who requested these routine estimations since they saw them as part of proper patient management. By contrast Bramwell, not strongly inclined to physiological problem solving, never requested a single estimation of alkali reserve in the whole decade.

Ammonia nitrogen, a significant presence in the urine in acidosis in non-renal conditions, was also present in blood in small quantities but it showed considerable variation and it was generally agreed there was no correlation of its levels with particular pathological states. A text of 1924 declared it "of little clinical interest."[102] None the less seven estimations of its blood levels were reported from the lab in 1921. Someone obviously saw them as necessary for good patient management. The number probably relates to Meakins's interests since forty-eight estimations of urine ammonia nitrogen were carried out in 1921, after which numbers fell to zero by 1924.[103] Similar considerations might explain attention to chlorides. Chlorides were present in great quantities in blood and their concentration was crucial to the performance of the vital functions. Changing gas tensions in the blood were known to be associated with changing chloride concentrations, which were thus central to the acid–base equilibrium. Chlorides were retained or excreted abnormally in conditions affecting the overall ion concentration in the blood, such as vomiting. Most workers seemed to agree that there was diminished excretion of chloride in fevers, notably pneumonia, and in nephritis.[104] In 1925 Meakins reported the "well-known retention of chlorine ions" in lobar pneumonia and added "much has yet to be done to elucidate these problems."[105] On the whole, however, estimating chloride concentration in blood or urine had no important diagnostic or monitoring function. Yet the lab reported sixty-nine blood chloride estimations in 1921, although after this interest in them generally lessened. (See Graph 7.8) It seems certain that the relatively large number of routine determinations carried out were related to Meakins's research interests.

As noted, after Meakins's departure measures of alkali reserve virtually disappeared from the statistics: very few were carried out in the late twenties, then numbers leaped up in 1930 and 1931 (See Graph 7.9). There was a definite research link here although, once again, since these

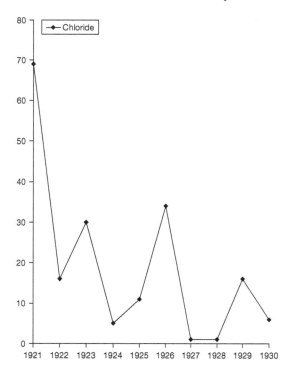

Graph 7.8: Blood chloride determinations 1921–30. Graph by author.

alkali reserve levels were reported as being done for the Infirmary, the physicians involved must have seen them as essential to patient care. In May 1930 Derrick Dunlop, a physiological assistant in the lab since 1929, applied to the MRC for a research grant. He reported he was carrying out studies on fat metabolism with the lab's biochemist C. P. Stewart on "the carbon dioxide combining power of the blood." He was also working on "acidosis in nephritis."[106] Dunlop, however, although medically qualified, had no clinical appointment at the Infirmary and Stewart obviously did not since he was a biochemist. That is, neither had access to patients. What were almost certainly the results of this research were published along with Murray Lyon in two papers in 1931, the first of which appeared in February. Presumably most of the biochemistry for this report was done in 1930. Briefly, patients with nephritis were given various acid and alkaline diets and in some instances medication. Each patient had the chemistry of his or her urine and blood monitored on

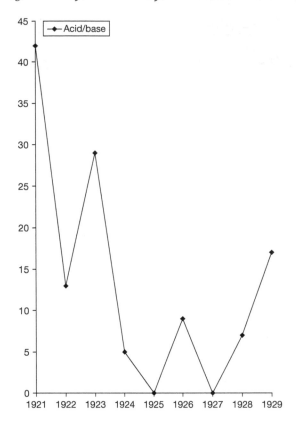

Graph 7.9: Tests related to the biochemistry of respiration and acid–base balance 1921–29. After 1929 numbers increase very sharply. Tests include those for "alveolar air" (carried out nine times in 1923 and once in 1924 only). Graph by author.

about eight occasions. Measures were made of, amongst other things, urine acidity, blood chloride and calcium, and the alkali reserve. What is impossible to figure out is which, if any, of these tests were deemed routine and reported accordingly. The lab reports for 1930 contain no record of urine acidity testing and only six blood chlorides. Calcium estimations, however, jumped to 88 from the 53 of the previous year, but most striking was the leap of alkali reserve from 16 to 151.[107] The final series included seventeen cases and was published in November 1931. Two "illustrative" cases described had, in the one instance, eleven, and in the other, ten alkali reserve estimations. In this year alkali reserve measurements rose to 195.[108]

Over the decade what emerges can scarcely be called a pattern, but on many occasions known research interests of lab workers were associated with a corresponding rise in routine test statistics, although never with an exact correlation. Andrew Doig was a student who started work in pathology in 1940 and remembers:

> If anybody is [sic] considering a research project involving the clinical laboratory's routine examination they would be asked to contact the head of the Clinical Laboratory. In my day, you would go and see Professor Whitby and ask him if you could do this and how many you intend to do. He would say whether it could be done. However, it if was a very expensive test and they wanted a lot carried out, he would ask you to try and get a research grant and reimburse the laboratory. Or, when you are applying to the MRC, for instance, tell them that we'll do it but we need the money to carry out the tests.[109]

There were thus various communities of physicians and others using the lab: some for "pure" research purposes at the infirmary, some for research which also constituted management, and others who seem to have used it in a limited way and solely for patient management. The exemplary case here is Edwin Bramwell, whom I discuss in Chapter 9. First, however, I explore the science done in the lab.

Notes

1. A. Logan Turner, *Story of a Great Hospital. The Royal Infirmary of Edinburgh 1729–1929* (Edinburgh: Oliver and Boyd Ltd., 1937), 329–30.

2. "Behind the Operating Theatre in the Surgical Clinic there is a Pathological Laboratory fully equipped for histological and bacteriological work." "University Clinic, Edinburgh: Surgery," [n.d., ? c.1923], folder 5, box 1, series 405, RG 1.1, Rockefeller Foundation Archives, RAC.

3. Richard Bright, *Reports of Medical Cases, Selected with a View of Illustrating the Symptoms and Cure of Diseases by a Reference to Morbid Anatomy*, 2 vols. (London: Longman, Rees, Orme, and Green, 1827–31).

4. Robert Kohler has explored some of the ways in which biochemistry was institutionalized at this time in Europe and America: in universities as an autonomous basic

science, or sheltered in chemistry and physiology departments; in other institutions such as hospitals and research institutes. By 1920, independent chairs were still rare; lectureships in physiology departments were the rule. Robert E. Kohler, *From Medical Chemistry to Biochemistry: The Making of a Biomedical Discipline* (Cambridge: Cambridge University Press, 1982).

5. W. D. Foster and J. L. Pinniger, "History of Pathology at St Thomas's Hospital, London," *Medical History* 7 (1963): 330–47. See also, Louis Rosenfeld, *Four Centuries of Clinical Chemistry* (Amsterdam: Gordon and Breach Science Publishers, 1999).

6. The novelty (and marginality) of the discipline can be measured by the fact that when laboratory assistants formed their association in 1912, it was called "The Pathological and Bacteriological Laboratory Assistants Association." Their first exams took place in 1921 and comprised pathological and bacteriological technique (including haematology and serology). It was not until 1929 that "pathological chemistry technique" was included. "Pathological Chemistry Technique," *The Laboratory Journal* 10 (1929): 271.

7. W. W. Taylor, *Practical Chemical Physiology* (London: Edward Arnold, 1922). Interleaved copy at EUL.

8. Professor A. R. Simpson, "Ward Journal, Ward 12," May 1875–July 1875, LHB1/129/6/11, LHSA, EUL.

9. Of albumen, the author of a clinical textbook of the period observed: "Where no test-tube is available at the bedside, it is useful to remember that the urine may be boiled in an iron spoon, and a little vinegar used instead of acetic acid." Thomas Dixon Savill, *A System of Clinical Medicine*, 5th ed. (London: Edward Arnold, 1919), 394. The author did, however, give small print instructions for quantitative detection.

10. Ibid., 391.

11. Andrew Fergus Hewat, *Examination of the Urine and other Clinical Side-Room Methods*, 6th ed. (Edinburgh: E. & S. Livingstone, 1921).

12. Savill, *A System of Clinical Medicine*, 912.

13. In Edwin Bramwell's case notes (see Chapter 9) records of Wassermann tests being done in the Bacteriology Department do not appear until 1926.

14. Andrew Doig, Edited transcript of interview with Helen Coyle, November 20, 1997.

15. Albert P. Mathews, *Physiological Chemistry: A Textbook and Manual for Students* (London: Baillière, Tindall and Cox, 1916), Preface [1915].

16. J. J. R. Macleod, *Physiology and Biochemistry in Modern Medicine*, 3rd ed. (London: Henry Kimpton, 1921), 571.

17. Ibid., 633.

18. Ibid., 647. The remainder was the so-called "rest N" or undetermined nitrogen. A good overview is Hugh MacLean, *Modern Methods in the Diagnosis and Treatment of Renal Disease* (London, Constable, 1921). MacLean has a slightly different classification of the constituents of NPN.

19. Macleod, *Physiology and Biochemistry*, 647–55.

20. James Campbell Todd, *Clinical Diagnosis: A Manual of Laboratory Methods*, 4th ed. (Philadelphia, London: W. B. Saunders, 1918), 242–48; William Osler and Thomas McCrae, *The Principles and Practice of Medicine*, 9th ed. (New York, London: D. Appleton and Company, 1920) 447.

21. Macleod, *Physiology and Biochemistry*, 724.

22. For some excellent examples of the use of instruments to change and embody disease concepts see Keith Wailoo, *Drawing Blood: Technology and Disease Identity in Twentieth-Century America* (Baltimore: The Johns Hopkins University Press, 1997).

23. Jonathan Meakins, "Autobiography," 68, 867/51, OLHM.

24. P. N. Panton, *Clinical Pathology* (London: J. & A. Churchill, 1913), Preface.

25. Ibid., 98, 99.

26. Olga Amsterdamska, "Chemistry in the Clinic: The Research Career of Donald Dexter Van Slyke," in *Molecularizing Biology: New Practices and Alliances, 1910s–1970s*, ed. Soraya de Chadarevian and Harmke Kamminga (Amsterdam: Harwood Academic, 1998), 47–82.

27. Todd, *Clinical Diagnosis*, 272.

28. R. B. H. Gradwohl and A. J. Blaivas, *The Newer Methods of Blood and Urine Chemistry*, 2nd ed. (London: Henry Kimpton, 1920), 17.

29. Raphael Isaacs and David S. Hachen, "Chemistry of the Blood," in *Clinical Laboratory Diagnosis: Designed for the Use of Students and Practitioners of Medicine*, ed. Roger Morris (New York and London: D. Appleton, 1923), 367.

30. "Scotland: Clinical Meeting of the Edinburgh Branch," *British Medical Journal* 2 (1922): 368. The demonstrators were the lab's biochemist, C. R. Harington and two Infirmary physicians, George Malcolm-Smith and John Comrie. H. W. Davies, the physiologist, also demonstrated estimations of basal metabolic rate.

31. Walter Langdon Brown, "Changing Standpoints in Metabolic Diseases: Diabetes, Nephritis, Jaundice," *British Medical Journal* 2 (1924): 1119–22.

32. This relative neglect of blood biochemistry around 1920 does not mean of course that biochemically-minded clinicians at the RIE were not carrying out blood analyses before the lab opened. In 1916 Harry Rainy, an Infirmary physician, had read a paper at the Royal Society of Edinburgh discussing the relative values of the various ways of estimating blood glucose. Harry Rainy, "The Significance and Treatment of Glycosuria," *The Transactions of the Medico-Chirurgical Society of Edinburgh* 36 (1922): 46–68. Murray Lyon reported a case admitted in November 1920 in which the blood fats were estimated. D. Murray Lyon, "Xanthoma Diabeticorum: With Report of a Case," *Edinburgh Medical Journal* 38 (1922): 168–73. These tests were stated to have been done by the Therapeutic Department's biochemist C. R. Harington in an unspecified place, possibly Barger's lab.

33. Taylor, *Practical Chemical Physiology*, 67–68.

34. Sydney W. Cole, *Practical Physiological Chemistry*, 6th ed. (Cambridge: Heffer, 1920), 249–64.

35. See Hewat, *Examination of the Urine*. Nothing had changed by the 7th ed., 1926.

36. Although MacLean seemed to consider estimation of blood urea a simple procedure. MacLean, *Modern Methods*, 40.

37. Todd, an American author, in 1918 had assumed that the blood biochemistry tests he described would be within the capability of the ordinary practitioner. No details of how to estimate substances were given, the reader being referred to the "printed matter" accompanying commercial colorimeters. Clearly, manufacturing companies had targeted GPs in America. Todd, *Clinical Diagnosis*, 372–73. Texts appeared in America describing blood tests that could be carried out by the general practitioner. See, for example, Willard J. Stone, *Blood Chemistry, Colorimetric Methods for the General Practitioner: With Clinical Comments and Dietary Suggestions* (New York: Paul B. Hoeber, 1923).

38. Hewat, *Examination of the Urine*, 17–18.

39. Frederick Taylor, *The Practice of Medicine*, 11th ed. (London: J & A Churchill, 1918), Preface, 865–74, 1029–33, quotes at 880, 871.

40. Ibid., 803, 1039, 804.

41. Osler and McCrae, *The Principles and Practice of Medicine*, 690, 703, 428.

42. O. Folin and H. Wu, "A System of Blood Analysis," *Journal of Biological Chemistry* 38 (1919): 81–110.

43. Osler and McCrae, *The Principles and Practice of Medicine*, 871.

44. Robert Hutchison and Harry Rainy, *Clinical Methods: A Guide to the Practical Study of Medicine*, 6th ed. (London: Cassell, 1916); 7th ed., 1920; 9th ed., Robert Hutchison and Donald Hunter, 1929.

45. Equivalent to 75p in decimal currency.

46. The staffing of the lab can be reconstructed from the Minutes of the Advisory Committee. "Scrap-Book of the RIE Biochemical Laboratory," boxes 1 and 2, RCPE.

47. In the following I give an overview of the amount and variety of work done in the lab 1921–30 derived from the Annual Reports, "Scrap-Book of the RIE Biochemical Laboratory," box 2, RCPE. There are anomalies. Sometimes Edwin Bramwell's case notes contain test results in years in which no such test was reported by the lab. The tests may have been done at the College of Physicians' lab or in the side room or simply not recorded in the lab's annual returns. The figures are so small compared to the number of tests done overall, that their absence is insignificant.

48. Presumably, however, the lab did not operate on Sundays and statutory holidays. Nor is there evidence of emergency "out of hours" determinations. The lab seems not to have routinely offered a service to patients other than those in the Infirmary. Tests were almost certainly done on out-patients. Monthly figures belie the figure of 396 that suggests an average arrival of slightly more than one specimen a day (without Sundays). Obviously the small number of specimens received (eight) in the lab's first operational month, January, is not surprising; but against the overall rising trend (peaking at seventy-one in November) numbers fell in June and July. In 1925, the only other year for which monthly figures exist, estimations, although gradually rising, were fairly consistent through the year.

49. In 1921, the numbers of blood specimens (217) and examinations (429) greatly outnumbered those for urine (61 specimens; 204 examinations). After 1921 only

numbers for the total of all specimens together (blood, urine, and others) exist, although it is clear blood specimens made up a large majority of that total.

50. This was not strictly a biochemical test but I include it here since it was done in the lab.

51. Clinicians collected the specimens and sent them to the lab with a biochemistry request form that had a blank space for specific requests to be inserted. No test was done routinely. Clinicians not only had the freedom to stipulate the determination they required but (in some instances) they could nominate the means to carry it out. For example, the 1926 laboratory statistics on cerebrospinal fluid (CSF) tests showed that there had been requests both for "globulin" and more specifically for "Pandy's reaction" (then usually regarded as the most delicate of several possible tests for globulin).

52. RIE, Minutes of Medical Managers' Committee, "Consideration of a Report from the Advisory Committee of the Bio-chemical Laboratory," August 7, 1922, LHSA, LHB1/1/58, EUL.

53. J. Fayrer [Superintendent] to Meakins, June 2, 1922, "Scrap-Book of the RIE Biochemical Laboratory," box 2, RCPE.

54. Minutes of the Advisory Committee of the Biochemical Laboratory, July 26, 1922, "Scrap-Book of the RIE Biochemical Laboratory," box 2, RCPE.

55. Report from the Advisory Committee of the Biochemical Laboratory, July 26, 1922, "Scrap-Book of the RIE Biochemical Laboratory," box 2, RCPE.

56. RIE, Minutes of Medical Managers' Committee, "Consideration of a Report from the Advisory Committee of the Bio-chemical Laboratory," August 7, 1922, LHSA, LHB1/1/58, EUL.

57. Archibald was taken over in November 1922; his wages increased to 30s. per week and, after six months, to 40s. The lab boy, John Flet, got 12s. 6d. per week and the Technical Assistant, Robert McMartin, got 20s. (£1). See "Technical Assistants," 1926, "Scrap-Book of the RIE Biochemical Laboratory," box 2, RCPE.

58. Minutes of the Advisory Committee of the Biochemical Laboratory, March 13, 1925, "Scrap-Book of the RIE Biochemical Laboratory, box 2, RCPE.

59. Hewat, *Examination of the Urine*, 17, 22.

60. This figure comprises blood: urea nitrogen 700, NPN 705, creatinine 443; urine: total nitrogen 118, urea nitrogen 133.

61. Todd, *Clinical Diagnosis*, 135.

62. Morris, *Clinical Laboratory Diagnosis*, 8.

63. Hewat, *Examination of the Urine*, 17; MacLean, *Modern Methods*, 53.

64. Ibid., 42; Hewat, *Examination of the Urine*, 16; 7th ed. (1926), 17.

65. Ibid., 7th ed. (1926), 17.

66. MacLean, *Modern Methods*, 53.

67. Ibid., 44.

68. Ibid., 40–41.

69. Folin and Wu, "A System of Blood Analysis," 91.

70. Gradwohl and Blaivas, *The Newer Methods of Blood and Urine Chemistry*, 274, 288, 289.

71. For a tabular taxonomy see ibid., 276–77.

72. MacLean, *Modern Methods*, 40, considered uric acid, urea and creatinine to accumulate, in that order, in chronic nephritis. Although urate deposition in joints was the agreed culprit in gout, blood uric acid levels, because of their variability, were not regarded as helpful diagnostically. See O. L. V. De Wesselow, *The Chemistry of the Blood in Clinical Medicine* (London: Ernest Benn, 1924), 177.

73. Gradwohl and Blaivas, *The Newer Methods of Blood and Urine Chemistry*, 278.

74. Figures on users are extant for 1921, the first half of 1922, the second half of 1925, and all the years thereafter.

75. See p. 46–47.

76. Besides Meakins, Francis Darby Boyd, Professor of Clinical Medicine, sent sixty-two specimens in 1921 and none in the first half of 1922, the year in which he died. John Eason sent none in 1921 and eighty-nine in the first half of 1922. Eason was an Ordinary Physician.

77. In 1929, for example, of the more than 2,000 specimens received, surgeons sent just over 200.

78. Murray Lyon, John Eason, and John Comrie. Murray Lyon's figures were presumably inflated by diabetic out-patient tests.

79. Rockefeller Meeting, February 5, 1925, "Scrap-Book of the RIE Biochemical Laboratory," box 1, folder 4, RCPE.

80. J. Meakins and H. W. Davies, "Basal Metabolic Rate: Its Determination and Clinical Significance," *Edinburgh Medical Journal* 28 (1922): 1–15.

81. Davies to Fletcher, August 19 [? mistake for October], 1922, FD1/1015, 49222, PRO.

82. J. Eason and G. L. Malcolm Smith, "Hereditary and Familial Nephritis," *The Lancet* 2 (1924): 639–46. Smith possibly hyphenated his name after this date.

83. Dorothy G. E. Potter, "Changes in the Blood in Anaesthesia," *Quarterly Journal of Medicine* 18 (1925): 261–73.

84. A. Logan Turner, J. Davidson, and A. C. White, "Xanthomatosis: Some Aspects of its Blood Chemistry and Pathology," *Edinburgh Medical Journal* 32 (1925): 153–74. As with so many published papers in these years, the exact numbers of tests done on the patients who are described are hard to quantify.

85. D. Murray Lyon, W. Robson, and A. C. White, "The Use of Intarvin in Diabetes Mellitus," *British Medical Journal* 1 (1925): 207–10.

86. G. H. Percival and C. P. Stewart, "Pathological Variations in the Serum Calcium," *Quarterly Journal of Medicine* 19 (1926): 235–48. The Fund was an endowment by the Earl of Moray for the promotion of original research.

87. Also known as the hydrogen ion or H-ion concentration.

88. Donald Dexter Van Slyke and Glenn E. Cullen in a much-cited paper defined bicarbonate concentration as alkaline reserve, "Studies of Acidosis. I The Bicarbonate Concentration of the Blood Plasma; Its Significance and its Determination as a Measure of Acidosis," *Journal of Biological Chemistry* 30 (1917): 289–346. Not everyone agreed this was a sufficient definition and since the 1920s other factors have been implicated.

89. Normal urine was acid in reaction. See, for example, Todd, *Clinical Diagnosis*, 5th ed. (1924), 136–37 for contemporary views of acid excretion in urine. A massive literature on acid–base balance appeared in the 1920s and cannot be recited here.

90. In fact the term acidosis had been coined at the beginning of the century to describe what was later called ketosis. One expert in 1921 described the term acidosis as being surrounded by "chaos." MacLean, *Modern Methods*, 10. An Edinburgh clinical tutor in 1921 described acidosis as an "obscure condition." Hewat, *Examination of the Urine*, 11.

91. A general medical text of 1918 only gave one reference to acidosis in the index to a chapter on "Rare Constituents of the Urine" but there was no discussion at the appropriate page. A revised edition of 1922 discussed it in some biochemical detail (albeit in the same place). Savill, *A System of Clinical Medicine*, 401; 6th ed. (1922), 401. Taylor in 1918 recognized the acidosis of diabetes and the concurrent rise in urinary ammonia. Taylor, *The Practice of Medicine*, 1038. Osler and McCrae in 1920 discussed acidosis at some length, *The Principles and Practice of Medicine*, 445–47, 702. For a volume with a chapter on metabolic disease see, J. J. Conybeare "Diseases of Metabolism," in *A Textbook of Medicine*, ed. J. J. Conybeare (Edinburgh: E. & S. Livingstone, 1929), 284–327.

92. MacLean, *Modern Methods*, 6–8.

93. Ibid., 10; Jonathan Meakins and H. Whitridge Davies, *Respiratory Function in Disease* (Edinburgh: Oliver and Boyd, 1925), 123.

94. Andrew Watson Sellards, *The Principles of Acidosis and Clinical Methods for its Study* (Cambridge, MA: Harvard University Press, 1917), 9–10; Medical Research Council, *The Acid–Base Equilibrium of the Blood* (London: HMSO, 1923); Meakins and Davies, *Respiratory Function*, 120–21.

95. See Poul Astrup and John W. Severinghaus, *The History of Blood Gases, Acids and Bases* (Copenhagen: Munksgaard, 1986).

96. For example he published a number of papers on oxygen saturation of human blood obtained by radial artery puncture. Among others these included one tabulating the data obtained in "various normal and abnormal conditions." J. Meakins and H. W. Davies, "Observations on the Gases in Human Arterial and Venous Blood," *Journal of Pathology and Bacteriology* 23 (1920): 451–61. I discuss this paper from a different perspective in the next chapter. In the same year he was also measuring the oxygen saturation of patients with pulmonary lesions (almost certainly on his wards) to determine the value of oxygen therapy. J. Meakins, "Observations on the Gases in Human Arterial Blood in Certain Pathological Pulmonary Conditions, and their Treatment with Oxygen," *Journal of Pathology and Bacteriology* 34 (1921): 79–90.

97. J. Meakins, Lucien Dautrebande, and W. J. Fetter, "The Influence of Circulatory Disturbances on the Gaseous Exchange of the Blood. IV. The Blood Gases and Circulation Rate in Cases of Mitral Stenosis," *Heart* 10 (1923): 153–78.

98. H. Whitridge Davies, Jonathan Meakins and Jane Sands, "The Influence of Circulatory Disturbances on the Gaseous Exchange of the Blood. V. The Blood Gases and Circulation Rate in Hyperthyroidism," *Heart* 11 (1924): 299–307.

99. This was the total of twenty-two tests for alkaline reserve and twenty for carbon dioxide combining power, which was considered the same thing.

100. The 1924 figures comprised one alkali reserve and three bicarbonate reserves.

101. "Blood gas analysis," [? August 1, 1923], "Scrap-Book of the RIE Biochemical Laboratory," box 2, RCPE.

102. Wesselow, *The Chemistry of the Blood*, 24.

103. Urine ammonia nitrogen peaked again in 1927–28 only to disappear at the end of the decade, suggesting a research interest.

104. However, this was detectable by fairly simple side room testing. See, for example, Todd, *Clinical Diagnosis*, 126.

105. Meakins and Davies, *Respiratory Function*, 237. Simplified methods for determining urine chlorides were being described about this time. Morris, *Clinical Laboratory Diagnosis*, 21.

106. Derrick Dunlop, "Application for a Research Grant," May 23, 1930, FD1/1017, 49222, PRO.

107. D. M. Lyon, D. M. Dunlop, and C. P. Stewart, "The Effect of Acidic and Basic Diets in Chronic Nephritis," *Edinburgh Medical Journal* 38 (1931): 87–108.

108. D. M. Lyon, D. M. Dunlop, and C. P. Stewart, "The Alkaline Treatment of Chronic Nephritis," *The Lancet* 2 (1931): 1009–13.

109. Andrew Doig, Edited transcript of interview with Helen Coyle, November 20, 1997.

8

A UNIVERSITY LABORATORY IN A HOSPITAL

The Department of Therapeutics used the lab to achieve high academic visibility in three ways: through the "pure" research of basic scientists, through the studies of clinicians who combined bedside observations with bench research, and through the joint investigations of both groups. By the 1920s a background in research was essential to constructing a career in academic medicine. It could also be used to further a future in private medical practice since it might enhance the possibility of obtaining a hospital appointment and hence a higher public profile. Creating a prestigious academic department of medicine in Britain was not easy in these years. Basic problems of administration and conditions of employment had to be sorted out. A model of collaborative work and attributions of seniority had to be agreed on. In Edinburgh, the Infirmary Managers and clinical staff had to be convinced that a powerful professorial unit was a good thing. The University would of course be sympathetic to promoting academic excellence but that did not mean it could be relied on for limitless economic support. Outside agencies, notably the RF and MRC, had to be enrolled.

Making an academic career in medicine at this time was extremely difficult and most of those clinicians using the lab probably did so to improve their prospects in regular practice. Money was the problem. By the 1920s scientific staff in non-clinical departments such as medical chemistry were paid by universities to teach and research. Meakins's scientific staff in the lab were paid by the University, in this case largely to do research. The University staff in clinical medicine, working on the wards of the Infirmary, were paid by the University to teach. The Infirmary paid no salaries. If Infirmary staff did research it was in their own time and largely at their own expense. A few funding possibilities, however, did exist. First, and most important, was the MRC which could be approached for personal expenses grants. These were used to free younger clinicians (almost invariably those active in the lab) from taking on additional duties such as extra-mural teaching. They were also used to supplement the University salary of full-time research workers in the lab. The MRC also provided equipment grants, usually of £100, for specific projects. The University had various fellowships, scholarships, bursaries, and grants in aid of research. A young man or woman wishing to spend a year or more in full-time academic medicine could apply for one of these scarce fellowships or one of the few offered by philanthropic organizations.[1] Even one of these might need to be supplemented by teaching.

The history of the lab in the 1920s was not one of the continual progress of academic medicine: far from it. In the first part of the decade, under Meakins, there was a broad but relatively coherent research programme. It turned on the investigation of physiological problems, especially of metabolism, in health and disease. Ambitious and able young workers were attracted. There seems to have been a good collaborative atmosphere in the lab. Meakins had the backing of the RF and the MRC. Under Murray Lyon the coherence of the research programme fragmented. Few workers with the interests or of the scientific calibre of those enrolled by Meakins were attracted. Indeed, most of Meakins's recruits left. Murray Lyon's programme was closer to the clinic than the lab and to pathological anatomy than to physiological chemistry. It is hard to disentangle these preferences from personality factors in the lab's relative decline. But decline there was. There were definite episodes of jealousy. The support of the Rockefeller and MRC withered: in fact it turned to hostility. Although some aspects of the change are attributable to Murray Lyon himself, the culture of Edinburgh medicine as a whole needs examining.

Certainly in Meakins's eyes, if the lab were to become prominent its mission was going to be research. Part of the lab's original remit was provision for "Organised investigations by members of the Honorary Staff, by the Assistants of the Professors of Therapeutics, of Clinical Medicine, and of Clinical Surgery, and by other persons nominated by the Honorary Staff." Meakins was to be responsible "for the allotment of places and providing ordinary facilities for workers." None the less he did not have autocratic power, since the rules decreed "a standing Advisory Committee shall be constituted which shall determine as to the suitability of applicants to work in the Laboratory." To gain access to the lab "All applicants for research places . . . shall be in writing, and addressed to the Director, accompanied by an outline of the work proposed, and by details regarding any special apparatus required." Although the "ordinary apparatus and material required in the Laboratory shall be supplied from grants made to the professor of Therapeutics . . . Any special apparatus or material required for a particular investigation shall be supplied by the worker."[2] As already observed, besides economic hindrances to research work the Infirmary Managers placed an "absolute ban . . . on experimental animals" within the hospital.[3]

Animal work, however, was important to Meakins in his push to develop a place for the lab in general (and his own lab in particular) as a major institution in the advancement of modern medicine. A great deal of animal experiment was done by members of the department either in the University or at the College of Physicians. Drug development and assessment was an important part of this work. In the 1920s this was done in several ways. Individual clinicians might try out new agents on one or many patients; several clinicians at one or many centres might collaborate in such "trials". In addition basic scientists might be enrolled to determine the chemical composition of drugs, to standardize them by chemical and biological methods, and to determine their mode of action by animal experiment. Pharmaceutical companies might also be involved. There was little consensus as to the best means to test and assess therapeutic efficacy, or universal recognition of authorities that might be trusted to carry out such testing.[4] The MRC made many attempts to regulate the introduction of new drugs and their testing and use. In the case of insulin it was remarkably successful (at least at first).

In Edinburgh Meakins was keen to draw attention to laboratory work as the basis of what was described as "rational therapeutics"—that is, therapy based on physiological knowledge primarily gained through animal experiment. This was an approach that had its critics, first among whom were the antivivisectionists; but doubts were also raised in medical scientific circles as to whether results obtained from animals could be extrapolated to humans. This criticism had a substantial history in clinical medicine and was often linked to anxieties about the importance that some attached to experimental physiology in general.[5] Although researchers in Meakins's lab seemed to have freedom to pursue their own interests it was not the site of random experimentation. Workers' interests overlapped with those of Meakins. A relatively coherent philosophy of drug evaluation was being created and presented to the medical, scientific, and, to some extent, the generally educated world at large.

Meakins was not slow off the mark to pursue his experimental work in Edinburgh. It is impossible to be exact but something like fifty plus papers appeared from the lab during his directorship. By the end of the decade well over 120 papers had appeared and of course many of these were studies done during Meakins's tenure but published after his departure. Much of the work that was done after he left was carried out by his appointees and perpetuated his concerns. In sum the lab had his imprint on it for much of the decade. Studies were carried out on normal subjects (lab workers and students) and on patients. In one apparently rare instance patients were thanked for their "willing co-operation" in undergoing procedures "knowing them to be of a non-therapeutic nature."[6] How often patients knew they were taking part in experimental procedures let alone thanked for doing so is obviously unascertainable. In one instance, patients who had no disorder of the circulatory system had their circulation rate measured but it is not recorded if they were informed of the procedure they were undergoing.[7] Meakins obviously enjoyed collaborating and encouraging it in others. To make a career in academic medicine then, just as today, it was necessary to publish. Papers from lab workers appeared in a range of journals, from high-powered research periodicals to more didactic works. It is notable that much of the research done by lab workers reappeared in different forms in different journals.

The work of the lab in the early years was stamped with Meakins's interests. Studies on respiration and its relation to the circulation and the acid–base balance of the blood poured out. The imperative behind this was the Oxygen Committee of the MRC. Related to these specific interests was a more general concern with how physiological integration was affected, especially by the endocrine system. Integration was a very important post-war concern for both scientific and more general cultural reasons. Speaking at a meeting on mental science in July 1920 Meakins observed it was difficult to see the way ahead in pathophysiology because "the function of no one organ can be considered an isolated phenomenon unto itself, but all the intimate and intricate co-ordinations which are so beautifully balanced in health must be considered in this light when we are dealing with disease."[8] Such an approach is scarcely surprising in a man who had endeared himself to J. S. Haldane, undoubtedly the most famous British exponent of a holist physiology even before the First World War.[9]

Not only was creating a sound research-based rationale for therapeutics important to Meakins and his team, preaching this message to clinicians was also significant. This theme was particularly pronounced in the case of oxygen therapy. Historians have shown that pre-war physicians thought little of oxygen therapy. During the war physiologists who had recently developed an expanded understanding of respiratory exchange began to have access to patients, that is, to gassed soldiers. These physiologists vigorously defended oxygen therapy on scientific grounds, devising new methods for administering the gas.[10] After the war the therapy was an important vehicle through which departments, like that of Meakins, actively promoted the place of clinical science in medicine, many older physicians still not being convinced of the value of the therapy. A paper by two of Meakins's disciples appearing from the department in 1925 made this version of the history quite clear: "During and since the war, owing to intensive study of anoxaemia in aviators and in gassed men, and to the introduction of efficient methods of oxygen administration, most of the older misconceptions have been swept away and the gas has attained an assured place as a valuable and life-saving therapeutic agent."[11] Meakins of course had been deeply involved in this wartime work.

From the beginning one of the most vociferous supporters of the new approaches to oxygen therapy was the Medical Research Committee and, in turn, its successor, the Council (MRC). Also interested was the

Department of Scientific and Industrial Research (DSIR) the MRC's equivalent for science. After the war the MRC set up the Clinical Uses of Oxygen Committee of which Meakins was a member. The first meeting of the Committee was held in March 1920 at the MRC's headquarters in Buckingham Street, off the Strand. It was agreed that Meakins would work on a number of things including oxygen saturation of the blood in various conditions, and the best means for administering oxygen.[12] The Committee provided grants to study the subject. Meakins had an expenses grant of up to £100 per annum.[13] Guy's Hospital Medical School and Glasgow University also received money. Rather than address the Edinburgh work on oxygen in one place I will unfold it gradually as I examine the work of Meakins and his successors.

Meakins, as observed, was keen on collaboration and significantly, nearly all of the twelve papers solely authored by him while in Edinburgh were addresses or pedagogical pieces and not strictly research papers at all. Having arrived in the second half of 1919 he began to collaborate almost immediately and sent off a research paper on gases in the human blood in May 1920.[14] It was jointly written with Harold Whitridge Davies, a recent medical graduate from Adelaide who was at this time a research student at New College, Oxford, working in J. S. Haldane's private laboratory.[15] The gaseous content of normal arterial and venous blood obtained by puncture was measured, as was the content under various artificial circumstances (such as during oxygen inhalation). The gaseous content in a number of diseases was also reported. The evidence suggests that this work was done in the two centres, Davies working on normal subjects in Oxford and Meakins studying infirmary patients.[16] Meakins had not met Davies, although he certainly knew of him for Haldane wrote to Meakins in December 1918 about some research and that he had written "at once to Davis [sic]."[17] In June 1919, perhaps having forgotten his earlier letter, Haldane wrote "Davis [sic], a young Australian medical officer, is now working with us."[18] Davies was obviously a young man of immense promise. It is not clear when he became committed to physiology (particularly respiratory physiology). Perhaps he never intended to gain a position as a physician (although he did practise medicine as a captain in the war in France). A medical degree, however, was still an important route into professional physiology. Recommendation by Haldane was high praise and perhaps the joint work with Meakins was, in effect, a trial for one of the University Assistant posts that were to be created in the Department of Therapeutics and based in the lab.[19] If it was a trial, Davies passed with flying colours, for in May 1920 the Medical Faculty approved Meakins's recommendation that Davies be appointed to such a position.[20] Meakins had begun to build around himself a cadre of physiologically-minded physicians and scientists. Davies's report to Fletcher in 1924 of his work in Edinburgh reveals the new approaches of this period. He said he was "investigating the physiological disturbances in clinical cases."[21]

Davies took up his appointment in January 1921. He was paid £300 per annum by the University. He had no clinical position in the RIE although he does seem to have had access to Meakins's patients. He probably did no private practice. He was a young man with no clinical reputation and would have had great difficulty attracting patients. Apart from routine estimations of BMRs he was engaged in full-time research. In mid-1921 Meakins described Davies's salary to Fletcher as "not what one would call munificent."[22] Meakins obtained a personal grant for him of £100 per annum from the MRC.[23] Fletcher was particularly keen to help in this respect, noting: "There is no direction in which [the MRC is] . . . more anxious to help than in getting scientific work done in laboratory wards."[24] In November 1922 Meakins left the lab until the following February, joining a high altitude expedition to study respiration in the Andes.[25] In his absence Murray Lyon took charge of his wards and the lab.

Davies, like his boss, was something of a powerhouse. His first two years at Edinburgh were extremely busy investigating respiratory, circulatory, and metabolic disorders in patients at the Infirmary. The respiratory work was done jointly with Meakins and they planned a monograph which in October 1922 they aspired to publish "shortly" although it did not appear until 1925.[26] They did, however, publish a paper together in April 1922.[27] It described a technique for determining the circulation rate based on the analysis of expired air. The paper exemplified the role that clinicians like Meakins envisaged for clinical science. The authors took a laboratory method which they found "difficult" to apply to patients and simplified it by experimenting (albeit only with tubes and bags of inhaled and exhaled air) on Infirmary inmates. Davies worked on the practical as well as the experimental side of oxygen therapy. At a meeting in July 1922 Meakins delivered a paper on the physiology of oxygen want and Davies presented one on methods for the therapeutic administration of oxygen. Significant here was Davies's rigorous quantitative approach to an agent often given in a casual fashion: "Oxygen," he wrote, "must be regarded as a drug and its dose regulated according to the needs of the patient."[28]

The following year, 1923, Davies published again with Meakins and another lab worker, Lucien Dautrebande. Davies and Dautrebande were the subjects in experiments on the carbon dioxide dissociation curve of the blood.[29] Work on the effects of external temperature on blood volume was carried out with Meakins and Meakins's old friend, Joseph Barcroft, who was Reader in Physiology at Cambridge and spent three days in Edinburgh in March 1923.[30] This work eventually appeared in 1923 as a part of the Report to the Peru High-Altitude Committee.[31] Besides this work, at the end of 1922 Davies reported he was constructing "a new apparatus for the quantitative estimation of carbon dioxide in blood."[32] In addition he published with Dautrebande on an oxygen administration mask made in the Edinburgh laboratory of the Oxygen Research Committee of the DSIR. The subjects used in the experiments were Dautrebande, Davies, Meakins, and the lab's biochemist, Charles Harington.[33]

All this work did not exhaust Davies's interests. His routine BMR measurements formed the basis of a paper published with Meakins.[34] He also published with an RIE physician and active lab user, John Eason, on BMR and blood pressure in thyroid disease using patients on the wards of Meakins and Harold Stiles.[35] The collaboration with Stiles was significant for Stiles was one of the clinicians targeted by Rockefeller. In December 1924 Davies published with Meakins and Jane Sands (see below) on blood gases and hyperthyroidism.[36] Part of the study involved eleven people who underwent thyroidectomy and presumably again these were Stiles's patients. Not all of Davies's work was clinical. Along with Dautrebande he researched and published on the chlorine interchange between corpuscles and plasma.[37] This work was related to the study of acidosis. Measurements were made in the lab of various biochemical constituents of the blood of both researchers, under a variety of conditions (carbon dioxide saturation for example). Davies was also involved in the insulin studies of 1923. This work, based on experiments on rabbits, could not have been done in the hospital's lab; perhaps it was carried out in Cushny's lab, where facilities were certainly extended to Meakins on one occasion.[38]

In 1923 Davies did what any ambitious medical scientist aspired to in the inter-war years. He gained (or at least Meakins obtained for him) a Rockefeller Fellowship to study in North America for a year.[39] He left Scotland in September 1923 and for most of his year he worked at the Hospital of the Rockefeller Institute, New York, studying respiratory and circulatory disturbances with Donald Van Slyke, Alfred Cohn, and Rufus Cole, the hospital's director.[40] A large part of Cole's research programme was centred on pneumonia and Davies's interest in blood gases and oxygen therapy would have dovetailed with this. Davies indeed, with two co-authors, published on his work at the hospital.[41] In addition to his stay in New York, Davies visited other prestigious North American medical schools.

While Davies was in America, Meakins acacepted the Chair in Montreal. It is a measure of Meakins's unique qualities that Davies obviously no longer found Edinburgh attractive. Shortly before he left New York in September 1924, Davies must have seen Pearce, for the latter wrote in his diary that Davies's future was "uncertain," and that he "May remain at Edinburgh and after a year go to Meakins at Montreal, and would consider a full time position in his home univ[ersity] at Adelaide, Australia."[42] Perhaps in an effort to keep him in Edinburgh, on his return promotion from research assistant to lecturer was recommended.[43]

On coming back from America Davies did not seem to be quite so busy. He was probably not, as it happens, quite as happy in his job. He produced a few papers, all but one jointly authored, and all devoted to aspects of respiratory function. When appointed as a lecturer, he said he intended to deliver "a short practical course in the use of modern physiological methods in the investigation of disease." This was "with a view to selecting and training men for research positions."[44] Attempts to keep him in Edinburgh were of little avail. In October 1926 Davies took up a position as Lecturer in Physiology and Pharmacology at the University of Leeds.[45] He eventually became Professor of Physiology in Sydney.

As noted, Meakins published most of his research jointly. Before he had been at Edinburgh long he was collaborating with the second and only other junior researcher employed in the lab besides Davies, Charles Harington. A descendant of an ennobled old English family which boasted the Royalist author James Harington in its stock, Charles Harington was born in 1897. He was up at Cambridge from 1916 until 1919, when he obtained a first in the Natural Sciences Tripos, Part I. He did not stay on to take Part II, but left for Edinburgh to work in Barger's Department of Medical Chemistry. Barger thought highly of him and, no doubt on Barger's recommendation, Harington was appointed University Assistant and biochemist in Meakins's department at a salary of £300 per annum.[46] Meakins considered him "a young but brilliant biochemist."[47] As in the case of Davies, the Faculty approved his appointment in May 1920 and by November he was certainly carrying out biochemical tests for clinicians, presumably in Barger's lab.[48] In November 1921, also like Davies, he gained a £100 per annum grant from the MRC "in respect of your work on liver function in relation to the fate of amino acids."[49] This work related to that of Meakins, for amino acid breakdown produced ammonia, a key chemical in acid–base balance. Once again Meakins had appointed a promising young scientist with interests overlapping those of his team. So promising was Harington, however, that Meakins could not keep him, for in June 1922 he departed for America for a year and then returned to fill the newly-created post of Lecturer in Chemical Pathology at University College Hospital Medical School, London. Harington went on to fulfil his promise, becoming Professor at the College and an FRS.

Harington may not have been in the lab long but by November 1921 he had submitted two papers for publication with Meakins which appeared the following year. As a pair these papers constituted "classic" clinical science. The first described experiments on patients, the second gave an account of the animal models utilized to explore further the human findings. The papers were biochemical investigations into the then accepted, fashionable even, condition of intestinal intoxication, a disorder the mechanisms of which were not understood but were generally agreed to involve bacteria and food residues in the large bowel producing toxic products that were then absorbed, leading to symptoms. Meakins and Harington (second author) set out to discover whether histamine might be one of these toxic products by determining its presence in the human colon. Histamine, a chemical synthesized early in the century, was the subject of much physiological work since it was suspected to be the cause of surgical shock. In their first paper Meakins and Harington reported that colonic washings and faeces were collected from seven infirmary patients with intestinal symptoms and from one with nephritis.[50] After filtration and chemical treatment the solutions were tested for physiological activity on the isolated uterus of the virgin guineapig, an organ extremely sensitive to histamine. Minute quantities of histamine were detected in six cases but not in a case in which there had been surgical bypass of the ascending colon, nor in the case of nephritis. The authors made no comments on their findings. Whether the use of guineapig uterus might have been thought by the Managers of the Infirmary to constitute animal experimentation is not known. The experiments may have been done in Barger's or Cushny's labs.

The second paper reported the experimental absorption of histamine.[51] These experiments, on cats, were done in Cushny's laboratory. A cannula was inserted into the intestine of an anaesthetized animal and histamine injected. Another cannula in the carotid artery recorded blood pressure. In female cats, tracings of uterine contractions were also made. In a second series of experiments the blood leaving the intestines was diverted directly into the systemic circulation, bypassing the liver using a device known as the Eck fistula.[52] In sum the authors found that the blood pressure fall after intestinal injection was much more rapid when the Eck fistula was in place. They attributed this effect to the liver being bypassed and therefore unable to play some chemical or mechanical protective role in mitigating the effects of histamine. They considered "the balance of evidence so far obtained is against the view that histamine is an active agent in causing intestinal intoxication," except possibly in cases where there was structural deficiency at the ileo-caecal junction.[53] Although these experiments seem at first sight a long way from the interests of either author, in fact they relate to Harington's work on the role of the liver in amino acid breakdown. While doing this work Harington was simultaneously performing almost identical experiments to determine the role of the liver in the fate of histidine.[54] Histamine, it was known, could be produced by the action of putrefactive organisms on histidine. Meakins was obviously directing aspects of Harington's "pure" research towards a clinical problem.

Harington published one further paper from the lab, although this did not appear until 1924. This was co-authored with Jessie M. Craig, who graduated in medicine in Edinburgh in 1921.[55] Harington became engaged to Craig in 1922 and they married the following year. Their joint paper was a study in variations in protein metabolism as indicated by sulphur excretion. The paper had a clinical dimension, being based on patients with exophthalmic goitre. Craig was funded from a scholarship from the Carnegie Post-graduate Research Fund. She ceased to practise medicine late in the 1920s.

A significant worker in the lab in 1920, in the light of the fact that he succeeded Meakins in the Chair of Therapeutics in 1924, was David Murray Lyon. Murray Lyon had graduated in 1910. For a while he seems to have considered a career as a pathologist for he was Assistant Pathologist to the Infirmary 1912–19. He had extensive clinical experience in France in the war and in 1919 was appointed Assistant Physician in the Infirmary. He worked on Meakins's ward and devoted extensive time to clinical teaching and to research in the Biochemistry Laboratory, for which latter he was not paid. He was a Junior Lecturer in Clinical Medicine and received a salary from the University of fifty guineas plus a bonus, making a stipend of £100 per annum. He added about £350 pounds to his income by, in Meakins's words, "eking out a living" teaching pathology in the Extra-academical School.[56] He was, said Meakins in 1922, the "type of man I must encourage here."[57] Meakins requested, probably in March 1923, £500 per annum from the MRC for Murray Lyon to continue his research.[58] It seems that he did not get this at this time for in October 1923 Meakins wrote to Fletcher asking for "four or five hundred pounds" for Murray Lyon, "the man who has helped me so much so far."[59] It is a measure of the dominance of the case history and pathological anatomical approach to research in Edinburgh that Meakins noted of Murray Lyon and one other clinician (Charles Lambie, see below): "They are almost the only workers in the clinical department of the University who are doing this [i.e. laboratory research]."[60] Murray Lyon, whose dedication to the laboratory was not as total as Meakins thought, got £400 per annum from the MRC from October 1, 1923, and £500 per annum from the following April. The condition of the award was that Murray Lyon was to undertake nothing other than teaching and research. Thanking Fletcher for the award, Meakins observed of Murray Lyon, "I think before long he will be taking a very important place in scientific Medicine."[61] Meakins was of course absolutely right in one sense since Murray Lyon, at the age of thirty-six, gained Meakins's Chair.

Murray Lyon published something in the region of thirty-five papers in the decade 1920–30. There were no books. There was a distinct tendency to collaboration in the second half of the decade, perhaps unsurprising in an established professor as opposed to a young researcher attempting to make his name and an academic career. In 1920 he received his M.D. for a thesis on the viscosity of blood, a subject on which he published the following year.[62] This was Murray Lyon's first clinical science paper, that is, it combined ward work with laboratory study, although the laboratory work was strictly haematological and probably done in the University's Pathology Department. It seems to have been started at least as early as 1911 when Murray Lyon was a Crichton Scholar in Pathology, 1911–13, since cases were provided by William Greenfield who retired as Professor of Pathology in 1912. Significantly the work was based on Murray Lyon's pathological expertise rather than biochemical knowledge. His first published paper including biochemical data was a case report. In April 1920 a twenty-six-year-old man developed symptoms of diabetes and was admitted to the Infirmary in November of that year. When blood was drawn it had a "curious opaque or cloudy appearance."[63] Harington (at this time still employed in Barger's lab) reported that the blood contained nearly 10 per cent of fat. The blood's viscosity was also determined, no doubt by Murray Lyon himself. The respiratory quotient was calculated. Murray Lyon probably carried out this relatively simple test on expired air using a Haldane apparatus too. The significance of this report is that he called on Harington's biochemical expertise and did not perform the fat test himself.

Murray Lyon published a good deal on insulin but in almost every instance he took on the role of explaining its use in the clinic and what knowledge the general practitioner needed to employ it. He also reported on the assessment of alternative agents to insulin, but these papers were overwhelmingly clinical and no animal experiments were involved. Around 1920 Murray Lyon embarked on a D.Sc. which was awarded in 1924 for "Some Observations on the Action of Adrenalin." Four papers on adrenalin based on this work appeared in 1923. In the first of these Murray Lyon published on what seems to have been the small amount of animal work he ever did. This study obviously grew from his earlier interest in blood pressure. Adrenalin was injected into decerebrate cats in increasingly large doses to discover whether blood pressure rose logarithmically (it did). The work suggested Murray Lyon had an interest in applying mathematics to physiology and medicine and later papers confirm this.[64] The study was done in Cushny's department. The second paper on adrenalin was signalled as being from the Department of Therapeutics. It was clinical but used the resources of the biochemistry laboratory. It was, however, typical of the simpler clinical science that characterized Murray Lyon's work. About twenty-five infirmary patients, several with thyroid disease, had their basal metabolic rates measured. They were injected with a small dose of subcutaneous adrenalin. Pulse and blood pressure measurements were made and BMRs measured again. The aim was to discover whether a more marked response to adrenalin occurred in mild hyperthyroidism, so that the injection might be used as a test for the condition by general practitioners. The results seemed equivocal. Whether the BMRs were included in the hospital returns or paid for out of Murray Lyon's research expenses is unknown.

The third paper, also from the Department of Therapeutics, was very similar to the second but far more detailed. It appears that it used the results reported in the second paper and included others. It was, however, tailored to the experimental journal it was published in (for it contained no reference to tests useful for GPs) just as the second had been tailored to the style of the *British Medical Journal*. The fourth paper, again from the Department of Therapeutics, confirmed Murray Lyon's mathematical interests. Based on the same sort of experiments as papers two and three (perhaps the very same experiments) its aim was to give a mathematical account of the rate of absorption of adrenalin. It was published in a premier experimental journal.

As noted, the biochemist Harington left in June 1922, and a replacement was found in William Robson. Born in 1893 he obtained a B.Sc. at King's College, London and then worked as an assistant in Barger's lab, where he started a Ph.D. in physiological chemistry. Meakins's eye for talent was once again evident, for Robson left Edinburgh in 1927 and eventually held the chair of biochemistry at his old college, King's in London. In Meakins's lab, like Harington, Robson was paid £300 per annum by the University and from April 1923 he received £100 per annum from the MRC.[65] He obtained his Ph.D. in 1924. Like the promising Davies, he also gained a Rockefeller

Fellowship, which he took up in September 1924. He arrived in the US the day Davies sailed back from Quebec. In Robson's absence, C. P. Stewart from Barger's Department of Chemistry in Relation to Medicine substituted.[66]

Like Davies too, most of Robson's time (ten months) was spent at the Rockefeller Hospital in New York with Donald Van Slyke. Unlike Davies's trip, however, Robson's generated some friction with the MRC which, since 1923–24, had been entrusted with the award of the Rockefeller Fellowships.[67] Besides its amusing features the relevant correspondence indicates how seriously the MRC expected researchers to take their science.

Robson applied for a Fellowship in the spring of 1924 and failed to mention he intended to marry in the summer. New York, it turned out, was rather expensive for a man on a single person's stipend to support a wife and in November 1924 Robson wrote to the MRC hoping the stipend might be "placed on a basis approximating that received by a married man."[68] Robson had opened a can of worms. Fletcher replied: "Your letter of the 11th November . . . puts the Council in much difficulty, and it would be hard for them to give favourable consideration to what you ask, unless you treat them with much greater frankness." He continued: "When you applied for the Fellowship, you knew from the regulations that the additional allowances might be made to men who were married at the time of application. You were also informed that married Fellows were advised, if they intended to work under the best conditions, to leave their wives behind." He then delivered the core of the Council's complaint: "After receiving the award, you married, and arranged to take your wife with you, without informing the Council. Dr. Thomson was put to much unnecessary trouble in changing the berths arranged for yourself and your friend whom he had naturally believed to be a man." He went on: "The Fellowship was awarded to you in order that you might devote yourself intensively during a period of months to research work in the United States . . . You will understand that the Council . . . must be put into a position to satisfy themselves that your unexpected use of your journey as a wedding tour is not conflicting with the objects for which the Fellowship was gained."[69]

On the same day Fletcher wrote to Barger about Robson: "May I ask you to tell me in confidence what you think of his personal character, and for the following reasons? When he applied he described himself as unmarried," later, however, Robson "asked us to take a berth for himself and a friend, who we naturally assumed to be a man friend. At the last minute we discovered he was newly married, and that the friend was his wife, and at great inconvenience we had to get berths in another ship because the first booking was for a man's cabin." Fletcher wondered: "Is Robson an honest fellow? If he is, I am afraid he must be called very stupid."[70] Barger replied: "Robson is an honest fellow . . . but I fully agree with you that he must be called very stupid."[71] Two days later, after further thought, he sent Fletcher a hand-written note saying: "Although at the time I supported his application I was not aware that he was anything but quite honest. I feel now that asking you to book a berth for a 'friend' was certainly not straight. He evidently wished to conceal that he was taking his wife with him." He added that he had "pointed out to Murray Lyon that the presence of a young wife would not be conducive to Robson's scientific studies, and Murray Lyon volunteered to write to Robson . . . giving him a hint that he must on no account neglect his work. We don't want Robson to let us down any further than he already seems to have done."[72] Fletcher replied: "To be quite fair, I must tell you he did not ask us to book a berth for a 'friend'. You added the quotation marks. He asked us to take another berth at his expense. We assumed it was for a man friend, and of course took the berth with his in a man's cabin. This was stupid of him, but I do not suggest that he wished deliberately to mislead."[73] Meanwhile in New York, suitably chastened, Robson wrote to Fletcher withdrawing his application for an increase.[74] Fletcher, however, did not see that as solving the problem since Robson could not work well if he was "financially embarrassed."[75] Further correspondence followed but Robson was adamant and the matter was closed.

While working in the lab when Meakins was there Robson studied the chemistry of insulin. He had a particular interest in insulin and lipaemia, which formed the second topic of his Ph.D. thesis. His first interest, however, was the metabolism of the amino acid tryptophane on which he published in biochemical journals.[76] He seems to have published only one paper between 1924 and 1928: the study of Intarvin in diabetes made with Murray Lyon and A. C. White published in 1925.[77] Presumably Robson was responsible for explaining the biochemistry and doing the laboratory tests while Murray Lyon did the clinical work. In

1925, however, the medical managers recommended to the Infirmary Board that Robson (not medically qualified) be allowed to visit the wards.[78] In 1929 Robson published on work done in the lab although the paper was perhaps written in London.[79] It centred on a patient of Murray Lyon's admitted in 1926 with cystinuria, the excretion of the amino acid cystine in the urine, a well-known but rare disorder of which the metabolic processes were still debated. This patient had abdominal pain and vomiting and was the focus of dietary experimentation with a therapeutic aim. For about a month her protein intake was varied daily and her cystine output was measured, also daily. Robson drew some technical conclusions about cystine metabolism but as far as therapy was concerned the only recommendation was to cut down daily protein intake.

Another newcomer to the lab in 1922 was Charles George Lambie. Born in Trinidad in 1891 he graduated in medicine in Edinburgh in 1914. After war service, one year of which was spent as a pathologist, he was appointed a lecturer in Cushny's department in 1919. In 1922 he was made an Assistant Physician to W. T. Ritchie. Like Murray Lyon he received a small salary of £100 from the University. Meakins thought highly of him: "the type of man we must encourage," he wrote to Fletcher in an effort to get the MRC to supplement Lambie's salary by £300 per annum plus a further £200 for research expenses.[80] Meakins set Lambie to study the pharmacology and physiology of insulin, which he did, publishing jointly with his colleagues on the subject. Lambie's "style" of science, as revealed in papers published later in the decade, looks much more like that of Meakins than that of Murray Lyon, but then Lambie was trained in experimental pharmacology. In 1923 Lambie was awarded a Junior Beit Memorial Fellowship. These were founded in 1909 by Otto Beit, residuary legatee of an extremely wealthy brother, Alfred, who had died in 1906. Fellowships were for three years at a stipend of £350 per annum.[81] They were one of the very few sources of funding which permitted medical men to engage in full-time laboratory research. Lambie presumably held his in Edinburgh. He seemingly used the time to study insulin and carbohydrate metabolism, working on patients in the infirmary and animals in an unspecified lab.[82] Lambie was awarded an Edinburgh M.D. in 1927 for his thesis "The Locus of Insulin Action."

When his Beit Fellowship expired in 1926 he applied to the MRC for a grant to fund a large four-pronged project. His post as Assistant

Physician, he wrote, left him about twenty hours a week for research. Lambie received £200 per annum from the University for his teaching, in addition he taught Systematic Medicine at Surgeons Hall and was trying to build up a consulting practice in Edinburgh.[83] With Murray Lyon's support he was granted £100 per annum by the MRC. In 1927 and 1929 he published a total of four papers co-authored with other lab workers on carbohydrate metabolism. These "Studies in Carbohydrate Metabolism" were published in the *Biochemical Journal*.[84] They involved normal subjects (students), diabetic patients, and animal experiments, the latter being done at the College of Physicians. All the experiments involved determining the effect of various chemical agents introduced into the circulation and extensive biochemical analysis was reported. No doubt these publications helped his career, for in 1929 he was offered chairs in medicine at Aberdeen and at Sydney. He chose the latter and left in 1930. Lambie was one of the few young Edinburgh medical graduates who worked in the lab who can be said to have internalized fully a style of clinical research based on chemical physiology.

Fourteen researchers other than paid employees were reported to have worked in the lab by July 1922, some of whom I have already noticed.[85] Not all have been easy to trace. Those that have been include the few infirmary physicians interested in lab work who asserted their right (suitably vetted) to use its facilities. John Eason graduated at Edinburgh in 1896 and showed an interest in pathological research in his M.D. thesis on haemoglobinuria which was submitted in 1905. From 1912 to 1923 he was an Assistant Physician to the infirmary and from then on until 1938 an Ordinary Physician. There is no detailed information on whether he used the lab for research after 1922. It is likely that he did so because throughout the decade he was a consistently high user of the lab's routine facilities. Eason had a keen interest in thyroid disorders, collaborating, as noted above, on a research paper with Davies published in 1924. He published a monograph on exophthalmic goitre in 1927 in which he stressed the value of BMR (along with clinical signs) in differential diagnosis. In his "Suggested Scheme for the Examination of Cases of Disease of the Thyroid," he also advised a glucose tolerance test.[86] This involved taking serial blood samples after a meal of glucose. Its significance is dealt with in the next chapter. If he did these regularly it would certainly help to explain his high routine lab usage. More significant is that all the evidence points to

Eason as a "biochemically-friendly" physician. Edwin Bramwell, discussed in Chapter 9, did no lab research nor did he do tolerance tests in thyroid disease.

A clutch of other workers was recorded as using the lab in 1922, five of whom it has proved difficult to trace. Some were relatively junior infirmary doctors keen to do some research but probably not looking for a career in academic medicine. George Malcolm-Smith was a clinical tutor whose interest in nephritis was noted in the previous chapter.[87] Presumably he used the lab to investigate renal function. Malcolm-Smith had a limited publication record and eventually went into general practice. John Struthers Fulton was Meakins's resident in summer 1922 and also worked in the lab.

The lab was scarcely the research powerhouse of the Rockefeller Institute Hospital of New York but Meakins obviously had sufficient reputation to attract researchers from abroad, at least two of whom who were in the lab in 1922 and went on to academic careers. Lucien Dautrebande was a Belgian with an M.D. obtained from the University of Louvain in 1919. He came to Edinburgh specifically to further an academic career by studying for a Ph.D. on acid–base balance under Meakins. This he gained in 1925.[88] He published at least four technical articles on respiratory physiology from his Edinburgh work. The Edinburgh experience stood him in good stead: he went on to become Professor of Pharmacodynamics at the University of Liège.

A student who had a rather different career was Shankar Hardiker. Born in India in 1880 he attended Hyderabad medical school between 1906 and 1911. He practised medicine in India until 1916 when he attended the Edinburgh Medical School, graduating in 1920. He was reported as working in Meakins's lab in 1922 and was Crichton Research Fellow in Materia Medica in the Pharmacology Department 1923–24. He was appointed Professor of Physiology at the Osmania Medical College, Hyderabad, in 1927.[89] He published papers on the action of quinine, the subject of his Edinburgh M.D. of 1924 for which he won a gold medal.

In the summer of 1923 when it looked as if Davies was going to gain a one-year Rockefeller Fellowship, Meakins began to cast about for a temporary replacement. Once again he was successful in attracting a worker from abroad, as was his intent. He wrote to Fletcher that he thought Davies's absence would be a good opportunity "of bringing a couple from the other side." He went on: "There is a woman who has been working with Bazett who is very anxious to come here."[90] Henry Cuthbert Bazett was Professor of Physiology at the University of Pennsylvania. He had written to Meakins in May 1923 about Jane Sands "who is working here with me on electrocardiographs on dogs with experimental aortic regurgitation."[91] Sands came to the Edinburgh lab as a Medical Fellow of the National Research Council, USA (which was supported by Rockefeller) and sent back weekly reports.[92] It is not clear what Meakins did with Davies's salary. In January 1924 the Dean of the University of Pennsylvania wrote to Meakins of "the excellent character of the opportunities which she is finding under your preceptorship."[93] It does not seem that Sands did routine chemical work. As noted, she published with Meakins and Davies on blood gases and hyperthyroidism, suggesting either she overlapped with Davies or carried on work with Meakins that Davies had started. She obviously continued her earlier haemodynamic interests for she published two papers, "Studies in Pulse Wave Velocity," from the Department of Therapeutics.[94] Experiments were done on healthy subjects and patients (but not for pathological research) and by modelling with rubber tubing. The work is best described as pure science for although correlations of pulse wave velocity and blood pressure were made there was no suggestion of diagnostic or therapeutic implications. One of the papers was co-authored with Murray Lyon and confined itself to the mathematical and physical science he seemed more comfortable with than biochemistry.

During this period, 1922–23, the names of two junior Infirmary staff appear in connection with the laboratory. Neither went on to a career in academic medicine. Alister Matheson, whose name crops up in 1922, was an Edinburgh graduate (1917) and a tutor in clinical medicine. He eventually became an Assistant Physician at the Leith Hospital (and presumably made his living in private practice). Sydney Ammon, also an Edinburgh graduate (1921), was a clinical assistant who became a District Medical Officer in Trinidad. They are an interesting pair in that they seem to be one of the few links between the University's Physiology Department and Meakins's lab. Jointly and with other authors in 1922–23 they published from Sharpey-Schafer's laboratory on the results of animal and human experiments on gastric secretion. The human subjects they studied were not patients. They were particularly interested in the effect of histamine and in developing new methods of gastric and duodenal aspiration. This was human normal physiology of the sort Sharpey-Shafer fostered. Their work was financed by grants from the Carnegie Trust and the Moray Fund. In 1923 they published from Meakins's department on the effect of histamine on human gastric secretion. By this time they were no longer working in pure physiology but had carried their interests over to clinical work. Their observations were made on twelve convalescent hospital patients "without any obvious disturbance of gastric function." Whether the patients' consent was obtained is unknown. Gastric juice, obtained by tube, was examined before and after the subcutaneous injection of histamine. Various chemical tests were done (no doubt in the lab) to determine total acidity, free hydrochloric acid, and the pepsin, mucus and bile content of the fluid. They concluded that histamine increased gastric secretion and it might therefore have a diagnostic or therapeutic use.[95] What is unusual about this work is that, at first sight, it is unlike the other work done in the lab. However, Meakins and Harington had worked on histamine. Moreover, Meakins, a year before Ammon and Matheson published, had worked on the use of the duodenal tube in the diagnosis of biliary diseases.[96] This was a departure for him since no biochemistry was involved. Meakins's role as the inspirer and co-ordinator of clinical research by bringing together various interests seems clear.

The year 1924 saw Davies return from America and the departure of Meakins for good. Their book manuscript had been delivered to the publishers by November. It appeared the following year (dedicated to J. S. Haldane).[97] New workers in the lab in 1924 included the recently-qualified Frances Redhead, who came on a voluntary basis to do BMR estimations.[98] In 1925 the medical managers recommended the Infirmary pay her an honorarium of £25, which it did.[99] When Davies left in 1926 she was taken on as a part time physiologist. She was still there in 1928 when, still part time, she was described as fourth assistant and physiologist, being paid £100 per annum by the University and the honorarium of £25 a year from the Infirmary.[100] Her main occupation, however, (certainly by 1926) was as an anaesthetist at two other hospitals in Edinburgh. None the less she found time to publish a technical physiological paper with Lambie in 1927 on dihydroxyacetone, a substance implicated in glucose metabolism. The respiratory metabolism of normal subjects was reported.[101] The paper was the third in a series in which various workers collaborated with Lambie. Others papers in the series reported experimental work on animals carried out at the College of Physicians.[102] Redhead's most important paper was published with Murray Lyon in 1927. Thyroxin, the active hormone of the thyroid gland, was isolated at the Mayo clinic in 1915. Renamed thyroxine, it was synthesized by the department's former biochemist, Harington, in the mid 1920s. Barger had been involved in some of this work and this is possibly from where Murray Lyon and Redhead got their "small quantity" before Harington had published. They tested it on two myxoedematous subjects, finding an immediate rise in the metabolic rate.[103] Harington cited this work as evidence of the success of his synthesis.[104] The other name that crops up in 1924 is that of Ruth Pybus, made Sister Dietitian that year, who worked closely with Murray Lyon caring for diabetic patients. She was thought of very highly and in 1926–27 secured a Rockefeller Fellowship to study on the wards and in the kitchens of various American hospitals.

Working in the lab in 1924, although his name does not appear until 1925, was Adam Cairns White, a young Edinburgh medical graduate and Lecturer in the department. He was funded by a University Stark Scholarship in Clinical Medicine. He studied patients, probably under the care of Meakins, publishing on bicarbonate reserve in febrile conditions in 1925, the year he received his Ph.D.[105] He also published a paper with Murray Lyon and Robson on diabetes in early 1925 and also in 1925 with C. P. Stewart (see below) on the estimation of fat in blood.[106] He was one of the few lab workers who went on to a scientific career, for he left the department to become an Assistant Pharmacologist at the commercial Wellcome Physiological Research Laboratories at Beckenham in Kent.

The year 1925 saw Murray Lyon's first full year in charge of the lab. Davies remained as Assistant Physiologist and Robson returned in October as biochemist after his Rockefeller Fellowship. He picked up his previous salary of £300 per annum and wrote to Morley Fletcher asking for a renewal of his £100 annual grant. He outlined his research programme, which centred on amino acid metabolism and a related study of insulin-induced convulsions.[107]

A significant figure in the department at this time (and eventually a major figure in Edinburgh medicine) was Andrew Rae Gilchrist. Although his name does not appear until 1925, he was a Meakins product and significantly, much of his work was done with Davies. The son of a minister, Gilchrist was born in Edinburgh in 1899. Graduating in medicine in his native city in 1921, he showed his ability by winning various prizes. His willingness to travel was signalled by his taking junior appointments in Cambridge and London. From April 1924 he served as Meakins's House Physician and in November of that year he was awarded the McCunn Scholarship, tenable for one year on the medical wards of the Infirmary. He spent the year in the Department of Therapeutics. As the Scholarship came to an end Murray Lyon sought to keep him in the department. There was no remunerative position of any substance open to him and Murray Lyon proposed to take him on as a Clinical Tutor teaching four hours a week for £75 per annum. To supplement this meagre stipend, Murray Lyon wrote to Fletcher in October 1925 asking for a grant of £200, on the understanding Gilchrist devoted his whole time to research. Pulling every string he could, Murray Lyon noted, "I may add that Professor Meakins had a very high opinion of Dr. Gilchrist's qualifications and ability."[108] How far the magical name Meakins worked is unknown but Fletcher wrote back ten days later with the MRC's blessing.[109] Gilchrist stayed, presumably for the year, until he went to the Rockefeller Hospital as a Resident, probably for a year. He returned to the department in 1927 taking over the second assistant's post at £300 per annum.[110] Murray Lyon applied, probably successfully, for Gilchrist's grant of £200 per annum from the MRC to be renewed.[111] When he returned to Edinburgh, however, Gilchrist's work became more orientated to clinical cardiology and did not have a marked laboratory dimension. Gilchrist's reputation steadily grew, such that in 1930 he was appointed Assistant Physician to the Infirmary at the age of thirty-one. He went on to accrue many honours and develop an international reputation in cardiology.

Gilchrist published at least nine papers from the department, several of them collaborative. He was quick off the mark too, publishing three papers in 1925. The first two were jointly written with Davies. Neither was exactly a research paper, rather both sought to inform a wider audience about oxygen therapy. The authors carefully credited J. S. Haldane for much of the transformation in the appreciation of the value of oxygen usage and Meakins for demonstrating, through research, the value of the therapy in pneumonia. All this was a prelude to describing an apparatus that could deliver oxygen in an "*efficient* and *quantitative*" manner.[112] In a paper published in the *Edinburgh Medical Journal* in the same month, their strategy for promoting the use of oxygen was to describe the pathophysiology of respiration and the *principles* on which the administration of oxygen was based.[113]

Gilchrist published again in 1925 on "Novasurol: A New Diuretic". This study did not involve lab analysis. Novasurol was an injectable mercury compound introduced by a pharmaceutical company for the treatment of syphilis. It was later noted to have diuretic side effects. Gilchrist used it in unresponsive cases of advanced cardiac failure and "As a means of comparing its effects" it was administered to "certain other cases." Various clinical parameters such as urine volume and the patient's weight were recorded. The drug was reported as effective in cardiac failure in three cases out of five. No report of its effect in "certain other cases" was given. Gilchrist concluded the drug was "a most suitable adjuvant to digitalis therapy." This paper has the appearance of an amalgam of an old and new medicine about it. On the "old" side it was based on a small number of cases and relied on the judgement of the individual clinician. It did not use any laboratory findings. On the "new" front, it cited measurements and an attempt at what can, anachronistically, be called control.[114]

The year 1926 had not long arrived and Gilchrist was in print again on "The Use of Massive Doses of Digitalis." This was a paper based on experimental work by Cushny.[115] The title was slightly misleading for the paper was devoted to determining how the optimum dose of digitalis might be given very quickly. Although the study was purely clinical, by pointing to Cushny's work attention was drawn to the laboratory as the basis of rational therapeutics. Shortly before he left for America in 1926 Gilchrist, along with Davies, submitted a paper to the premier clinical science publication *Quarterly Journal of Medicine* and it was published the following April. It described a relatively simple and painless method for determining the circulation rate by inhaling ethyl iodide. Davies applied to the MRC for a grant (which he got) for a "large 200-litre spirometer" to be manufactured by a local company.[116] The method was also used by Murray Lyon's summer resident of 1926, J. G. Kininmonth, to investigate the circulation rate in various disorders. He made 163 determinations but no strong correlations emerged, nor suggestions for the use of the test in everyday practice.[117]

Various other figures worked in the lab in 1925: residents, clinical assistants, tutors, and the distinguished surgeon Arthur Logan Turner.

Dorothy Potter was another who used the lab as a stepping stone to a scientific career. An Edinburgh graduate, Potter worked as a house surgeon in the Royal Maternity Hospital in 1924. In November of that year she submitted a paper to the *Quarterly Journal of Medicine* from the Department of Therapeutics. "Changes in the Blood in Anaesthesia" appeared the following year.[118] It is not clear when this work was done but it was initiated at Meakins's suggestion and focused on bicarbonate reserve. By 1927 she had become Assistant Professor of Physiology at the Women's Medical College in Philadelphia.

In 1926 the first signs of dissatisfaction in the lab began to appear among the full-time research workers. In the summer Davies accepted the Leeds job at double his salary: £600 per annum seems to have been about the going rate for an academic in medicine in early to mid-career. Davies wrote to Fletcher at the MRC about the "excellent facilities" he would have at Leeds. Although the facilities at Edinburgh were "good and likely to improve" he felt "there seems to be little encouragement for research workers and no money to pay them."[119] Fletcher thought Davies "wise to take this new opportunity."[120] Puzzling is that Davies was not replaced. A departmental memorandum of 1928 noted that "The post of physiological assistant is at present vacant"[121]

Davies's good fortune was probably not lost on Robson. In this year, 1926, he was awarded a University of London M.Sc. At this time his £300 salary from Edinburgh University remained unaltered and it was not subject to increments. His £100 annual grant from the MRC since 1923 had not been increased either. Aged thirty-three and married, he probably felt his qualifications as a professional scientist were not fully appreciated. In July 1926 he wrote to Fletcher to see if there was any chance of a grant increase.[122] Fletcher saw his point of view but avoided a direct response. Whether safeguarding MRC money or out of indignation (or both) Fletcher wrote to Murray Lyon that Robson's salary was "scandalously small for a well-qualified man" adding, "Can we get the University to do more for him . . .?"[123] Fletcher, it turned out, had walked into a minefield. On October 20 Murray Lyon wrote Fletcher a revealing letter about Infirmary and University attitudes to medical chemistry:

> As you are aware, Medical Chemistry is pretty well served in this University. Barger's Department has four Assistants on the staff, and deals

only with First-Year Medical Students. Second-Year Students are taught Physiological Chemistry by a non-medical member [Taylor] of Professor Schafer's staff. There is also a non-medical Chemist on the staff of the Department of Pathology serving the Third-Year Students. Clinical Chemistry is taught in the wards by eight medically qualified Clinical Tutors, so that Robson finds no place as a Teacher.

He continued:

It was hoped that the Board of Managers of the Infirmary would be quick to recognize the advantage to be gained from employing a qualified Chemist in this capacity, and that they would take over the responsibility for his salary. Instead, they contented themselves with paying the salary of one Chemical Technician. In practice, it turns out that the Qualified Chemist in this Department is engaged during practically his whole time in doing Research Work, and I have had difficulty in continuing the appointment as other Departments object to whole-time non-teaching Researchers being supported from University Funds in certain favoured Departments only. To apply directly for an advance in salary, would, I feel certain, lead to a discontinuance of the office altogether.[124]

There was obviously no arguing, although how far Murray Lyon was not prepared to push Robson for other reasons is not clear. A few days later Robson received a letter from the MRC telling him his grant had been increased to £200.[125] It was obviously not enough to keep him in Scotland, for he left for London the following year. There were, however, almost certainly frictions in the department that encouraged his departure.

On September 1, 1926, John Hamilton Crawford started work in the lab. Crawford had originally studied in Edinburgh but was whisked off to the war before he could complete his degree, which he did in 1918. He left the Navy in 1920 to be resident under Meakins, in the winter 1920–21. For two academic years, 1921–23, he was an assistant in Cushny's department and at the same time a Clinical Tutor. On the advice and recommendations of Meakins and Cushny he went to New York as an Assistant Resident Physician at the Hospital of the Rockefeller Institute. He intended to stay for two years but, as he wrote to Fletcher in 1926: "The departure of Professor Meakins for Montreal altered this scheme so I remained another year."[126] It is not clear whether Edinburgh without

Meakins was not attractive or whether Meakins had promised Crawford a position but obviously could no longer fulfil such a promise. Both explanations of course might apply. This was not the whole story anyhow, for Murray Lyon had tried to induce him back in 1925. Crawford was interested in heart disease, the capillaries, and oedema and by 1925 had an impressive publication record. Cushny had "a very high opinion of his ability as an investigator."[127] Murray Lyon thought him "a very able clinician" and that he had had "thorough scientific training," adding that he was "a type we would like to develop and eventually add to our staff."[128]

There was evidently no position vacant in Murray Lyon's department however. Murray Lyon obtained a £300 a year grant for Crawford from the MRC and said he could supplement this by a "small sum."[129] Murray Lyon wrote to Crawford with this offer. Crawford declined. A year later, writing to the MRC, Murray Lyon reported that when Crawford received the offer "about the same time, a colleague in New York was returning to one of the units in London to receive a much bigger salary, and this fact, more than anything else, determined his refusal of the offer."[130] Crawford, however, told Fletcher that what Murray Lyon "was able to offer would have made it impossible for me to support myself in Edinburgh as I am engaged be married and have no private income."[131] Murray Lyon was less generous: "I feel that Dr Crawford's sojourn in America has had the unhappy effect of making him over-rate his worth, and feel that he would be conferring a favour by his return."[132] Still, in May 1926, Murray Lyon to all appearances felt Crawford remained a desirable commodity and was prepared to find him £300 if the MRC could match the sum. This would "put him on a par with the medical units in London."[133] The MRC was prepared to do this if Crawford devoted himself whole time to teaching and research and did not engage in professional practice.[134] Crawford took up a position as a Senior Clinical Assistant on these terms on September 1, 1926.[135] There is still something of a mystery about why Murray Lyon, who clearly did not care for Crawford, took him on board. It may be significant, however, that he was well liked by Cushny and Meakins, and Pearce thought highly of him and had told Fletcher so.[136] Murray Lyon may have known this and felt obliged to take Crawford.

As might have been guessed, Murray Lyon and Crawford were not made for each other and the following spring Crawford left for America for good. A "private and confidential" letter from him to Fletcher revealed Crawford's dismal perception of the department's affairs. He began: "When I returned to work with Prof. Murray Lyon I understood that my position was to be next to him in his department. However, this did not prove to be so. I was also to have all the material that I wanted for my work placed at my disposal. Here again, things did not turn out as expected." Friction had begun early: "What cases I obtained in his wards were only got after a struggle and with little co-operation. When I obtained cases from some of my friends on the staff to work on, this did not meet with approval." Collaboration was seemingly disapproved of: "Dr Robson and I started *with his consent* [Murray Lyon's] on a problem which was very interesting and were getting very good results when the combination was split up and we were not allowed to continue." Crawford saw his own interests stifled: "As you know I am particularly interested in cardio-vascular disease and have worked on it for several years but last week was the first time since I returned that I have been asked my opinion or to do anything in regard to heart cases." He continued: "Before I returned to this country he [Murray Lyon] even told Drs Davies and Gilchrist that I was not to be allowed to touch the apparatus for estimating circulation rate by the ethyl iodide method." He concluded: "I have really had no position in the department and it looks as if he did not want me back. I have gone on all winter hoping things might improve but little change has taken place so I have decided to clear out as things are most unsatisfactory." His final thought in this respect was a chilling indictment of departmental frictions: "My position is not peculiar but applies to other members of the staff also particularly those who were there in Prof. Meakins' time." Crawford, however, had obviously found the other two medical professors, Gulland and Bramwell, and the senior clinician W. T. Ritchie supportive.[137] Fletcher replied to Crawford's lament with a sympathetic but unrevealing letter although he obviously wanted to keep in touch.[138] This they did: Crawford thanked Fletcher in 1928 for his "personal kindness" while Crawford was in Edinburgh.[139]

Within just over a year three researchers of proven quality, two of them clinically qualified and products of the loose alliance of Meakins, Barger, and Cushny, had left.[140] This, coupled with Crawford's explicit criticisms, suggests that all was not right with the lab. Murray Lyon had been appointed in 1924. Meakins's role in this is not fully clear. It was certainly not a promotion greeted with all-round delight. On hearing of Meakins's acceptance of the McGill post, Fletcher confessed himself "perturbed" and admitted to being "greatly depressed" at the thought of Meakins leaving Edinburgh.[141] In July 1924 Fletcher told Meakins that he was "startled" at the rapidity of Murray Lyon's appointment a week, he thought, after the post was announced as vacant. Fletcher obviously considered Murray Lyon's record not impressive enough yet and he had hoped that Murray Lyon would have had "a few undisturbed years in which to make his mark in research work and fit himself for promotion to a Chair there or elsewhere." He considered Murray Lyon was at an age "most fitted for research work and least fitted for responsibility." Fletcher hoped "I may be wrong."[142]

Murray Lyon's appointment embodied Edinburgh's traditional values. Here was a man who was an Edinburgh graduate, a faithful servant of the University and Infirmary who had served his apprenticeship for a modest salary in junior positions. The time had now come to reward him fully. Meakins tendered his resignation on June 9, 1924.[143] Ten days later Murray Lyon applied for the post.[144] By July 11, the Therapeutics Committee of the Faculty had made up its mind and unanimously appointed Murray Lyon because of "circumstances of difficulty resulting from his extended period of War Service" and because he "has for the last five years devoted himself to the work of the Therapeutics Department" and contributed to its success. The only other candidate considered with Murray Lyon "best fitted to take undertake [*sic*] the duties of the Chair" was John McNee of University College, London.[145] In retrospect, and probably to Fletcher at the time, this was a remarkable decision. McNee, a Scot but a Glasgow graduate (a matter possibly of importance), had shown himself by this time to be one of the most gifted young researchers in clinical medicine. He had travelled widely, working in Germany and the United States. His work on the etiological classification of jaundice published in 1923 was much admired. He went on to fulfil this early promise, becoming Regius Professor of the Practice of Medicine at Glasgow. He was knighted in 1951.

At no point did Meakins indicate in writing to Fletcher that Murray Lyon had his backing although he obviously did since Meakins was on the appointment committee. However, in reply to something Fletcher had probably said, rather than put on paper, Meakins wrote cryptically the same month: "As you say practically all the links [of the MRC] with this clinic will be broken next year." Meakins saw Davies as the only strong ongoing contact.[146] Certainly Murray Lyon's relations with Fletcher were quite different from those the latter had with Meakins. Whereas Murray Lyon's letters to Fletcher were always formal, Meakins and Fletcher obviously enjoyed a friendship. On at least one occasion Fletcher sought Meakins's opinion of MRC "general policy and development."[147] The families were intimate and the Fletchers stayed at Meakins's home on visits to Edinburgh.

If Fletcher knew McNee was a candidate, which he surely did, he would have backed him, but, strangely, his opinion does not seem to have been asked. The truth was that if, perhaps, Fletcher did not think Murray Lyon was a suitable person for the Chair at the time he certainly did not think so a few years later. Neither did Pearce at the RF. As noted, by 1928 ideas for reconstruction of the Medical Department in Edinburgh were being bandied about in earnest. In May of that year Pearce wrote to Fletcher about the end of Murray Lyon's RF subvention: "The real problem before us will be Murray Lyon a couple of years from now. Frankly I do not see how we can capitalize our present aid to his department."[148] In December 1928, Fletcher was very frank with Pearce, explaining how he had told Ewing: "Murray Lyon was quite unfit for his position, and three promising young men (paid by us) had already left him in despair." Fletcher implied Murray Lyon was unable to attract researchers, observing that "there was still unused space in the Rockefeller building for at least 35 workers." He concluded: "The real difficulty is how to get rid of Murray Lyon." Startlingly he added, "I have never been able to forgive Meakins for selling the pass as he did when he made that appointment." He finished calculatingly: "What part of your bargain with him is terminable in about two years?"[149] Six months later Fletcher was still talking about it. In a conversation with Pearce, Fletcher said he "Agreed that Murray-Lyon has not lived up to . . . expectations and that he is likely to resign shortly and go into general practice."[150]

One of Fletcher's other allies in Edinburgh was Barger. What Barger thought of Murray Lyon is not known but a letter from Barger to Fletcher in 1929 is suggestive. In this letter, outlined in Chapter 6,[151] Barger described how "Some of us are furious" that Principal Ewing would continue to supplement Murray Lyon's salary after Rockefeller support for it had ceased and Murray Lyon was returning to private practice.[152] This hardly suggests a Professor of Therapeutics that the supporters of academic medicine were anxious to keep.

The perception that Fletcher and others had of Murray Lyon was, no doubt, grounded in their view of his management of departmental affairs but other things were probably at work. Murray Lyon had shown an interest in clinical research early in his career but, perhaps because of the early interest in pathology, his research publications always evidenced a greater emphasis on clinical issues, especially therapeutic ones, than on the sort of technical, physiological, and biochemical problem-solving approach of Meakins. He had not, of course, had the same rigorous apprenticeship in these subjects as Meakins. He showed an interest in mathematics but not animal experiments. He was accused of not encouraging collaboration. He enjoyed private practice. In the eyes of those promoting the new academic medicine he was not in their mould. Indeed in 1936 he was appointed to the Moncrieff-Arnott Chair of Clinical Medicine. On his death in 1956 one obituarist noted "he was never at his best or really happy" in the Christison Chair.[153] Another obituary noted of his move to the clinical chair that "he found he could not meet the twofold demands of the laboratory and the hospital wards . . . The benefit to himself was in the enrichment and the wider range of his clinical teaching." More significantly it went on to reveal that in 1956 the way that laboratory medicine was introduced into Edinburgh in the 1920s was perceived as having produced an imbalance in the School. The obituary stated: "The benefit [of Murray Lyon's move] to the whole medical school was in the rehabilitation and restoration of clinical teaching in Edinburgh towards its primary position in the medical curriculum."[154] Perhaps that was a sentiment generated at the time and which had endured until at least Murray Lyon's death. Murray Lyon's orientation, shared by many of the Edinburgh teachers, was preserved in a vignette drawn by his son: "My father was very much of the suggestion that you need to teach students basic medicine. Then when they qualify with a MB ChB, they are basic doctors and they can go and do anything they like. He was rather against all this specialist teaching." Consistent with this position was Murray Lyon's long term advocacy of the view that the Edinburgh Municipal Hospitals should be brought into the teaching circuit.[155]

When, in 1927, Robson the biochemist left for London, his place was filled jointly, part time, by two assistants from Barger's department, C. P. Stewart and Fred P. Coyne, who continued to keep that connection. Corbet Page Stewart was born in 1897 and graduated in chemistry from the University of Durham. From there he went to Edinburgh, obtaining his Ph.D. in Barger's department. He held a Beit Memorial Fellowship between 1923 and 1926 and spent some of this time in Cambridge studying with Gowland Hopkins though seemingly, with Meakins's backing, also filling in for Robson as the lab's full-time biochemist while the latter was in America 1924–25.[156] Stewart received no salary from the Department of Therapeutics although he received £350 per annum from the Department of Medical Chemistry.[157] He also had a grant of £200 from the MRC and a newly-agreed contribution of £200 per annum awarded by the Board of Managers of the Infirmary after a request from Murray Lyon. If all these were received concurrently he was comparatively well paid.[158] In 1929 he was offered a Carnegie Teaching Fellowship which did not augment his salary but paid for another assistant and released Stewart from his teaching duties, permitting him more time for research.[159] Stewart, called the "Infirmary Bio-Chemist," remained in the University for the rest of his career.[160] Fred Coyne, occupying the other half of the lab biochemist's post, was designated Chemical Assistant. He was paid £150 by the Department of Therapeutics and £100 by Medical Chemistry.[161] He left for a post with Imperial Chemical Industries in 1929.

Stewart published regularly from the lab, jointly and as sole author, mainly on the estimation of various substances in blood and urine. He seems to have been able to strike up relationships with the relatively junior inhabitants of the lab. Indeed his first paper, on phosphorus and magnesium estimation, was jointly published in 1925 with William Archibald, the lab's technical assistant (Stewart himself of course was relatively junior at this time).[162] He published several pieces with G. H. Percival, who had been Murray Lyon's resident in winter 1924–25 and went on to become the first holder of the Chair of Dermatology at Edinburgh established in 1929. Their first paper, published in 1926, was a study of blood urea changes in thirty-six cases (mainly children) with scarlatina at the City Hospital (the fever hospital). They had seemingly hoped to discover that urea levels might give an indication of impending nephritis, but the results were negative.[163] Likewise a study by them that appeared in 1926 of serum calcium and the administration of parathyroid hormone yielded no consistent result.[164] Stewart published on his own in these years too, notably on amino acid metabolism. This study was based on dietetic experiments on rats and carried out in Barger's laboratory.[165] As noted, Stewart stayed on in the department, eventually becoming Reader in the newly-created Department of Clinical Chemistry in 1946.[166]

William Lamb, a 1926 medical graduate, joined the department as the whole-time third assistant in 1927. He was paid £200 per annum by the department and £75 by the University for being a Tutor in Clinical Medicine. The other, and more senior, whole-time second assistant, Gilchrist, was paid £300 and also had a medical research grant of £200.[167] Lamb came to the lab with no connection to Meakins. He was a Murray Lyon appointment and his interests, connections, and career all demonstrate this patronage. He had no advanced training in basic science. For Lamb, time spent around the lab was probably a stepping stone to a prominent clinical career rather than an academic one. He became an Assistant Physician to the Infirmary in 1936 and an Ordinary Physician—twenty-five years later—in 1961. Two papers he published while in the department no doubt facilitated this eventual promotion. The first, co-authored with Murray Lyon (Lyon and Lamb!), on lobar pneumonia, appeared in 1929.[168] This paper adds weight to the view that Murray Lyon's outlook was often at odds with that of the research style backed by Meakins for it suggests he was not as warm a proponent of oxygen therapy as Meakins had been. Indeed Murray Lyon had not been party to any of the literature by Meakins and his handpicked colleagues on this subject that poured out of the department during the 1920s.

Pneumonia, Murray Lyon and Lamb acknowledged, "continues to be one of the most serious diseases with which the medical man is called to deal." They noted that the "startling suddenness of its onset and the dramatic improvement at the crisis attract special interest." Its frequency and fatal issue at that time made it particularly important. A vast and contradictory literature on therapeutics had grown up around it. Murray Lyon and Lamb argued that the disease was so variable in course and outcome that therapies could only be meaningfully tested in very large series of cases. None the less their conclusion also seemed to reveal that they made no distinction between statistical and individual evidence: "Looking to the evidence of statistics," they wrote, "and to the individual experience of careful observers, it must be admitted that medicinal interference and active treatment are, collectively speaking, of but little influence, either in shortening the duration in, or diminishing the mortality of, pneumonia."[169] Perhaps deliberately breaking with the department's past, they did not record that in 1921 Meakins had written forcefully on the value of oxygen therapy. He had observed:

> In pneumonia with cyanosis there is a clear indication for the administration of oxygen, and it is most important that it should be given early. I am certain more cases would recover if the cyanosis were not allowed to develop, or if it has developed if it were removed immediately by effective oxygen administration. In all pulmonary lesions, such as lobar pneumonia . . . proper administration of oxygen is imperatively indicated.[170]

Murray Lyon's work on pneumonia was part of a wider MRC study of vaccine therapy for the disease. T. R. Elliott dismissed it as "fallacious."[171]

Meakins cast a long shadow. In 1927 a jointly-authored paper on blood coagulation appeared in the *Quarterly Journal of Medicine*.[172] The work must have been done in the first half of 1926. The authors were Davies, Stewart (then assistant in Medical Chemistry) and Ronald V. Christie. Born in 1902, Christie graduated in medicine at Edinburgh in 1925. He had his house officer appointment in the Department of Medicine in winter 1925–26 when the paper was written. Christie was a young high-flyer in academic medicine. To carry out work of a quality publishable in such a prestigious journal while still a resident showed promise indeed. The details of the paper are unimportant except that a great deal of it centred on the acid–base balance of the blood. This made the paper something of a swansong for the Meakins regime, for this aspect of the study was clearly Davies's domain and he was to leave in the summer of 1926. More significant is that the bright young Christie also left in 1926, to spend two years at the Rockefeller Institute for Medical Research. At some point, possibly even in Edinburgh, Christie developed an interest in respiratory medicine. Meakins had him spotted and in 1928 he was invited to McGill to become a research assistant. Christie went on to fulfil his promise, becoming Professor of Medicine in the Unit at St Bartholomew's Hospital, one of the few full-time academic chairs of medicine in Britain. The point is that only briefly did Edinburgh figure in Christie's career, but it would probably have done rather more so had Meakins remained.

The year 1928 was of course a momentous one in the laboratory's life, for the new Clinical Laboratory opened. Nineteen requests for rooms or space were made by members of the senior Infirmary staff but only three, jointly, indicated they wished to work on biochemistry.[173] Histology was the over-riding interest of the remainder. In the event, no one who was not in the Department of Therapeutics seems to have done biochemical work in the lab. As noted in previous chapters, Pearce and Fletcher repeatedly lamented the lack of use of the lab. Although the opening of the lab enlarged the Director's responsibilities it made no difference to the academic structure of the department. In October 1928 Murray Lyon sent a memorandum to the Secretary to the University asking permission to appoint a whole-time assistant trained in physiology. Authority was given in January 1929.[174] Aside from the move to the new lab, 1928 was a quiet year on the research front with no evidence of new workers in the department.

Departmental staff changed and expanded in 1929. Coyne, the part-time chemical assistant, left but was soon replaced by Robert Gaddie, a man who had attained a first class honours degree in chemistry at the University that year. Gaddie worked on his Ph.D. while in the department, gained a Beit Memorial Fellowship and went on to an extremely successful career as a biochemist in England. Two new clini-cally-qualified assistants were appointed. The appointment of Derrick Dunlop to the vacant position of assistant physiologist at the unchanging salary of £300 was scarcely one the department would regret for it had just selected its next Professor. It was an inspired choice. Dunlop gradu-ated B.A. in physiology at Oxford in 1923, studied in medicine at Edinburgh and in 1926 "winning the Allan Fellowship for best in Clinical Medicine and Surgery in the Final Examinations."[175] He took his M.D. a year later. Dunlop progressed rapidly in the department, being made lec-turer in 1930 and attaining the chair in 1936 aged thirty-four. He retired from the chair in 1962 aged sixty, by which time his immense experience of therapeutics had been put to wide use by governmental bodies.[176] He had scarcely been in the department a year when he published with its biochemist, Stewart, *Clinical Chemistry in Practical Medicine*.[177] Dunlop's research at this time has been described in the previous chapter. His interest in acid–base balance harked back to the days of Meakins, although his prime concern was with nephritis, not respiration. He also worked with C. P. Stewart on fat metabolism in relation to obesity. He published in all these areas in the early 1930s.

The other new appointment in 1929 was to the assistantship vacated by William Lamb (of Murray Lyon and Lamb fame). Ranald Malcolm Murray Lyon, a relation of the Director, had graduated in 1926. He was Murray Lyon's resident in summer 1927 and gained his M.D. the year he became an assistant in the department. Ranald Murray Lyon published a number of papers but they were all rather more clinical than clinical science.[178] Not unexpectedly his future was as a clinician and not in academic medicine. Indeed he rose to become Senior Physician at the Infirmary.

In 1929 Lambie, still the senior assistant, was awarded £100 from the MRC for the expenses of work on parathyroid hormone administration and chemical and histological changes in bone.[179] This was purely experimental work on rats to be carried out at the College of Physicians. The expensive item in the research was parathyroid extract (Parathormone) costing 16*s*. for 5 cc. Simultaneously with this study the industrious Lambie was working on a variety of projects in the new lab. Apart from Murray Lyon and Gilchrist, Lambie represented the last link with the Meakins years and in many ways was the only physician still working in that tradition. Early in 1930 he was offered the Chair of Medicine in Sydney and, not surprisingly, he took the job. His departure fittingly rounds off the decade.

Notes

1. For a list of various awards made by the University in the 1920s see the appropriate edition of *Edinburgh University Calendar* (Edinburgh: James Thin).

2. "Regulations for the Conduct of the Laboratory" [January 1, 1921], "Scrap-Book of the RIE Biochemical Laboratory," box 1, folder 11, RCPE.

3. D. Wilkie to R. Pearce, June 2, 1925, folder 34, box 3, series 405, RG 1.1, Rockefeller Foundation Archives, RAC.

4. For a description of the American scene see Harry M. Marks, *The Progress of Experiment: Science and Therapeutic Reform in the United States, 1900–1990* (Cambridge: Cambridge University Press, 1997). For a specific challenge to new authority see Martin Edwards, "Good, Bad or Offal? The Evaluation of Raw Pancreas Therapy and the Rhetoric of Control in the Therapeutic Trial, 1925," *Annals of Science* 61 (2004): 79–98.

5. For a "classic" statement by a senior medical figure of the centrality of the clinician and the objection to animal models see Samuel Gee, "Sects in Medicine," in *Medical Lectures and Aphorisms*, ed. Samuel Gee (London: Smith Elder & Co., 1902). Gee was a much-admired London medical teacher of the late nineteenth and early twentieth centuries.

6. R. V. Christie, H. W. Davies, and C. P. Stewart, "Studies in Blood Coagulation and Haemophilia. II. Observations on Haemic Functions in Haemophilia," *Quarterly Journal of Medicine* 20 (1927): 481–98.

7. H. W. Davies and A. R. Gilchrist, "Observations upon the Circulation Rate in Man by the Ethyl Iodide Method," *Quarterly Journal of Medicine* 20 (1927): 245–64.

8. J. Meakins, "Some Chemical Influences in Regard to the Endocrine Glands and the Central Nervous System," *Journal of Mental Science* 68 (1922): 367–74.

9. Steve Sturdy, "Biology as Social Theory: John Scott Haldane and Physiological Regulation," *British Journal for the History of Science* 21 (1988): 315–40.

10. Steve Sturdy, "From the Trenches to the Hospitals at Home: Physiologists, Clinicians and Oxygen Therapy, 1914–30," in *Medical Innovations in Historical Perspective*, ed. John V. Pickstone (Basingstoke, Hampshire: Macmillan, in association with the Centre for the History of Science, Technology, and Medicine, University of Manchester, 1992), 104–23; Steve Sturdy, "War as Experiment: Physiology, Innovation and Administration in Britain, 1914–1918: The Case of Chemical Warfare," in *War, Medicine and Modernity*, ed. Roger Cooter, Mark Harrison, and Steve Sturdy (Stroud: Sutton, 1998), 63–84.

11. H. W. Davies and A. R. Gilchrist, "A New Outfit for Oxygen Administration," *The Lancet* 1 (1925): 916–17.

12. Minutes of the Clinical Uses of Oxygen Committee, March 20, 1920, FD1/5310, 49252, PRO.

13. A. L. Thomson (Assistant Secretary MRC) to Dr. Hunt, May 10, 1921, FD1/5310, 49252, PRO.

14. J. Meakins and H. W. Davies, "Observations on the Gases in Human Arterial and Venous Blood," *Journal of Pathology and Bacteriology* 23 (1920): 451–61.

15. Davies had already published with Haldane: J. S. Haldane, J. G. Priestley, and H. W. Davies, "The Response to Respiratory Resistance," *Journal of Physiology* 53 (1919): 60–69.

16. One of the tables reported tests on "JSH" [Haldane], and Davies had no access to patients.

17. Haldane to Meakins, December 11, 1918, 867/36/6, OLHM.

18. Haldane to Meakins, June 2, 1919, 867/39/39, OLHM.

19. On Haldane's recommendation of Davies see J. Meakins, "Autobiography," 107, 867/51, OLHM.

20. University of Edinburgh, Faculty of Medicine, "Minutes of a Meeting," May 5, 1920. Shelf ref. DA43, EUA.

21. Davies to Fletcher, November 15, 1924, FD1/1015, 49222, PRO.

22. Meakins to Fletcher, June 3, 1921, FD1/1015, 49222, PRO.

23. A. L. Thomson (Assistant Secretary MRC) to Davies, November 22, 1921, FD1/1015, 49222, PRO.

24. Fletcher to Meakins, June 9, 1921, FD1/1015, 49222, PRO.

25. For Meakins's experiences in South America see Meakins, "Autobiography," 112–120.

26. J. Meakins and H. W. Davies, *Respiratory Function in Disease* (Edinburgh: Oliver and Boyd, 1925).

27. J. Meakins and H. W. Davies, "The Influence of Circulatory Disturbances on the Gaseous Exchange in the Blood. II. A Method of Estimating the Circulation Rate in Man," *Heart* 9 (1922): 191–98.

28. J. Meakins, "Oxygen-Want: Its Causes, Signs and Treatment," *Edinburgh Medical Journal* 29 (1922): 142–61; H. W. Davies, "Methods for the Therapeutic Administration of Oxygen," ibid: 161–68.

29. L. Dautrebande, H. W. Davies, and J. Meakins, "The Influence of Circulatory Changes on the Gaseous Exchanges of the Blood. III. An Experimental Study of the Circulatory Stasis," *Heart* 10 (1923): 133–52.

30. Meakins to Fletcher, March 3, 1923, FD1/1015, 49222, PRO.

31. J. Barcroft et al.,"On the Relation of External Temperature to Blood Volume," *Philosophical Transactions of the Royal Society Series*, B, 211 (1923): 455–64 (Appendix to Peru Report). W. J. Fetter, one of the co-authors, was another worker in the Edinburgh lab.

32. Davies to Fletcher, August 19 [? mistake for October], 1922, FD1/1015, 49222, PRO.

33. L. Dautrebande and H. W. Davies, "Variations in Respiratory Exchange with Masks of Different Types," *Edinburgh Medical Journal* 29 (1922): 127–35.

34. J. Meakins and H. W. Davies, "Basal Metabolic Rate: Its Determination and Clinical Significance," *Edinburgh Medical Journal* 28 (1922): 1–18.

35. H. W. Davies and John Eason, "The Relation between the Basal Metabolic Rate and the Pulse-Pressure in Conditions of Disturbed Thyroid Function," *Quarterly Journal of Medicine* 18 (1924): 36–61.

36. H. W. Davies, Jonathan Meakins, and Jane Sands, "The Influence of Circulatory Disturbances on the Gaseous Exchange of the Blood. V. The Blood Gases and Circulation Rate in Hyperthyroidism," *Heart* 11 (1924): 299–307.

37. L. Dautrebande and H. W. Davies, "A Study of the Chlorine Interchange between Corpuscles and Plasma," *Journal of Physiology* 57 (1923): 36–46.

38. J. Meakins and C. R. Harington, "The Relation of Histamine to Intestinal Intoxication. II. The Absorption of Histamine from the Intestine," *Journal of Pharmacology and Experimental Therapeutics* 20 (1923): 45–64.

39. Meakins to Fletcher, June 6, 1923, FD1/1015, 49222, PRO.

40. For Davies's itinerary see "Rockefeller Foundation Fellowships (Davies), NY," Rockefeller Foundation Archives, RAC.

41. H. W. Davies, George. R. Brow, and Carl A. L. Binger, "The Respiratory Response to Carbon Dioxide." *Journal of Experimental Medicine* 41 (1925): 37–52.

42. Pearce's Diary, September 3, 1924, in Rockefeller Foundation Fellowships (Davies), NY, Rockefeller Foundation Archives, RAC.

43. Davies to Fletcher, November 15, 1924, FD1/1015, 49222, PRO. Davies is first recorded as a Lecturer in Therapeutics for the academic year 1925–26. Edinburgh University Calendar, 1925–1926 (Edinburgh: James Thin, 1925).

44. Davies to Fletcher, November 15, 1924.

45. Davies to Fletcher, August 3, 1926, FD1/1016, 49222, PRO. It is not at all clear what happened to Davies' salary.

46. On Barger's "warm recommendation" of Harington see, Royal Society, "Charles Robert Harington, 1897–1972," *Biographical Memoirs of Fellows of the Royal Society* 18 (1972): 267–308.

47. Meakins, "Autobiography," 106.

48. University of Edinburgh, Faculty of Medicine, "Minutes of a Meeting," May 5, 1920. On testing in 1920 see D. Murray Lyon, "Xanthoma Diabeticorum: With Report of a Case," *Edinburgh Medical Journal* 28 (1922): 168–73.

49. A. L. Thomson (Assistant Secretary MRC) to Harington, November 22, 1921, FD1/1015, 49222, PRO.

50. J. Meakins and C. R. Harington, "The Relation of Histamine to Intestinal Intoxication. I. The Presence of Histamine in the Human Intestine," *Journal of Pharmacology and Experimental Therapeutics* 18 (1921): 455–65.

51. Meakins and Harington, "The Absorption of Histamine."

52. Nikolai Vladimirovich Eck, Russian surgeon.

53. Meakins and Harington, "Absorption," 63.

54. C. R. Harington, "The rate of destruction of Histidine in Relation to the Functional Activity of the Liver." This paper, unpublished in this form, is part of Harington's annual report, 1921–22, to the MRC. Harington to MRC, September 1, 1922, FD1/1015, 49222, PRO.

55. Jessie McCririe Craig and Robert Harington, "Disturbances in Metabolism. I. Variations in Protein Metabolism as Indicated by Sulphur Excretion," *The Biochemical Journal* 18 (1924): 85–92.

56. J. Meakins, "Statement re Remuneration," [n.d. ? 1923], FD1/1015, 49222, PRO.

57. Meakins to Fletcher, July 25, 1922, FD1/1015, 49222, PRO.

58. Meakins, "Statement re Remuneration."

59. Meakins to Fletcher, October 16, 1923, FD1/1015, 49222, PRO.

60. J. Meakins, "Statement re Remuneration."

61. Meakins to Fletcher, October 10, 1923, FD1/1015, 49222, PRO.

62. D. Murray Lyon, "Blood Viscosity and Blood-Pressure," *Quarterly Journal of Medicine* 14 (1921): 398–408.

63. Lyon, "Xanthoma."

64. D. Murray Lyon, "Does the Reaction to Adrenaline Obey Weber's Law?" *Journal of Pharmacology and Experimental Therapeutics* 21 (1923): 229–35; "The Reaction to Adrenaline in Man," *Quarterly Journal of Medicine* 17 (1923): 19–33; "The Absorption

of Adrenaline," *Journal of Experimental Medicine* 38 (1923): 655–65; "The Influence of the Thyroid Gland on the Response to Adrenaline," *British Medical Journal* 1 (1923): 966–67.

65. Robson to Fletcher, July 14, 1926, FD1/1016, 49222, PRO.

66. University of Edinburgh, Faculty of Medicine, "Minutes of a Meeting," July 1, 1924. Shelf ref. DA43, EUA.

67. A. Landsborough Thomson, *The Medical Research Council: Half a Century of Medical Research*, 2 vols. (London: HMSO, 1973–1975), 1, 168.

68. Robson to A. L. Thomson (Assistant Secretary MRC), November 11, 1924, FD1/2636, 49313, PRO.

69. Fletcher to Robson, November 21, 1924, FD1/2636, 49313, PRO.

70. Fletcher to Barger, November 21, 1924, FD1/2636, 49313, PRO.

71. Barger to Fletcher, November 25, 1924, FD1/2636, 49313, PRO.

72. Barger to Fletcher, November 27, 1924, FD1/2636, 49313, PRO.

73. Fletcher to Barger, December 3, 1924, FD1/2636, 49313, PRO.

74. Robson to Fletcher, December 2, 1924, FD1/2636, 49313, PRO.

75. Fletcher to Robson, December 17, 1924, FD1/2636, 49313, PRO.

76. William Robson, "The Metabolism of Tryptophane. I. The Synthesis of Racemic Bz-Methyltryptophane," *Journal of Biological Chemistry* 62 (1924): 495–514 was published when Robson held his appointment in the Department.

77. D. Murray Lyon, W. Robson, and A. C. White, "The Use of Intarvin in Diabetes Mellitus," *British Medical Journal* 1 (1925): 207–10.

78. RIE, "Minutes of Medical Managers' Committee, Consideration of a report from the Advisory Committee of the Bio-chemical Laboratory," October 19, 1925, LHSA, LHB1/1/61, EUL.

79. W. Robson, "Protein Metabolism in Cystinuria," *The Biochemical Journal* 23 (1929): 138–48.

80. Meakins to Fletcher, July 25, 1922.

81. Beit Memorial Trustees, *The Beit Memorial Fellowships for Medical Research 1909–1959* ([London]: Privately Printed for the Trustees, 1960).

82. C. G. Lambie, "Insulin and Glucose Utilization: Effects of Anaesthetics and Pituitrin," *The British Journal of Experimental Pathology* 7 (1926): 22–32.

83. Lyon to Fletcher, September 8, 1926, FD1/1016, 49222, PRO; Lyon to Fletcher, October 1, 1926, FD1/1016, 49222, PRO.

84. C. G. Lambie and Frances Agnes Redhead, "Studies in Carbohydrate Metabolism. III. The Influence of Dihydroxyacetone upon the Respiratory Metabolism and upon the Inorganic Phosphate of the Blood," *The Biochemical Journal* 21 (1927): 549–59; W. O. Kermack, C. G. Lambie, and R. H. Slater, "Studies in Carbohydrate Metabolism. IV. Action of Hydroxymethylglyoxal upon Normal and Hypoglycaemic Animals," *The Biochemical Journal* 23 (1929): 410–15; W. O. Kermack, C. G. Lambie, and R. H. Slater, "Studies in Carbohydrate Metabolism. V. The Effect of Administration of Dextrose and Dihydroxyacetone upon the Glycogen Content of Muscle in Depancreatised Cats," ibid., 416–21; C. G. Lambie and F. A. Redhead, "Studies in

Carbohydrate Metabolism. VI. The Antagonistic Action of Pituitrin and Adrenaline upon Carbohydrate Metabolism with Special Reference to the Gaseous Exchange, the Inorganic Blood-Phosphate and the Blood-Sugar," ibid., 608–23.

85. "Minutes of the Advisory Committee," July 26, 1922, "Scrap-Book of the RIE Biochemical Laboratory," box 2, RCPE.

86. John Eason, *Exophthalmic Goitre* (Edinburgh: Oliver and Boyd, 1927), 191.

87. See p. 209.

88. Lucien Dautrebande, "Blood and Circulatory System: The Acid Base Equilibrium of the Blood in Circulatory Stasis" (Ph.D. thesis, University of Edinburgh, 1925). "Dr Nolf" of Brussels jointly supervised him. The RF had strong and good relations with Belgium and particularly the University of Brussels. These relations were seen by the RF as a circuitous route to reform, sequentially, Parisian, French, and Latin medicine. See William H. Schneider, "The Men who Followed Flexner: Richard Pearce, Alan Gregg, and the Rockefeller Foundation Medical Divisions, 1919–1951," in *Rockefeller Philanthropy and Modern Biomedicine: International Initiatives from World War I to the Cold War*, ed. William H. Schneider (Bloomington: Indiana University Press, 2002), 7–60, 24.

89. *University of Edinburgh Journal* (1927): 177; *The Medical Who's Who*, 8th ed. (London: Grafton, 1927), 353. The latter identifies him as Professor of Pathology but Physiology seems more likely.

90. Meakins to Fletcher, June 8, 1923, FD1/1015, 49222, PRO.

91. Bazett to Meakins, May 15, 1923, 867/33/6, OLHM.

92. Bazett to Meakins, January 24, 1924, 867/32/4, OLHM; Pearce to Meakins, February 13, 1923 [but must be 1924], 867/37/3, OLHM.

93. Bazett to Meakins, January 24, 1924, 867/32/4, OLHM.

94. Jane Sands, "Studies in Pulse Wave Velocity. III. Pulse Wave Velocity in Pathological Conditions," *The American Journal of Physiology* 71 (1925): 519–33; D. Murray Lyon and Jane Sands, "Studies in Pulse Wave Velocity. IV. Effect of Adrenaline on Pulse Wave Velocity," *The American Journal of Physiology* 71 (1925): 534–42.

95. A. R. Matheson and S. E. Ammon, "Observations on the Effect of Histamine on the Human Gastric Secretion," *The Lancet* 1 (1923): 482–83.

96. J. Meakins, "Observations on the Duodenal Tube in the Diagnosis and Treatment of Biliary Diseases," *British Medical Journal* 1 (1922): 483–87.

97. "The Monograph. 'Respiratory Function in Disease', written in collaboration with Professor Meakins, is at present in course of publication by Messers. Oliver and Boyd." "List of Published Papers by Dr. H. Whitridge Davies," appended to letter from Davies to Fletcher, November 15, 1924, bibliography, FD1/1015, 49222, PRO.

98. [Murray Lyon] to William Caw [Infirmary Treasurer], August 13, 1925, "Scrap-Book of the RIE Biochemical Laboratory," box 2, RCPE.

99. RIE, "Minutes of Medical Managers," April 15, 1925, LHSA, LHB1/2/48 EUL.

100. "Memorandum re the New Clinical Laboratory," [July 3, 1928], Secretary's File, DRT 95/002., pt. 1, Faculty of Medicine, box 27, EUA.

101. Lambie and Redhead, "Studies in Carbohydrate Metabolism."

102. Ibid.

103. D. M. Lyon and F. A. Redhead, "Synthetic Thyroxine-Clinical Tests," *Edinburgh Medical Journal* 34 (1927): 194–99.

104. "Charles Robert Harington, 1897–1972."

105. A. C. White, "The Bicarbonate Reserve and the Dissociation Curve of the Oxyhemoglobin in Febrile Conditions," *Journal of Experimental Medicine* 41 (1925): 315–26.

106. Lyon, Robson, and White, "The Use of Intarvin"; C. P. Stewart and A. C. White, "The Estimation of Fat in Blood," *The Biochemical Journal* 19 (1925): 840–44.

107. Robson to Fletcher, October 10, 1925, FD1/1015, 49222, PRO.

108. Lyon to Fletcher, October 9, 1925, FD1/1015, 49222, PRO.

109. Fletcher to Lyon, October 19, 1925, FD1/1015, 49222, PRO.

110. "Memorandum re the New Clinical Laboratory."

111. Lyon to Fletcher, October 4, 1927, FD1/1015, 49222, PRO.

112. Davies and Gilchrist, "A New Outfit for Oxygen Administration."

113. H. W. Davies and A. R. Gilchrist, "Oxygen Therapy: Indications, Principles and Methods," *Edinburgh Medical Journal* 32 (1925): 225–44.

114. A. R. Gilchrist, "Novasurol: A New Diuretic," *The Lancet*, 2 (1925): 1019–23.

115. A. R. Gilchrist, "The Use of Massive Doses of Digitalis," *Edinburgh Medical Journal* 33 (1926): 65–73. For the experimental work see, Arthur R. Cushny, *The Action and Uses in Medicine of Digitalis and its Allies* (London: Longmans, Green, 1925).

116. Davies and Gilchrist, "Observations upon the Circulation Rate"; Davies to Fletcher, January, 20, 1926, FD1/1015, 49222, PRO.

117. J. G. Kininmonth, "The Circulation Rate in some Pathological States, with Observations on the Effect of Digitalis," *Quarterly Journal of Medicine* 21 (1928): 277–96.

118. Dorothy G. E. Potter, "Changes in the Blood in Anaesthesia," *Quarterly Journal of Medicine* 18 (1925): 261–73.

119. Davies to Fletcher, August 3, 1926, FD1/1016, 49222, PRO.

120. Fletcher to Davies, August 10, 1926, FD1/1016, 49222, PRO.

121. "Memorandum re the New Clinical Laboratory."

122. Robson to Fletcher, July 14, 1926, FD1/1016, 49222, PRO.

123. Fletcher to Murray Lyon, October 18, 1926, FD1/1016, 49222, PRO.

124. Murray Lyon to Fletcher, October 20, 1926, FD1/1016, 49222, PRO.

125. A. L. Thomson (Assistant Secretary MRC) to Robson, October 25, 1926, FD1/1015, 49222, PRO.

126. Crawford to Fletcher, April 29, 1926, FD1/1016, 49222, PRO.

127. Cushny to A. L. Thomson (Assistant Secretary MRC), March 18, 1923, FD1/1015, 49222, PRO.

128. Application on behalf of Dr. J. H. Crawford, March 30, 1926, FD1/1015, 49222, PRO.

129. Murray Lyon to A. L. Thomson (Assistant Secretary MRC), May 14, 1926, FD1/1015, 49222, PRO.

130. Ibid.

131. Crawford to Fletcher, April 29, 1926, FD1/1016, 49222, PRO.

132. Murray Lyon to Thomson, May 14, 1926.

133. Ibid.

134. Unsigned [? A. L. Thomson (Assistant Secretary MRC)] to Murray Lyon, May 31, 1926, FD1/1015, 49222, PRO.

135. Crawford to Fletcher, September 18, 1926, FD1/1016, 49222, PRO.

136. Pearce to Fletcher, May 4, 1926, FD1/1015, 49222, PRO.

137. Crawford to Fletcher, April 30, 1927, FD1/1016, 49222, PRO.

138. Fletcher to Crawford, May 23, 1927, FD1/1016, 49222, PRO.

139. Crawford to Fletcher, March 26, 1928, FD1/1016, 49222, PRO.

140. Davies at the end of September 1926, Crawford in spring 1927, and Robson in October 1927.

141. Fletcher to Meakins, June 20, 1924, FD1/1015, 49222, PRO.

142. Fletcher to Meakins, July 16, 1924, FD1/1015, 49222, PRO.

143. Meakins to Secretary of the University Court [W. Wilson], June 9, 1924, Secretary's File, DRT 95/002, pt. 1, Faculty of Medicine, box 27, EUA.

144. Lyon to [J.] Alfred Ewing, June 19, 1924, Secretary's File, DRT 95/002, pt. 1, Faculty of Medicine, box 27, EUA.

145. J. Lorrain Smith to Principal [J. Alfred Ewing], July 11, 1924, Secretary's File, DRT 95/002, pt. 1, Faculty of Medicine, box 27, EUA.

146. Meakins to Fletcher, July 18, 1924, FD1/1015, 49222, PRO.

147. Fletcher to Meakins, March 7, 1923, FD1/1015, 49222, PRO.

148. Pearce to [Fletcher], May 21, 1928, FD1/1841, 49222, PRO.

149. Fletcher to Pearce, December 20, 1928, FD1/1841, 49222, PRO. The three "promising young men" were Davies, Crawford and Robson.

150. R. M. Pearce, "Edinburgh, W. Fletcher talking to RMP, Aug. 27, 1929," folder 10, box 1, series 405, RG 1.1, Rockefeller Foundation Archives, RAC.

151. See p. 177.

152. Barger to Fletcher, April 28, 1929, FD1/1842, 49252, PRO.

153. "Obituary," *British Medical Journal* 2 (1956): 1309–10.

154. "Obituary," *The Lancet* 2 (1956): 1167–68.

155. Rae Llewelyn Lyon, Edited transcript of interview with Helen Coyle, August 12, 1997.

156. University of Edinburgh, Faculty of Medicine, "Minutes of a Meeting," July 1, 1924. Shelf ref. DA43, EUA.

157. Stewart to Fletcher, October 21, 1929, FD1/1016, 49222, PRO.

158. Superintendent of the Infirmary [G. St. C. Thom] to Lyon, July 27, 1927, "Scrap-Book of the RIE Biochemical Laboratory," box 2, RCPE; "Memorandum re the New Clinical Laboratory."

159. Stewart to Fletcher, October 21, 1929, FD1/1016, 49222, PRO.

160. "Memorandum re the New Clinical Laboratory."

161. Ibid.

162. C. P. Stewart and William Archibald, "The Estimation of Phosphorus and Magnesium," *The Biochemical Journal* 19 (1925): 484–91.

163. G. H. Percival and C. P. Stewart, "A Note on Renal Function in Scarlet Fever," *Edinburgh Medical Journal* 33 (1926): 53–57.

164. G. H. Percival and C. P. Stewart, "Pathological Variations in the Serum Calcium," *Quarterly Journal of Medicine* 19 (1926): 235–48.

165. C. P. Stewart, "Studies on the Metabolism of Arginine and Histidine. Part II. Arginine and Histidine as Precursors of Purines," *The Biochemical Journal* 19 (1925): 1101–10.

166. Elliot Simpson, *People who Made Scottish Clinical Biochemistry* (Airdrie: Sponsored by Mannheim Boehringer Diagnostics, 1995), 7.

167. "Memorandum re the New Clinical Laboratory."

168. D. M. Lyon. and W. L. Lamb, "Difficulties in Comparing Methods of Treatment for Lobar Pneumonia," *Edinburgh Medical Journal* 36 (1929): 79–92.

169. Ibid.

170. Meakins, "Oxygen-Want." Lyon and Lamb noted, without comment, that in the RIE oxygen was administered in a few of the more severe cases, "Difficulties in Comparing Methods of Treatment."

171. F. H. K. Green to John Ryle, July 21, 1931. FD1/2369, PRO. Cited in Martin Edwards, "Control and the Therapeutic Trial 1918–1948" (M.D. Thesis, University of London, 2005).

172. R. V. Christie, H. W. Davies, and C. P. Stewart, "Studies in Blood Coagulation and Haemophilia. II. Observations on Haemic Functions in Haemophilia," *Quarterly Journal of Medicine* 20 (1927): 481–98.

173. "Accommodation list," November 19, 1928, "Scrap-Book of the RIE Biochemical Laboratory," box 1, folder 6, RCPE.

174. "Memorandum re the New Clinical Laboratory"; W. A. Fleming [Secretary to the University] to Lyon, January 16, 1929, "Scrap-Book of the RIE Biochemical Laboratory," box 1, folder 7, RCPE.

175. D. M. Dunlop, "Form of Application for a Research Grant," FD1/1017, 49222, PRO.

176. "Obituary," *The Lancet*, 1 (1980): 1425–26.

177. C. P. Stewart and D. M. Dunlop, *Clinical Chemistry in Practical Medicine* (Edinburgh: E. & S. Livingstone, 1930).

178. For example, D. M. Dunlop and R. M. Lyon, "A Study of 523 Cases of Obesity," *Edinburgh Medical Journal* 38 (1931): 561–77.

179. A. L. Thomson (Assistant Secretary, MRC) to Lambie, March 13, 1929, FD1/1016, 49222, PRO. See C. G. Lambie, W. O. Kermack, and W. F. Harvey, "Effect of Parathyroid Hormone on the Structure of Bone," *Nature* 1234 (1929): 348.

9

BENCH AND BEDSIDE

How did physicians who were not laboratory researchers use the lab? This question does not admit of a full answer. Original case records for the medical wards do not exist except for the physician Edwin Bramwell. There is an almost full set of his patient records for the period 1919–1935. In addition a complete register of all of Bramwell's in-patients exists, so it is usually possible to know the names, diagnoses, admission, and discharge (or death) dates of those few patients whose notes are missing. Further, in surgery, there is virtually a complete set of case notes from 1925–1946 of Professor John Fraser. There are various problems in using the records of Bramwell. The major one is that they are frequently written up long after admission and for the most part contain virtually no progress notes or discharge summaries. The records are often in duplicate or even triplicate and are occasionally contradictory, seemingly having been written up by student clerks. Temperature charts, presumably kept by the nurses, sometimes with daily entries and comments have often proved vital sources of information. It is frequently difficult, often impossible, to work out who is using the lab and for what purpose. Even when this is clear the clinical reasoning behind lab usage is rarely recorded.

If there are general conclusions they are two very cautious ones. First, the lab was not a major resource for Bramwell and by extrapolation from the figures of lab usage this holds true for many other clinicians at the Infirmary. In the light of the overwhelming centrality of laboratory testing to modern medicine this is an extremely difficult chapter to write without seeming critical of Bramwell and other clinicians who might have availed themselves of the lab's facilities more frequently. They were, however, devoted to preserving their clinical skills and, in a way that might make the best teachers of medicine today jealous, they sought to show how valid conclusions might be arrived at without recourse to laboratory data. Perhaps too, they were, as they saw it, perpetuating a great clinical tradition tuned to the production of general practitioners who would not have easy access to laboratory tests. Further, although this is more difficult to reconstruct from case notes, clinicians such as Bramwell were assessing their patients' sickness through the subjective data of symptoms rather than the objective data of the lab. The second conclusion is an ironic one that seems to sustain Bramwell's criticisms of the way medicine around him was changing for the worse. Too often, he recurrently complained, students and juniors were rushing to laboratory tests before thorough bedside investigation had been carried out. In many of the cases cited here there is little or no evidence to show why a test was done or whether it changed clinical management. A good number, perhaps most, tests seem not to have been initiated by Bramwell at all but by baffled residents. Bramwell, after all, had a large private practice and was not paid to be on the wards as a full-time physician. Much must have gone on without his supervision. In his absence, residents were using tests as a blunderbuss. Andrew Doig remembered: "The senior clinical staff were responsible for requesting the laboratory tests but often delegated this duty to the clinical tutor or the resident."[1] Bramwell's support of a system—individualism and voluntary service— that he said was the safeguard of clinical skill fostered the very subversion he feared.

Bramwell's wards—numbers 31 and part of 33—had a sizeable intake of patients. Over the year 1921, 494 cases were admitted and by 1925 this figure had risen to 623. Numbers continued to rise and by 1930 they had reached 744. Patients were of both sexes, varied quite widely in age and occasionally included youngsters (Edinburgh had its own children's hospital). Patients were almost invariably from the lower income groups and from a range of occupations: manual workers, clerks, shop assistants, and a very large number of housewives. Bramwell was a neurologist and the population of his ward reflected this. There were many cases, roughly a third, of stroke, encephalitis lethargica, cerebral tumour, myopathy and so forth.[2] But his case load also included heart and lung disease, nephritis, and endocrine disorders. With few exceptions, however, notably occasional cases of scarlet fever, acute infectious diseases were not admitted. These were sent to the City Hospital.

Bramwell's case notes confirm that, as in theory so in practice, stress was laid on training the unaided senses and making judgements without recourse to laboratory assistance. For example, the notes contain records of estimations of blood pressure made by feeling the pulse. These were sometimes checked by the use of a sphygmomanometer.[3] In 1920, a patient with a pulse "characteristic of auricular fibrillation" did not, apparently, merit EKG examination.[4] In the same year, in a patient with a thirty-year history of valvular lesions of the heart, it was concluded that in "the absence of Babinski and other signs of specific affection of the nervous system, we may exclude a diagnosis of primary syphilitic disease with secondary affection of the circulatory system."[5] There is no record of a Wassermann test which, presumably, was deemed superfluous.

A large number of Bramwell's patients, after routine urine tests in the side room had been carried out, were managed entirely by their bedside symptoms and signs. When outside help was resorted to, as it increasingly was in the 1920s, it was the assistance of the Pathology and Bacteriology Departments that was most often requested. Scarcely surprising on a neurological ward was the extensive number of blood specimens sent to these departments for Wassermann reactions. Sampling of records suggests that the use of this test increased during the decade so that by 1930 more than half the patients were being tested. Very few results were positive. Bramwell also relied on these departments to culture bacteria, notably in renal disease and suspected tuberculosis of the lung or meninges. The next most extensively used facility was the Radiological Department. By 1930 roughly a third of patients were being X-rayed. Apart from biochemical investigations, which are discussed next, the only other examination requested that required external expertise was electrocardiography. Even by 1930, however, only a handful of EKGs was requested each year.

In 1920, the year before the lab was available to him, 456 patients were admitted to Bramwell's wards. The side room was employed in various ways. All patients had qualitative urine analysis. Blood counts were done in cases such as suspected anaemia and when the diagnosis was obscure. In two cases faeces were examined microscopically for fat globules. Quantitative estimations of substances in the urine, such as albumin, urea, ammonia, and sugar were occasionally performed in patients with nephritis. Another analysis carried out in the side rooms was the "test meal." After a meal, gastric juice was obtained by a stomach tube and its hydrochloric acid content measured. The juice could also be examined microscopically.

Two cases admitted in 1920 merit particular notice. Together they are unique for having the biochemistry of their blood investigated. Elizabeth C., a 48-year-old housewife from Edinburgh, was admitted on January 6, 1920, after a four-week history of itching and yellowing of skin.[6] On examination there was tenderness in the hypochondrium. She was diagnosed, at some point, as having obstructive jaundice, possibly caused by gallstones or malignancy. The case was obviously puzzling since she underwent a battery of side room tests including a blood count, microscopy of the faeces and urine, tests for occult blood and bile in the faeces, and a test meal. She also had a Sahli's test of pancreatic function in which a capsule containing iodoform was swallowed, and the urine and saliva later tested for iodine. Other departments were recruited: a radiographic examination after an opaque meal and a Wassermann reaction were carried out. Nine days after admission, the notes record that the ammonia nitrogen, urea, total nitrogen, and the acidity of the urine were measured *quantitatively*. These estimations were surely done in the side room. Most probably at the same time, the non-protein nitrogen (NPN) in the blood was estimated. It is possible that the blood test was done in the side room but it is more likely that the laboratory of the College of Physicians was asked to carry it out.[7] The notes contain no comment on the significance of the test nor do they provide anything but minimal access to the clinical reasoning behind the management of the case. They do contain an observation, probably by a student, on the ammonia nitrogen in the urine, which was about double its normal level.[8] The writer reasoned that "this is most likely to be due to deficient liver functioning" and observed that this was a more probable cause "than . . . acidosis to which this upset in the ammonia nitrogen co-efficient in jaundice is so frequently attributed."[9] What is significant about this remark (which seems incorrect by the criteria of the day) is the student's analysis of the urine's constituents in terms of the hotly-debated biochemical concept of acidosis. No final diagnosis was ever indicated in the notes. Not much can be said about this case either medically or otherwise. There was no account of the patient's condition after discharge. There was no record of who ordered the blood test and it may just have been a shot in the dark by a junior doctor—the very thing Bramwell was so concerned to prevent. The notes only show that blood biochemistry was an option when investigating a puzzling case.

The rarity of biochemical blood testing on Bramwell's wards in 1920 is highlighted by its happening only once more in that year. On September 3, 1920, William C., a 28-year-old baker from Edinburgh, was admitted. He stayed in hospital nearly four months.[10] He had a three-year history of head pains and giddiness and, over the previous year, fits and double vision. On examination he was "a fat 'nephritic' looking young man." There was no sugar in the urine. The notes, as usual, are not much of a guide as to how a diagnosis was made or to his management. At an early stage, because of the neurological symptoms and his general appearance a pituitary disorder (a special interest of Bramwell's) seems to have been suspected. Diabetes was undoubtedly ruled out because of the absence of sugar in the urine. Three weeks after admission he was given a glucose test meal (tolerance test). This required that the fasting subject should ingest glucose and have several estimations made of urine and/or blood sugars: customarily, one estimation before ingestion and three or four afterwards at half-hourly intervals. William was given 50 g of glucose at 8:00 A.M. and the next six specimens of urine were examined *qualitatively* for sugar (it was present in the first four). Far more interesting is that his notes also contain a graph recording two tolerance tests in which the *blood* glucose was measured; one estimation being made before 100 g of glucose were given orally, a five further being carried out during the following hour and a half. There was no indication of where the glucose estimations were made: perhaps on the ward, perhaps at the College of Physicians. A note on the graph records that glycosuria appeared on both occasions and, describing the curves,

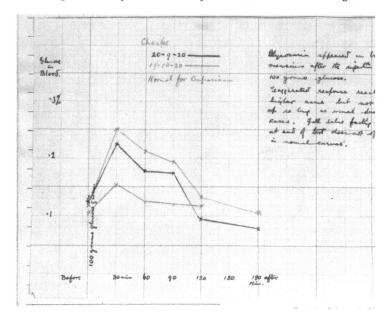

Fig. 9.1: Glucose tolerance curve from the case notes of
William C. in "Case notes of medical patients under the care of Edwin
Bramwell, 1919–35." (Vol. 13, case 467, LHB1, CC/37a, LHSA, EUL.)
Photograph courtesy of LHSA.

explained: "Exaggerated response reaching a higher acme but not remaining up so long as usual ductless gland cases. Fell below fasting level at end of test does not often appear in normal curves." (see Figure 9.1) The case notes make no reference to this graph. A glucose tolerance test was regarded as valuable in some endocrine disorders and atypical cases of glycosuria.[11] For biochemically-minded clinicians this test was particularly important in the diagnosis and particularly the assessment of diabetes. Bramwell, however, seemed to value it, certainly here but also elsewhere, as a general indicator of a pituitary disorder. The test in this instance seems to have been used to support rather than make the diagnosis. The patient was operated on and cerebrospinal fluid was drained off "under great pressure." The final diagnosis (made presumably on clinical and surgical grounds) was internal hydrocephalus with pituitary symptoms. As in the previous case there is no record of the patient's subsequent history.

On the eve of the opening of the biochemistry laboratory then, Bramwell appears as a clinician versed in the use of modern medical laboratory aids but committed to the primacy of experience and individual clinical judgement. Since the hospital had no lab, perhaps the almost certain difficulty of having tests performed contributes to this appearance. Did the opening of the new lab change Bramwell's practice? Bramwell used the new biochemistry lab little in its first year. He sent thirteen specimens to the lab in 1921. There are, however, only seven biochemical forms in the cases notes, but case notes are also missing, including, perhaps significantly, those of a diabetic.[12] Of the seven forms present, five were requests for blood sugar tests from a single patient. Of the nearly 500 patients admitted that year then, *at most* Bramwell only carried out lab tests on nine of them, and possibly only four if the missing notes of the diabetic contained multiple requests for blood sugars. Given that one of the patients had five tests the appearance, as in 1920, is of a clinician prepared to use tests in a difficult case but by no means ready to employ the resource with any frequency and certainly not in a routine way. Did familiarity change habit?

Bramwell's use of the lab did increase but not by a great deal over the decade. In the first six months of 1922 he requested seven tests of the lab: four were for Basal Metabolic Rate (BMR), two for blood sugar, and one for urine lead. The next time there is a record of how many requests he sent is the latter six months of 1925, when forty-one were received. In the same six months the new head of the Department of Therapeutics, Murray Lyon, requested 343, but these figures probably indicate the number of diabetics having their blood sugars measured at out-patient clinics. A better comparison might be the 212 requests made by John Eason, a physician with a keen interest in biochemistry. William Ritchie, to become Professor of Medicine in 1928, sent eighty-three requests in the same period. In the whole of 1926 Bramwell sent only thirty-five. None the less over the decade Bramwell did become a more frequent lab user than he was initially (although his patient population increased too, but not quite proportionately). Some of this increase can be accounted for by rising requests for blood sugar tests due to the introduction of insulin, but other factors were at work. Bramwell's figures rose to ninety-one in 1930. In this year approximately one in eight patients had biochemical tests, carried out in the lab.[13] Bramwell's figures also show the general reliance on the lab for blood rather than urine testing. Of course the judgement "Bramwell sent . . ." begs the question of whether it was Bramwell, the resident, or the clinical tutor who initiated testing. There is evidence that they all did.

Because of missing forms and notes and other factors, exact tabulation of Bramwell's employment of tests is difficult. There were four major categories of use: in diabetes, in renal disease, in diseases of the central nervous system, and in thyroid disorders. The principal tests in these categories were, respectively, estimations of sugar in blood, of protein metabolites in blood, and of cerebro-spinal fluid (CSF) constituents, and determinations of BMR. Throughout most of the decade blood sugar estimations were roughly equal to the other three categories put together. By 1930, however, protein metabolite tests and sugar estimations were about equal in numbers and jointly comprised about 70 per cent of tests carried out. By this time CSF examinations made up a further 15 per cent, BMRs constituted 10 per cent, with a remaining 5 per cent in a miscellaneous category.

Diabetes was the condition in which the laboratory most obviously made itself a participant in clinical work. In no other disorder was there any therapeutic or diagnostic innovation associated with biochemical management that was as transforming as the introduction of insulin into general use in 1923. Perceptions of diabetes at this time lay on a spectrum with an emphasis on its clinical features at the one end and concern with its biochemical nature at the other. A good example of a clinical perception is found in the third edition of the medical textbook of Robert Fleming, physician at the RIE, published in 1919. Fleming began his survey of diabetes (which he included under "General Diseases") with a clinical definition. The disorder was the "persistent excretion of sugar in the urine with definite deterioration of health." The detection of sugar in the urine, either by taste (as was once the case) or by chemical means, was a clinical skill. Discussing the possible pathophysiological mechanisms producing the disease Fleming noted that the liver, pituitary, pancreas, and suprarenal glands possibly all had a role in producing glycosuria. That is, he stressed the clinical end point and not hyperglycaemia. The sorts of blood levels of sugar that might appear in diabetes were described in a single sentence. However a whole paragraph was devoted to changes in the urine. He then noted that "as a rule" the diagnosis of diabetes was "easy," adding that it was important to distinguish diabetes from simple glycosuria. This could be done by the "method of giving 25, 50 and 100 g of glucose on consecutive days and noting the tolerance of the patient by estimating the amount of sugar excreted [in the urine]."[14] This was a test easily carried out by GPs but Fleming gave no indication as to whether more technically-demanding tests (for instance of blood) might produce better results.

During the 1920s physiologically-minded clinicians began to take a view of diabetes as a metabolic disease and in doing so gave hyperglycaemia, rather than glycosuria, a defining role in the disorder. In these accounts, in which blood sugars were given a diagnostic function and a central place in ongoing management, a laboratory test began to being privileged over clinical skill. In such accounts, blood tests were portrayed as accurate and essential guides to diagnosis and treatment. The sugar content of the blood was described as a more sensitive indicator of diabetes than urine tests, for it could register the severity of the disorder in the absence of urinary symptoms (when, say, the patient was fasting). Urine tests were thus demoted from the centrality accorded them by clinicians such as Fleming. Blood glucose tolerance tests were also promoted as crucial for distinguishing renal diabetes (or simple glycosuria in which the blood sugar was normal) from diabetes mellitus. That there was, however, a middle way, will be seen in the writings of Murray Lyon. Although Murray Lyon promoted knowledge of metabolism and blood biochemistry as the key to understanding of diabetes, his management of the disease was usually based on simpler bedside approaches (such as urine testing). These, he said, skillfully used, could give access to the desired biochemical knowledge in an indirect way. The goal of clinical medicine, he explained, was the achievement of normal blood sugar levels but these, however, did not need to be measured in everyday practice. Here was the initial working out of compromise between new medical theory and traditional clinical art. The all-encompassing imperialism of the laboratory and technology was being resisted in the name of irreducible human characteristics.

In 1921 Murray Lyon and Meakins published "The Treatment of Diabetes Mellitus," a paper revealing a markedly metabolic or biochemical view of the disorder.[15] The treatment of diabetes by diet was the source of immense satisfaction in the early 1920s, being regarded as a triumph of modern scientific therapy. Endorsing these sentiments, Murray Lyon and Meakins recorded how a "remarkable advance" had occurred in 1913 when the Harvard researcher Frederick Allen introduced his "starvation" treatment.[16] This "fasting method," they observed, had met with "universal approval" and was "a triumph for carefully conducted laboratory research." They explained the rationale of the method in terms of the physiology of carbohydrate absorption, glycogen formation, and glucose uptake by the muscles. Central to their account was a description of the "Glucose Test Meal" (the tolerance test used by Bramwell in 1920 to assess pituitary function). In diabetics, after ingestion of glucose an "abnormally high and greatly prolonged" curve of sugar in the blood was produced. The meal was suitably illustrated by a graph, an important rhetorical and practical tool of academic medicine (see Figure 9.2). The aim of dietetic treatment, it was explained, was to present glucose to the body in complex carbohydrate form, slowing its absorption and preventing it appearing in the urine.[17] Meakins and Murray Lyon warned: "*Too much weight should not be put on the presence of sugar in the urine*, since glycosuria of itself is only a harmless symptom. It is the continued hyperglycaemia and the underlying functional difficulty in assimilating carbohydrates which are of importance."[18] Significant here, then, is centrality of the tolerance curve. Glycosuria was no certain guide in diabetes: serial blood measurement was the only sure test. Murray Lyon was to modify pragmatically his position on this maxim.

Knowledge of the physiology and biochemistry of diabetes, Murray Lyon and Meakins argued, provided a basis for sound therapy. The authors explained how the Allen treatment "consists in rapidly reducing the patient's diet, then fasting him till the urine becomes sugar free, and later building up the diet slowly." The first stage of treatment was "Preliminary Observation," at which point "the patient presents himself for treatment." During this stage, lasting several days, the patient was to be put on a "standard full diet." Twenty-four-hour urine samples were to be tested for acetone and di-acetic acid, and an estimation made of the total sugar excreted. At the end of the paper the case of a hospital patient, "an average case", was included as an illustration. This diabetic was given a test meal in the stage of "Preliminary Observation" and the authors employed the test as integral to the routine management of diabetes.[19] In the second stage of the Allen treatment the patient's diet

The Treatment of Diabetes Mellitus

fats should be at once stopped while the carbohydrates are
continued or even increased.

Ordinate = percentage of glucose in the blood.
Abscissa = time in minutes after ingestion of glucose.

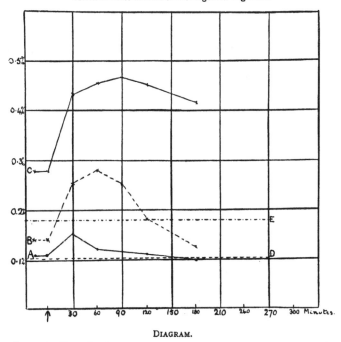

DIAGRAM.

Glucose Test Meal.   Blood-sugar reaction to ingestion of 100 grams of glucose (at ↑).

in A = Normal person.
  B = Hyperthyroidism.
  C = Diabetes Mellitus.
Line D = Average fasting level of blood-sugar.
  E = So-called renal threshold.

Glycosuria occurred in cases B and C.

The modern treatment of diabetes has no need for *drugs*
except in acidosis, but the dietetic course should be supplemented
by certain general measures.   The patient ought to live a quiet
life as far as possible, avoiding all causes of worry, excitement,
etc.   Glycosuria can be readily induced in some cases by

Fig. 9.2: The Glucose Test Meal as described by Lyon and Meakins in D.
Murray Lyon and Jonathan Meakins, "The Treatment of Diabetes
Mellitus," *Edinburgh Medical Journal* 27 (1921): 270–85. (LO027469BOO.)
The Wellcome Library, London.

was reduced and a 24-hour urine sugar was measured. After this came a fasting stage to render the urine sugar free. The illustrative case had a blood sugar estimated on the third day of his fast. Next came a stage of building up the patient's diet and finally there was the stage of "Maintenance." The "average case" returned to a "practically normal" diet without the return of glycosuria or hyperglycaemia.[20] It is clear that other blood sugar estimations had been done on this patient and regarded as part of normal monitoring but the report was unspecific as to details. Underlying the fasting method of treatment was the presumption that the pancreas was being rested and might recover its normal function. Startling though the introduction of insulin was, fasting still remained a key to therapy until the mid-1920s, when some clinicians began to institute regimes of dietary liberalization.[21] In Edinburgh strict dietary rules remained the norm, certainly into the 1930s.[22]

Bramwell did not treat many diabetics. In 1930, for example, only 18 of the 744 case records pertain to diabetes.[23] Presumably Murray Lyon treated most diabetics. Blood sugar tests were certainly carried out on one of Bramwell's diabetic cases in 1921, the year the lab opened. Catherine B., aged 20 years, was a typist from Linlithgow.[24] She was admitted on January 10, 1921, and discharged just over a month later. She had an eighteen-month history of thirst and polyuria and had been treated by her GP since the previous October for diabetes, having been given, she reported, "rather vague instructions as to diet." On the ward she was managed by the Allen method and a close record was made on the temperature chart, presumably by a nurse. Curiously the chart made provision for entering various urine tests, but not sugars. In Catherine's case these were recorded in the space for noting respiratory rate (see Figure 9.3). Tests for urine sugar were certainly done in the side room. The sugars were recorded by minus and plus signs and as "trace." There were no blood tests and her urine was free of sugar on discharge, when she left with dietetic instructions. Bramwell obviously saw no reason to utilize the new laboratory in the management of this diabetic patient at this time.

Catherine B. was readmitted ten moths later on November 11, 1921, with general weakness, loss of weight, some thirst and hunger, and a great deal of sugar in the urine.[25] Three days later she became the first recorded diabetic of Bramwell's to have a blood glucose carried out in the lab. Fergus Hewat, the Clinical Tutor, made the request. Murray Lyon

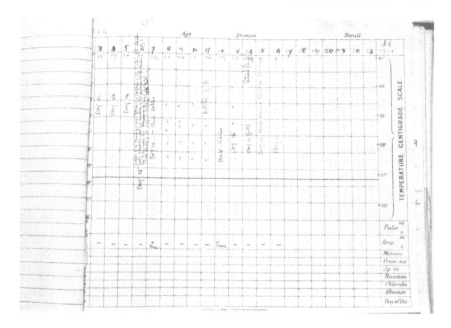

Fig. 9.3: Temperature chart of Catherine B. in "Case notes of medical patients under the care of Edwin Bramwell, 1919–35." (Vol. 17, case 622, LHB1, CC/37a, LHSA, EUL.) Photograph courtesy of LHSA.

signed the report with a comment written in red ink: "Time after meal & character of meal must be taken into consideration here." Perhaps he considered that clinicians needed educating in the significance of blood testing. A second blood test was done two days later. Presumably there had been some verbal communication between ward and lab over this specimen since the report, signed by Murray Lyon, stated that the analysis had been done on "B[loo]d sugar fasting." Catherine was treated by diet. Three further blood tests were done over the next three weeks. Most interesting is that a graph was drawn plotting her blood and urine sugars during her entire stay. This was probably a student's record including his or her own side room urine tests.[26] It was not a record of a tolerance test—it was presumably a means to monitor the effect of diet. On January 13, 1922, nine weeks after admission, Catherine B. was discharged. Blood tests here seem to have been marginal to clinical care in Catherine's case and to have been an almost random check on the usual form of clinical management, although such an approach would have been far from compatible with Bramwell's views. Perhaps they were used to determine whether the carbohydrate content of the diet might be increased. Without knowing exactly the conditions under which blood was taken no final judgement is possible. There is certainly no evidence that the test results were acted on to change therapy in any way. Catherine B.'s life after leaving the ward is unrecorded. She was presumably instructed as to her diet and seen at out-patients.

A case admitted in 1921 and another in 1922 are of interest in that they had glucose test meals carried out. However, in both instances it was the simple clinical test of measuring the sugar in the urine, not in the blood, that was performed. In the first case the test was presumably carried out as part of an assessment of general pancreatic function. William R., aged 22 years, a chartered accountant from Kirkaldy, was admitted on October 18, 1921, and diagnosed, eventually, as suffering from pancreatic infantilism.[27] Striking in this case, if the notes are anything to go by, was the apparently late employment of laboratory resources in diagnosis. William had a history of abnormal stools, inability to eat fats, and failure to thrive. Nine days after admission he had "a glucose reaction" test. Glucose was given at 8:30 A.M. and its concentration in the urine was measured over the next four hours. These estimations were almost certainly done in the side room, as was the Sahli's test carried out the next day. Nearly four weeks later a sample of faeces was sent to the pathologist. Over a week later, on December 1, a sample of faeces sent to the biochemistry lab was reported on, the form giving the results of estimations of total fat, neutral fat, and "fatty acid and scraps." William was discharged for Christmas, "Improved," on December 9. William had his test meal to probe for signs of either general endocrine deficiency or inadequate pancreatic function or both, but not as an assessment of diabetes. It was not a diagnostic test.

William L., aged 35 years, a ploughman from Colingham and a known diabetic, was admitted on May 13, 1922.[28] He discharged himself four weeks later, the cover page of the record stating that the "patient left Hospital without giving any warning and of course without doctor's permission." Two days after admission the very muddled notes recorded a side room test that showed "large amount of sugar [in urine]."[29] At the end of the record on a separate, undated sheet (but which states "Before treatment was started") was recorded a quantitative urine sugar test, then the administration of 100 g of glucose followed by six urine sugar estimations, presumably done in the side room. No useful comments about diagnosis, treatment, or outcome can be found. On Bramwell's ward patients were not managed according to the Murray Lyon–Meakins protocol: blood sugars were only occasionally estimated and glucose tolerance tests, when performed, were done using urine. In the one instance of a graph of the blood sugar levels being drawn, the record was more like a picture of the patient's whole illness while in hospital for it visualized several *days* of testing, not the hourly sequelae of a test meal.

Lyon and Meakins were not alone in considering blood sugar measurement proper in all cases of diabetes. At a meeting of the Medico-Chirurgical Society of Edinburgh in February 1922, Harry Rainy, an Infirmary physician, gave a paper on "The Significance and Treatment of Glycosuria."[30] He opened by noting how recent "fuller knowledge" of the cause of glycosuria had led to "so great an advance in treatment" that there could be no doubt of the patient's improved prospects. In Rainy's view, "any patient who has a demonstrable quantity of sugar in the urine is suffering from diabetes mellitus unless the contrary can be clearly proved." Nevertheless, he observed that distinguishing among "different types of glycosuria" was of "considerable importance." To do this it was of "first importance" to be able to estimate blood sugar with "considerable accuracy."[31] After outlining a taxonomy of glycosurias, Rainy confined his further remarks to "true diabetes," a disease in which "it may be asserted with some confidence that the essential factor in its production is pancreatic insufficiency." If that was so, he added in a conclusion which did not mirror Bramwell's approach, "one can hardly over-emphasize the importance of correlation between laboratory and clinical workers in carrying out treatment" because "[a]t every stage of treatment it is necessary that the clinical findings should be checked by somewhat elaborate tests in the chemical laboratory" and these could "hardly be performed" by the clinician who could not command the time for such work. Rainy advocated the fasting method of treatment and for the best results he observed that patients "should be under hospital observation for at least a couple of months." They should be weighed daily, their urine examined daily, and the "occasional" blood sugar estimated.[32]

In a discussion of this paper Murray Lyon described forty cases treated over the previous two years, observing "the outlook of the diabetic patient has entirely changed since the introduction of modern methods of treatment." After diagnosis, he observed, an estimate of severity could be helped by "a number of methods of laboratory examinations" including 24-hour urine sugar measurements, fasting blood glucose, and a test meal. The best indication of prognosis was a test meal after treatment, just before the patient left hospital. All but two of the forty cases treated by Murray Lyon were, he said, made aglycosuric. The two exceptions turned out not to be failures of treatment. In the first a boy with a fulminating type of diabetes and acidosis became homesick and "was removed from hospital." The second had features that suggested it was "really" a case of "renal diabetes" or innocuous glycosuria. It is noteworthy that after the introduction of insulin this meeting was remembered for the "strain of pessimism [that] coloured the discussion."[33]

In May 1922 Murray Lyon published in the *Lancet* on "Prognosis in Diabetes Mellitus." This was a paper originally given to senior medical students. In it Murray Lyon observed it was "important to decide whether a case should be diagnosed as mere glycosuria or as diabetes," adding, in a manner that might have seemed confusing, "in this extremely difficult matter it is probably best to accept the more serious view and treat accordingly." Presumably in support of the latter opinion, he offered the view that "No hard-and-fast line exists between 'simple glycosuria' and diabetes; they are merely grades of the same condition."[34] He was not referring here to renal glycosuria, which he recognized among the "mechanisms" by which sugar appeared in the urine and which in the following year he would call a "rare condition."[35] Murray Lyon agreed with the opinion that cure could not be expected when the pancreas was grossly affected, but in "functional" cases and in "mild organic conditions" there was no reason why "complete restitution may not be possible." In general in adequately-treated cases, with "modern methods . . . the outlook of the patient has been vastly improved." Murray Lyon then described how an analysis of a series of cases had been made "with a view to discovering the prognostic value of symptoms." The degree and rapidity of body wasting was a valuable index of the severity of the disease. A 24-hour urine sugar estimation was a good guide as to how the patient was at that moment but gave no indication of future response to treatment. Blood examinations were "helpful in giving an idea of the severity of the disease but a single examination fails to show whether the damage is temporary or permanent." It was more valuable "to investigate . . . the fasting level of the blood sugar, and the response to ingestion of a standard test meal."[36] The best possible guide to prognosis, however, was response to treatment (a clinical aphorism and not the biochemical one he had adopted two months earlier in February).

In spite of the methods advised by the experts and the laboratory resources now available, by and large at this time Bramwell's approach did not rely on blood chemistry. John T., aged 34 years, a "lorryman" from Coldingham, was admitted on December 4, 1922, after a three-and-a-half-month history of weight loss.[37] In November his GP diagnosed diabetes and cut down John's food but, the GP wrote, the urine was "still full of sugar" and he wanted the patient admitted to "see if his diet could be standardised." John was put on the Allen diet and had six quantitative urine sugar estimations done in the side ward. No blood tests were done. In spite of his GP's insistence that "he's an awfully good patient," he discharged himself ten days later. Similarly in January 1923 William M., aged 18 years, a clerk from Portobello, was admitted.[38] He had a twelve-month history of weight loss, polyuria and polydipsia. On admission his height was 5 ft 9½ in (1.77 m) and his weight a mere 8 st 9¾ lb (55.3 Kg). The notes recorded: "on admission it was found that his urine . . . contained a great deal of sugar, acetone and diacetic acid." He was treated by the Allen diet and his urine became sugar free. The notes indicated that the patient's "general health improved considerably, although he lost about 7 pounds in weight." John was discharged after two months. Control of diet for skilled physicians outweighed any considerations of patient well-being. To ease up on dietary restriction was to court death.

The history of the introduction of insulin into clinical medicine in 1922–23 has often been recounted.[39] Significant here is that insulin provided the opportunity for the proponents of academic medicine to control a valuable therapeutic agent, and in so doing give a lesson to the medical community on the organization and practice of what was deemed scientific drug assessment. The isolation of insulin in a physiological laboratory led, through personal and professional contacts, to the MRC having, initially, complete control of its use. The MRC ensured insulin was assessed by co-ordinated teams of basic scientists and clinicians in university centres. Individual practitioners who claimed a right to test it by virtue of their clinical experience were rigorously excluded.

Later, as insulin became more freely available, controversy would break out as doctors with their own ideas of its use and its monitoring fell outside the MRC's authority.[40] In response some academic physicians modified the rigid criteria they had created to govern insulin's employment.

A pancreatic extract, later called insulin, was prepared in the physiology laboratories of J. J. R. Macleod in Toronto and injected in patients in early 1922. The first publications of trials on patients appeared in March of that year.[41] On June 17 Meakins wrote to Macleod ("Dear Professor Macleod") asking if he could spare some pancreatic extract so that Meakins could treat a colleague, Norman Walker, who had glycosuria.[42] On July 8 Macleod, regretting that they had not worked out the deterioration curve for "insulin," declined, but he sent typed directions for its preparation, from a paper scheduled to appear a few months later. Meakins was sworn to secrecy for fear of commercial exploitation.[43] In spite of the formality of the communications, Macleod obviously held Meakins in high esteem. To other similar enquiries, of which he had many, Macleod only promised reprints of the paper when it appeared. It is quite likely that on the basis of Macleod's reply Meakins initiated work on the isolation of insulin in Edinburgh. In his autobiography he recorded:

> So we started with our grinding stage, using pig pancreases in a basement of one of the wards of the Infirmary as our "workshop". It was not long before Harington had what he believed to be a potent insulin, but we had to try it. We dared not do this on man and we could not house rabbits in the Infirmary. But we got a few into Banger's [*sic*] laboratory and a few more with Professor Cushny. Our first batch was so potent that we killed the rabbits. But by dilution we came to a level that both Banger and Cushny thought was safe.

After this, Meakins remembered: "we quietly—almost surreptitiously—sought for volunteers. Among the first to respond was Professor Norman Walker. He entered the public ward and after standardisation of his fasting blood sugar we gave an injection with our hearts in our mouths and intravenous solutions of glucose at hand. The result was perfect."[44] Infirmary records confirm that Norman Walker was admitted under Meakins between July 27 and August 31, 1922.[45] Oddly, Meakins does not seem to have mentioned these activities to Fletcher.

On July 25, 1922, Meakins wrote to Fletcher that he was in communication with Macleod. Meakins had also discussed insulin with J. G. Fitzgerald, Director of the University of Toronto's Anti-Toxin laboratories, who had collaborated on the insulin work and had recently been in Edinburgh. Meakins wanted Charles Lambie, who had worked with Cushny, to study the pharmacology and physiology of insulin. He also wanted William Robson, the physiological chemist in the department, to isolate the active chemical. Barger, Meakins felt sure, could be relied on for help and advice.[46] This is odd since, if Meakins's autobiography is accurate (see above), Barger was already doing just that.[47] It had been agreed Lambie would go to Toronto and he was prepared to travel at his own expense.[48] In August Macleod said he would be "very glad to see Dr. Lambie."[49]

By autumn 1922 insulin was in use in several centres in North America. In September, Henry Dale of the MRC visited Toronto and was impressed by the insulin work. On September 22 a Dr. J. G. Fraser of Essex, obviously an old acquaintance of Macleod's, wrote asking him if pancreatic extract might be available for Fraser's brother-in-law in Perthshire.[50] Macleod suggested the brother-in-law communicate with Meakins, advice indicating Meakins had isolated insulin.[51] None the less on October 17 Meakins wrote again to Fletcher reporting Lambie had returned from America and that they were "all prepared to go on with the insulin work."[52] On November 18 the British medical press announced that the University of Toronto had offered the MRC the patent covering the preparation of insulin.[53] A week previously, on November 10, Fletcher had written formally to Meakins ("Dear Professor Meakins" instead of his usual "Dear Meakins") telling him of the MRC's patent rights and inviting his "unit" to be one of the "selected centres" to take part in work of "great urgency" on the production, standardization, and therapeutic use of insulin. A precondition of centre selection was the presence of a biochemist to extract and prepare insulin and to assist in the "analytical control of the effects produced in the sugar-content of the blood and urine." Fletcher considered it "obvious" that the biochemist "must look forward to giving his whole time to this work." The Council was to defray the "special expenses" of the work but hoped the "ordinary resources" of the lab would provide "the further necessities." The Council was prepared to consider a special grant for the biochemist. Meakins was to use the insulin only on his own wards and the Council was to be recognized as being in final control and the channel of all communication between centres.[54] Meakins accepted five days later, adding, "since the early spring we have been preparing our department towards the present end." He reported that he had some forty diabetic cases under his care. Murray Lyon would take charge of the clinical work and carry out the lab tests with the help of Lambie, although the latter would mainly spend his time on the pharmacology and standardization of insulin. Robson would work on improving the extraction technique and on the chemistry of the hormone. A large supply of pancreas, Meakins said, was available from the Edinburgh abattoir, since the organ was not used as "sweet breads" but classified as offal.[55]

Fletcher replied on November 22 and reassured Meakins that in one way or another money for apparatus would eventually be forthcoming, but since the treatment was necessary for certain patients some of the costs "should fairly be borne out of general hospital funds given for charity." Fletcher wished Meakins would "sound" his "people in Edinburgh."[56] On the same day Meakins wrote to Fletcher about a potential conflict of interests. Meakins was treating privately a diabetic patient in a nursing home and had been approached by the patient's wealthy brother, who had asked if lack of funds was delaying the introduction of insulin. The brother had said to Meakins, if so, " 'can you give me an idea of what sum would be useful . . . [and] I shall be glad to see what can be done towards providing it'." He tentatively offered Meakins £500 to £1,000, assuring the latter it was "not given with any definite qualification that his brother should be necessarily treated." Meakins told him that any qualified offer was unacceptable and that any patients treated with insulin must be on the wards of the RIE. Meakins observed to Fletcher: "Of course I feel perfectly certain that he hoped, if the offer were accepted, that I would select his brother to be one of the early cases to be treated *in the Royal Infirmary*." Meakins asked Fletcher's advice.[57] Fletcher was quite clear and his reply reveals the distinction between the management of private and public patients: "If his brother is a man whom you could normally take into your wards, *and use for experimental treatment*, I do not myself see why you should not do so, so long as the donation is made entirely free of any stipulation to that effect." It was important you "guard yourself against any suggestion that rich men can buy the first results of your work." Fletcher considered the "only decent thing for a rich man to do . . . is to give money to help the work by which alone large scale production . . . may be made possible and easy."[58] In his autobiography Meakins recorded that a benefactor had donated "several ? [*sic*] hundred pounds" on condition that "no charge was to be made to any patient receiving our product." This was probably very early in the work but the exact time of donation is not clear.[59]

By December 6, 1922, Meakins could report that they were "pushing on" with insulin and hoped to have it "in full swing" by the time he and Fletcher met for lunch at "the Club" (either the Athenaeum, Brooks's, or the United University) a week later.[60] Meakins wrote to Fletcher on January 30, 1923: "We began treatment in the early part of January."[61] On February 24, 1923, the MRC issued a statement to the effect that at "various hospitals where the necessary facilities existed for biological and chemical work in the laboratories, and for scientific clinical studies . . . Insulin is being produced, standardised, and used in treatment for the relief of patients." Four London hospitals, Sheffield University and the Sheffield Royal Infirmary, and the Royal Infirmary of Edinburgh (but not the University) were named. Glasgow would later be added to this list. In all the institutions chosen there was a senior figure with a strong biochemical background involved in the trial. The Council was hopeful about the prospects of large-scale production of insulin in the near future. However, "some weeks must pass before laboratory tests and clinical use under special safeguards" could justify its general introduction.[62]

On March 5, at Fletcher's request, Meakins reported to him the results of treatment thus far. According to this version the first patient treated with insulin was in diabetic coma and the drug was used "without any material result," although Meakins admitted it was a first product and there were doubts about its strength. The second patient treated was also in coma and insulin was used with "spectacular results." She recovered, improved, and gained weight. She had been taken off insulin and Meakins's group were "working up her diet" to determine her tolerance before giving insulin again. Two other "severe" cases had responded well. Insulin had "cleared up" their acidosis and permitted a large amount of carbohydrate to be given. A number of isolated observations on blood sugar curves in different grades of diabetes had also been made.[63]

On March 17, Fletcher wrote to Meakins telling him that at "a very early date" his supply of insulin "may be supplemented and perhaps later superseded, by supplies from large scale manufacture." Fletcher also wished to know about any "particular clinical investigations" Meakins was pursuing and about "ill-results" of insulin use.[64] Meakins replied that, clinically, his group was working on whether insulin increased carbohy-drate tolerance, whether it influenced ketosis and the oxidation of fat, and on its effects on respiratory metabolism, blood sugar curves, and alkaline reserve. This work was linked to experimental investigations of the blood sugar curve in rabbits and respiratory parameters "in animals and man."[65] The group was also studying, experimentally, insulin hypo-glycaemia with special reference to the liver. All this was physiological problem solving at the bedside.

By the middle of April, British firms were selling insulin commer-cially manufactured from ox pancreas. After production it was tested for potency on rabbits and distributed in sealed capsules of twenty units. It was being produced in sufficient quantities to be distributed to "various large hospitals."[66] In April 1923, 100 units cost 25s. A year later the cost had fallen to 6s. 8d. (66p). By 1929, 100 units cost 2s. (10p)[67] On April 14, 1923, Fletcher wrote to Meakins querying the value of local pro-duction of insulin for clinical use.[68] On April 30 Meakins cabled Macleod: "LYON WRITES YOU CAN SPARE INSULIN DELIGHTED TO HAVE IT REGULARLY."[69] On receiving this, Macleod asked the Anti-Toxin laboratories to dispatch 5,000 units. The laboratories could furnish as much as Meakins needed at 3¢ to 4¢ per unit.[70] It was obviously cheaper than the British product but whether Meakins was purchasing it solely for research is not stated.

The first account in print of the use of insulin in Edinburgh was a report in the *British Medical Journal* of a meeting of the Edinburgh Medico-Chirurgical Society on May 2, 1923, when a communication was delivered by Meakins in collaboration with Robson, Lambie, and Davies.[71] A full report of this meeting later appeared in the Society's *Transactions*. The significance of this publication lies as much in its form as in its content. Here was a model of therapeutic assessment. A medical professor with a second clinician, a physiologist, and a biochemist pre-sented an account of drug use that embodied the ideal of academic med-icine. Meakins began with some introductory remarks on "the romance of the discovery of insulin." Robson then described the laborious process by which they prepared insulin from the pancreas of the ox, the material being obtained from the slaughterhouse. He made no mention of the commercial product. Lambie followed with an account of how the insulin was standardized by biological assay that required injecting it into rabbits and measuring blood sugars. He then described the normal and diabetic blood sugar curves with and without insulin. Davies then addressed the ways in which insulin influenced other phenomena in severe diabetes, namely disturbances of fat metabolism associated with acidosis. Attempts to create animal models of these disorders had been unsuccessful but they were "fortunate, however, in having several patients in whom it was possible to correlate changes in blood sugar and respiratory metabolism with changes in ketone bodies and bicarbonate reserve in the blood." Interestingly, he felt it necessary to explain what acidosis was. Davies described the case of a female diabetic with occasional acetonuria in whom an episode of acidosis with high blood sugar, a falling bicarbonate reserve, and rising levels of ketone bodies in the blood was successfully treated with insulin and glucose. Two rather more severe cases were described, the third in the series having acetone bodies "abundantly present" in her blood and urine. These patients alone had several (precise numbers not ascertainable) determinations of bicarbonate reserve. Interesting here is that the laboratory returns for 1923 showed eighteen determinations of "alkaline reserve." There were, however, no returns for determinations of ketone bodies in 1923. Because of MRC funding, tests in the insulin trial were probably not counted as part of routine lab work but it is not possible to be sure, perhaps some were, some were not.

Meakins followed Davies's account with five "typical" case histories, noting first that they had worked out a rule that one unit of insulin took care of about 2 g of carbohydrate. The first four cases were all known to be moderately severe diabetics in whom dietetic management proved unsuccessful, an interesting admission in the light of Murray Lyon's claimed success with diet alone. All were managed with insulin monitored by regular blood sugar estimations. The fifth case illustrated the dangers of insulin. Severe hypoglycaemia had been produced in a man who had had glycosuria earlier in the day. Meakins then described the successful treatment of a patient in diabetic coma but made no reference to any laboratory tests. The most notable feature of the discussion was the opinion of the Infirmary physician Chalmers Watson (a man with a keen interest in laboratory medicine) "that too much importance was at present attached to blood sugar as a guide to treatment."[72] Watson was propounding a view to which even some proponents of academic medicine were later to subscribe.

Presumably the MRC had privately given this presentation the green light, since three days after the meeting the *Lancet* published a statement of the MRC's guidelines on the clinical uses of insulin based on observations from the eight centres of study. The Edinburgh experience was typical. The *Lancet* reported that workers in all centres had been asked to select a small number of cases and to measure blood sugar and general metabolism "in great detail" with reference to a precisely calibrated diet. In all fifty patients had been treated, including seven in coma. The statement recommended that, initially, most patients should be managed with the Allen diet or some similar plan. But if the disease was of long standing with "proved excess of blood sugar," insulin should be given. Blood sugars were also essential to ensure excessive insulin was not given and if they could not be estimated then slight glycosuria was the preferred clinical state.[73]

A little over two weeks after this statement, on May 19, 1923, Davies, Lambie, Murray Lyon, Meakins, and Robson published a preliminary communication in the *British Medical Journal* on "The Influence of Insulin upon Acidosis and Lipaemia in Diabetes." This paper, like its predecessor, embodied a model of academic practice. It presented the result of the authors' joint researches on the effect of insulin in severe diabetics with studies of "lipaemia, ketone bodies in the blood, reduction of the bicarbonate reserve together with hyperpnoea and mental disturbances." Noteworthy is the undifferentiated listing of clinical and biochemical disturbances although, perhaps as an indication of priorities, biochemical changes came first. Four case histories (all female) were given, two of the patients being admitted on the verge of coma. Repeated tests were done for blood sugar and ketone bodies and the bicarbonate reserve. Lipaemia was estimated by visual inspection and "where possible" the hourly metabolism and respiratory quotient were determined. In all instances impressive results were reported and displayed graphically. The authors described the effect of insulin as "spectacular."[74]

The following week the *Lancet* reported that the supply of insulin had considerably increased and restrictions were no longer necessary. However, the MRC reminded doctors who wished to use insulin "of the great importance of making accurate blood sugar determinations, of correlating the diet, the blood sugar changes and the insulin dosage in each case." The *Lancet* observed that "a study of blood-sugar reactions is necessary for scientific therapeutics."[75] This point was an endorsement of Hugh MacLean's paper in the same issue in which he observed that for everyone treating a patient with insulin "it is imperative that . . . [the] blood changes be understood."[76]

Bramwell's use of insulin did not at any point consistently conform to the sorts of rigorous rules being worked out in the academic arena. Rather, the reverse is the case. As academic medicine gradually relaxed its rules by dint of practical necessity, its prescriptions increasingly looked like Bramwell's eclectic practice on the ward. Bramwell first used insulin in 1923 to treat Angus M., a postman, aged 23 years, admitted in June of that year and discharged just over three months later.[77] Angus came from Taynult, Argyllshire, and had been discovered to be diabetic eighteen months previously. He was admitted to the Glasgow Royal Infirmary in April 1922 and again the following February. He was treated by the Allen diet but his urine could not be cleared of sugar. He weighed but 7st 3½lb (45.8 Kg) on admission to the RIE. He was given an "ordinary diet" and the sugar in a 24-hour urine sample was estimated (in the side room). Two days after admission a fasting blood sugar was also estimated. He had no tolerance test. He was started on a starvation diet a week after admission. His urine was rarely sugar free. Just over a week later a blood sugar estimation, done on a starvation day, was raised and four days later, on June 26, 1923, insulin (ten units twice daily) was started (see Figure 9.4). Over the next two months the insulin dose was increased and decreased in response to urine tests and occasional fasting blood sugars. It appears, however, that management was largely by urine sugar estimations. Blood sugar measurements seemed to have had rather more of a policing role. The meagre progress notes recorded:

> He was a very severe case of Diabetes, with no carbohydrate body tolerance. He could only metabolize carbohydrates for which an equivalent of Insulin was given . . .He did not improve as much as expected on Insulin but this was due to the severity of his case and to the fact that on many occasions he did not stick strictly to the prescribed diet. He was found to be eating both fats and carbohydrates on the quiet. He was severely reprimanded and threatened with instant dismissal. At first he denied all

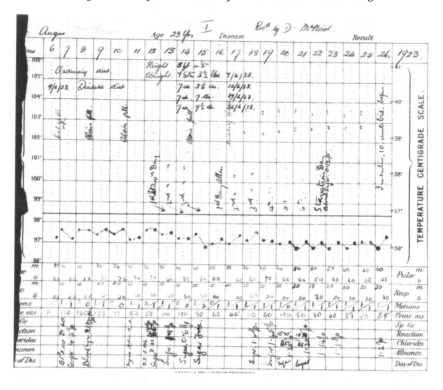

Fig. 9.4: Temperature chart of Angus M. showing start of insulin therapy on June 26, 1923 in "Case notes of medical patients under the care of Edwin Bramwell, 1919–35." (Vol. 43, case 1897, LHB1, CC/37a, LHSA, EUL.) Photograph courtesy of LHSA.

extra food but this could be proved 1) by the fluctuations on sugar output on a constant diet, 2) by the fact that he had been sugar free on the same diet, 3) by the difference in his blood sugar reports, 4) by his lack of response to extra insulin. It was not until he was rigidly confined to bed behind screens and without a locker and not allowed up for any purpose that he became sugar free.

He was discharged on a diet and twenty units of insulin to be injected half an hour before breakfast and tea. The notes state: "This diet was barely sufficient for hard manual work but was as much as the insulin allowed would utilise." This comment illustrates an important point about early insulin therapy. Presumably Angus was allowed only twenty units twice a day because of cost. Cost was a major consideration when high dosages might seem to be indicated. In November 1923 Murray Lyon wrote of diabetes: "In severe cases where the glucose tolerance is extremely low, daily quantities of 80 to 100 units [of insulin] might be necessary to keep the patient going, but such doses are prohibitive except for the wealthy. Where expense is a consideration, the amount of insulin to be employed has to be restricted, and this necessitates limitation of the food intake as well."[78] Costs for paying patients of course might include not only the drug but also blood tests when the doctor considered them necessary. By 1924 pharmacists, who charged anything between 5s. and one guinea[79] a sample, were doing these estimations.[80]

In Angus's case, payment for insulin was from the Scottish Board of Health, arranged through the patient's doctor. His GP was asked to send specimens of blood for sugar estimation in three months and six months, although whether the GP was told under what conditions the blood was to be drawn is not explicit. On discharge he was put on a fairly severe regime, which on precedent he was unlikely to follow. The notes record: "The patient was instructed in testing his urine daily with Fehling: given a diet with a variety of equivalents, a list of articles which were the same carbohydrate value; forbidden to take white bread; instructed in hypodermic technique, and insulin dosage, and given 2 sets of hypodermic syringes; told what to look out for if symptoms of Insulin poisoning, and how to treat these."

Shortly after Angus's admission a patient was admitted who had a glucose test meal. In accordance with Bramwell's practice at this time this was done "to eliminate the possibility of renal glycosuria" rather than to assess diabetes. Ana M., aged 66 years, a storehouse keeper from Dunfermline, had been discovered by her GP to have glycosuria and was admitted on June 7, 1923, and discharged about seven weeks later. The test here consisted of a *single* blood sugar estimation after a glucose meal. This was hardly recommended academic practice. She was diagnosed as diabetic.[81] The test meal probably confirmed a diagnosis that had already been made. A similar test meal was done on another patient, Evelyn P., a 58-year-old pianist from Edinburgh, shortly afterwards.[82] In this case the final diagnosis was temporary renal glycosuria. Such testing was fully in line with Bramwell's clinical agenda. Bramwell seemed to consider that the diagnosis and management of most diabetics did not require the use of a test meal.

Blood sugar estimations, however, but not test meals, were done with more frequency from now on. A patient receiving insulin would usually have three or four fasting blood sugar estimations over a period of a couple of months. For example, on September 24, 1923, Thomas R., aged 21 years, a joiner from Edinburgh, was admitted.[83] A known diabetic, the notes record: "He states his reason for coming now is to avail himself of the new insulin." He had no test meal but was put on insulin and occasional fasting blood sugars were estimated. By now records of blood sugar tests also began to appear in the records of patients managed by diet alone.

In September 1923 Fletcher wrote to Meakins about "vague and conflicting" information he had been receiving about skin reactions to various batches and brands of insulin.[84] Meakins replied four days later saying that he had made enquiries and found such reactions "practically unknown with us" in spite of some 5,000 doses having been given in the previous three months.[85] Alert to possible problems, Meakins reported to Fletcher in November 1923 that an Edinburgh patient had "suddenly gone backwards." Lambie tested the "Wellcome Insulin" on rabbits and found "it had practically no efficacy." Another sample from Allen & Hanbury had seemed to let them down in a case of coma. Meakins had "heard rumours" of such occurrences from other doctors in the district.[86] Immediately the letter arrived Fletcher sent a copy of it to Dale. As he did so Meakins wrote again about the differing results of the experimental injection of insulin from adjacent batches from British Drug Houses, notably pointing to lack of activity. This information too was forwarded to Dale. On the November 13 Dale advised Fletcher that he had written to Meakins asking for more information. Dale was not "impressed" by the complaint about the British Drug Houses product. The same batches had, elsewhere, been the source of comment because of their "*high* activity." Meakins's statement that he almost lost a case with "batch 239" did not "impress [Dale] . . . as conclusive."[87]

As noted, in May 1923 Hugh MacLean from the Medical Unit at St. Thomas' had argued that the understanding of blood sugar changes in diabetes was very important, but his interpretation of tests and the use of them in diagnosis and treatment seem different to those of Murray Lyon. Although, like Murray Lyon, he recognized renal glycosuria, unlike him MacLean considered it "by no means a rare condition." Glycosuria in general, which Murray Lyon seemed to regard as one end of a diabetic spectrum, MacLean considered "relatively common" and having "no essential relationship to diabetes." Diabetes on the other hand was "a comparatively rare disease." MacLean regarded a tolerance test as mandatory in any patient with glycosuria but "no definite symptoms of diabetes." Blood testing he regarded as "almost essential in treating patients with insulin." While acknowledging that many of the methods for determining blood glucose were "elaborate," MacLean described how he had devised a method for estimating blood sugar that required "the minimum of chemical knowledge and laboratory equipment" and he advocated its use by ordinary practitioners. In treatment, he wrote, it was important that modern dietetic principles be used "in conjunction" with insulin.[88] Expert opinion differed. In the Medical Unit at St. Bartholomew's Hospital in London at this time, the aim of insulin treatment was to keep "the fasting value of the blood sugars within normal limits" in order to rest the pancreas. Thus during treatment it was "essential that a certain number of determinations of the blood-sugar should be made." It was a goal that required "rigorous dietetic restrictions."[89] In the longer term, however, the St. Bartholomew's Unit did not deem blood sugar determinations "absolutely necessary."[90] In the Edinburgh Department of Therapeutics, diabetes seems to have been seen more as a disorder at the end of a physiological spectrum than the distinct disease that it seems to have been considered in the professorial units of London.

In November 1923, Murray Lyon, published other views on diabetes and its management that differed from those of London workers and were possibly not in line with those of his department. He began by noting that the "revolution in the treatment of diabetes, which followed the introduction of Allen's fasting methods, has been quite eclipsed by the discovery of insulin." He reported that insulin of high purity was now being produced on a commercial scale. Discussing treatment he observed that when insulin was first introduced its administration required monitoring of blood sugar levels. This was a "tedious" and "technical" task requiring "considerable apparatus" and was "impracticable for the average practitioner." However, he added, these restrictions no longer applied and "for the satisfactory handling of a case . . . blood sugar examinations are quite unnecessary" and insulin therapy "can now be undertaken by any medical man." Good control could be obtained by the informed use of urine testing. He made no mention of the simple blood test that MacLean had devised for the ordinary practitioner. This move from the laboratory as a source of authority may relate to the Edinburgh sense (or at least Murray Lyon's) that the Medical School's vocation was training large numbers of general practitioners.[91] Murray Lyon's use of insulin does not conform to the view of one historian who has claimed: "The introduction of insulin in 1922 marked a sharp break with past therapeutic practice."[92] Whereas for MacLean insulin was to be used "in conjunction" with diet, Murray Lyon explained that the physiological principles behind dietetic management of diabetes meant that insulin should be looked on "merely as an aid to dietary control of the disease."[93]

The insistence on the importance of blood testing that accompanied the early use of insulin and a move from regarding it as less than essential may also have arisen from familiarity with the new drug. In February 1924, writing from the Medical Unit of University College Hospital, K. S. Hetzel noticed this phenomenon saying: "Blood sugar measurements are, therefore, not essential . . . though they cannot be neglected if the best results in treatment are desired." Hetzel's paper discussed diet and insulin therapy and it is noteworthy that the single case he described had a full glucose tolerance test before starting treatment. Indeed after the patient commenced insulin, in one 24-hour period he had eight blood sugars estimated to gauge the drug's effectiveness.[94]

On March 1, 1924, the *Lancet* reported that a diabetic out-patient clinic had been started under Murray Lyon at the Royal Infirmary. This added to two other RIE special clinics: for lupus and for tuberculosis. After a few weeks there were about seventy patients on the diabetic clinic's list and about thirty patients attending weekly. Severe cases requiring insulin were put on a diet and later admitted. A test meal was probably an obligatory part of their assessment. Clinic patients brought a 24-hour urine sample which was tested for sugar and acetone; presumably if sugar was present it would have been quantified. Dietetic management was chiefly employed. Insulin was not used except in cases "previously investigated."[95] Whether new cases were seen and whether they had test meals as out-patients to rule out renal glycosuria is not clear.

In July 1924 Murray Lyon published "Observations on the Use of Insulin" in the *Lancet*, a week after the journal announced his appointment as Christison Professor. Murray Lyon recognized the clinical expediency of estimating urine sugar in managing diabetes but his explanation of the effect of insulin was given in terms of blood biochemistry. After meals, he observed, "the supply of insulin in normal individuals is such that the blood sugar remains about 0.1 per cent." In mild cases of diabetes "a sample of blood taken before breakfast will give a normal reading." In severe cases the blood sugar on awakening was already above the renal threshold and would rise further after each meal. Thus a morning blood sugar test was a good guide to the severity of the case at that moment. When insulin treatment had been introduced it was found that early morning glycosuria was troublesome but "Frequent blood-sugar examinations" explained why this happened. After describing the curve formed by plotting blood sugars from diabetics during the day, he noted that it was desirable to use insulin to maintain blood sugars at about the normal level at all times, adding, how best to do this "has not been decided."[96] However, always the bedside physician, Murray Lyon observed that theoretical knowledge of insulin's action was not enough: "Clinical experience has shown that other factors must be taken into account." He then noted that although glycosuria and hyperglycaemia following a meal might be reduced by simultaneously administering insulin and reduced further by larger doses "this would add greatly to the expense of treatment." In Edinburgh, he observed, insulin was administered two hours before a meal, a practice justified by plotting blood sugars in patients in whom insulin and food were given at different intervals. Murray Lyon iterated how important it was to ensure the optimum interval because of expense. Questions of management were "often decided automatically by the economic situation, when it is necessary to obtain the maximum result with the smallest outlay." The drug's "action on the blood sugar," he noted, could be monitored by blood or urine testing and the latter plan was the more generally acceptable.[97]

In August 1924 Murray Lyon jointly published "A Table of Standard Diets for Use in Diabetes." His co-author was Ruth Pybus, "Sister Dietitian" at the Infirmary, whose Rockefeller Fellowship was noted in the previous chapter.[98] To a great extent the paper was a rewrite of the *Edinburgh Medical Journal* paper of the previous year. The authors observed that all writers agreed that the introduction of insulin had made dietary control more important than ever because of the dangers of hypoglycaemia. The best chance of improvement in diabetics lay in balancing diet and insulin so that "the blood sugar level is kept approximately normal." By 1924 it was accepted by many within academic medicine that blood sugar measurement need not be part of the management of normal diabetes. For Murray Lyon, talk of the physiological aims of diabetic management was always structured in terms of blood sugar but practical advice was always clinical. The attending physician should "avoid acidosis and glycosuria (*or rather hyperglycaemia*)." The result would be that the blood sugar level remained "approximately normal."[99] Good clinical management in other words could achieve the desired, but unmeasured, biochemical end.

By 1925, blood sugars were nearly always estimated at some point during a diabetic's stay on Bramwell's wards although by no means immediately. Nor were glucose test meals the rule. Thomas C., aged 54 years, a blind organist from Oban, was admitted on January 12, 1925, with a twelve-month history of polydipsia and polyuria.[100] He was 5 ft 5 in (1.65 m) tall and weighed only 7 st 9 lb (49 Kg). On admission he had sugar in the urine and this was estimated quantitatively. Acetone was also present. Thomas was in heart failure. He had a blood sugar (probably fasting) estimated three days after admission and another one (definitely fasting) five days later. The progress notes record that he responded well to insulin and five weeks after admission he had gained seven pounds in weight. Unfortunately "the progress of the heart condition was . . . in the other direction" and the symptoms indicated that the patient "was approaching the last stages of heart failure." Thomas was discharged at the end of the first week of March, presumably to die at home.

Midway through Thomas's stay, a 63-year-old housewife, Margaret B., was admitted.[101] She had a four-year history of polydipsia and polyuria. Her urine contained sugar. Four days after admission she had a blood sugar estimated. This gave a normal reading but she still had sugar in the urine. Five days later a blood sugar was slightly raised. Finally, two weeks after admission, she had a glucose test meal and the case notes recorded a diagnosis of renal glycosuria. Someone, probably a student observed: "This diagnosis is made chiefly in view of the low percentage of sugar in the blood while the kidneys were still excreting sugar in a small percentage, and also on account of the mildness of the symptoms and the presence of thirst without any hunger." She was discharged and told to avoid excessive carbohydrates.

In some cases assessment and management were based almost entirely on urinalysis. Bernard M., a 25-year-old labourer from Edinburgh and a known diabetic, was admitted in July 1925. He had only had one blood sugar estimation (with a very high reading) five days after admission.[102] He failed to improve on diet and insulin and the notes record:

> Patient proved to be eating on the evidence of several other patients, although he himself strenuously denied it. Was placed behind screen on 14th August 1925 and sugar in urine steadily dropped to nothing 3 days before dismissal. Patient became very restless behind screens, insisted on going out of hospital one afternoon and returned with urine loaded with sugar. He was immediately dismissed. The mental condition was rather weak and the prognosis is exceedingly bad.[103]

In at least one patient treated with insulin no blood tests at all were recorded. Robert L. aged 63 years, an ex-serviceman from Duns, a known diabetic, was admitted on December 30, 1925, with paralysis of the right arm and leg.[104] He was managed by diet and insulin and monitored solely by urine sugars.

By 1925, Bramwell's use of a tolerance test in diabetics was still rare and, as formerly, it was usually employed to assess endocrine disorders. Samuel W., from Dunfermline, was a 27-year-old described as an "electric motor man" in the mines, was admitted in late August 1925.[105] He was a former Bramwell patient and suffered from muscular atrophy. A commentary in the notes runs: "There is here the question of endocrine deficiency. There was no evidence of pituitary or thyroid deficiency and the testes were not atrophied." Samuel had a blood sugar test meal done the day before he left and fully a month after admission. Presumably it was used here to discover if there was any insulin deficiency to support the general conclusion of endocrine deficiency.

By 1930 things had changed somewhat. Test meals using blood were more frequent. Of the twenty-two cases admitted that year with diabetes or renal glycosuria, fifteen had test meals. Equally significant, the tests were usually done shortly after admission. The test, although not an obligatory routine assessment, seems to have been something more than a resource to be used in very doubtful cases—its initial use on Bramwell's wards. The aim of managing the diabetic patient by diet as far as possible was still evident. The following case is typical except for the patient's extreme anxiety based on the apparent delusion of his wife's "misbehaviour with the young man who is courting the daughter."[106] James D. aged 49 years, a tailor from Edinburgh, was admitted March 17, 1930. He had a five-week history of agitation, worrying, sleepless- ness, and trembling after a friend told him "his daughter's young man was never out of the house." On examination there was sugar in the urine. A tolerance test based on blood sugars was done the day after admission. He was put on a diet but sugar was still present in the urine. No further blood tests were done. The diet was restricted further and he was put on five units of insulin daily. The diet was built up and he continued on insulin. He was discharged after a three-week stay, on a diet and no insulin. Diabetic treatment obviously did little for his anxieties for he assaulted the troublesome suitor and entered Bangour lunatic asylum in West Lothian shortly afterwards.

One further case merits closer attention. Janet H., a farm labourer aged 65 years, was a known diabetic. She was admitted in February 1930 complaining of increasing weakness. The notes record she was "on the verge of coma." On admission the urine was strongly positive for sugar. No blood sugar was done. She was given 30 mg of glucose and twenty units of insulin hourly. A full test meal was carried out two days after admission.[107] The notes, however, contain a plotted curve of urine sug- ars, seemingly estimated on the ward, and measured at the same time as those of the blood taken during the test meal (see Figure 9.5). A good guess would be that this curve was drawn by a student as an educational exercise to compare urine and blood sugar changes (although there is no blood curve in the notes). After all, most general practitioners were going to have to rely on older, simpler clinical tests. Certainly Bramwell would have expected his students to have mastered all the basic bedside techniques for managing diabetes.

One of the obvious ways in which the laboratory established itself in routine use was in the measurement of the BMR. In the same way that Meakins had published a general paper with Murray Lyon in 1921 on dia- betes, stressing the importance of blood sugar measurement so, in 1922, he published a paper with Davies on the value of estimating BMR.[108] By the use of such papers placed in less specialized journals, academic physi- cians no doubt hoped that clinicians were being educated in the value of laboratory tests and new ways of thinking about disease. Measuring the body's rate of metabolism by determining the concentrations of gases in

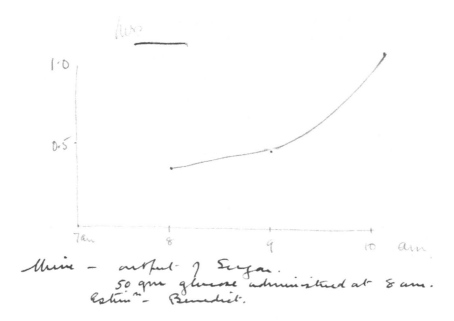

Fig. 9.5: Hand-drawn graph from the case notes of Janet H. in "Case notes of medical patients under the care of Edwin Bramwell, 1919–35." (Vol. 150, case 6456, LHB1, CC/37a, LHSA, EUL.) Photograph courtesy of LHSA.

inspired and expired air can be traced to the eighteenth-century French chemist Antoine Lavoisier, but it was in nineteenth-century Germany that precise apparatus for measuring this physiological indicator was developed. By 1900 studies of metabolic rates in a large number of diseases had been published. About this time the centre of gravity of metabolic studies shifted to America. Here simpler apparatus was devised and the value of basal metabolism measurements in thyroid disease investigated.[109] The Edinburgh technique was based on the analysis of expired air using a modification of the "Douglas bag" method, devised by Meakins. The lab reported 101 estimations in 1921 and numbers climbed through the 1920s to 613 in 1930.

Meakins and Davies's paper detailed the value of the test in thyroid disorders and referred to twenty-eight cases that had had sixty-four tests in all. Patients had more than one estimate done since the test was regarded as being of value in monitoring therapy.[110] It is important to note that the authors did not endorse BMR estimation to the exclusion of other means of assessment. They appreciated, however, "its great value in certain cases especially in those of disordered function of the thyroid and pituitary glands, where it may be useful both in diagnosis and in giving an accurate quantitative index of progress and of the effects of treatment." Noticeable about their attempt to persuade clinicians of the value of knowing the BMR was their use of figures in tabular form. Cases of thyroid disease were numbered and grouped into categories such as exophthalmic goitre. The patient's BMR and pulse rate were entered in columns alongside the case number. In the instance of exophthalmic goitre Meakins and Davies observed: "It will be noted that there was a conspicuous increase in the B.M.R. in every case." The reader could scarcely deny the correlation, and hence the value of the procedure. Conclusions such as these, the authors said, allowed them to make the judgement that in estimating the course of the disease, compared to the "customary" reliance on "the variation of pulse-rate . . . it has been found that changes in basal metabolic rate are much more reliable." Something very subtle was happening here. As in the instance of diabetes a familiar clinical disorder was being discussed largely in metabolic terms and in consequence a laboratory test was being raised to definitional status or co-definitional status along with clinical findings.[111]

Bramwell had a fair number of thyroid cases and drew increasingly on the lab in their management. In 1921 he treated eight cases of thyroid disease. None had a BMR test. Nor was one carried out in any other condition. In 1922, however, of fourteen cases diagnosed as having thyroid disease four had BMR estimations. The following year he had eight cases of possible or definite thyroid disease, six of which had BMR determinations. Of the eighteen thyroid cases seen in 1925, twelve had BMR estimations. Perhaps significantly, his first request for a patient's BMR was sent in February 1922, the month following Meakins and Davies's publication. The case, however, was not of thyroid disease but that of a 41-year-old miner diagnosed as having myotonia atrophica, a wasting disease of the muscles. It is quite likely that Bramwell suspected an underlying endocrine disturbance, possibly of the pituitary which he considered had a role in some of the myopathies. The pituitary was also thought by some to have a place in regulating metabolism and thus a BMR would detect any loss of pituitary function. In this case the BMR was -30 per cent. Davies wrote on the form "This result is very low but agrees with what one would expect from the low pulse rate and blood pressure."[112] A second BMR two days later was also low. Presumably Bramwell finally concluded that some loss of pituitary function was at the root of this case although the notes do not make this clear.

The second BMR estimation performed in 1922 was used to rule out any possibility of hyperthyroidism in a patient with an otherwise classic clinical picture of myasthenia gravis, a muscle-wasting disease. James R., aged 43 years, a shale oil worker from Midcalder was admitted on March 16, 1922.[113] He had a long history of weakness and on examination he was discovered to have "some exophthalmos," the bulging eyes characteristic of a hyperactive thyroid. However, he had no other physical signs of this disorder. Two days after admission a BMR was estimated. The request form stated myasthenia gravis as the diagnosis but also included the brief, "? exophthalmos." The BMR was reported as -10 per cent with the remark: "Patient rather apprehensive hence probable true result slightly lower. Pulse at time 97. Blood Pressure 140–102."

This was to be the general role of an assessment of the BMR for Bramwell. It was a test for ruling out thyroid dysfunction rather than for diagnosing or monitoring thyroid disease itself. Typical cases were diagnosed by bedside methods alone. Evelyn W., a 33-year-old milliner from Leith, was admitted for treatment on July 7, 1925.[114] A clerk wrote in the notes: "The diagnosis of hyperthyroidism is made on the history of nervousness, swelling in the neck, protrusion of the eyes and attacks of palpitation." As with diabetes, Bramwell remained faithful to his precepts about bedside practice. Clinical rather than laboratory concepts informed his practice. He did not shun the lab but it only ever played a fine-tuning role in patient management.

A similar picture can be painted of his management of neurological disorders. Lumbar puncture was introduced into clinical medicine as a *therapeutic* procedure in 1891.[115] Removing cerebro-spinal fluid for diagnostic purposes was initiated a few years later. Some clinicians were hostile to the technique.[116] The biochemistry of the CSF in health and disease was the subject of research from early in the century. By 1920 there was agreement in some areas over which chemical changes were valuable diagnostic signs but in others dispute ruled. Without detailed case notes it is impossible to know why some tests on CSF, such as that for cholesterol, were carried out on Bramwell's patients. In this and other instances there was no consensus as to the significance of the results.

Testing for proteins in the CSF (any more than a minute trace was considered abnormal) and associating them with pathological disorders was an early source of interest. In 1910 Thomas Horder, a London physician whose text on clinical pathology was aimed at the independent practitioner, reckoned that in addition to microscopy of the CSF the ordinary doctor could carry out tests for albumin, sugar, and urea.[117] Around this time albumin, which could be quantified, was synonymous in the clinical literature with protein. In 1909 specialized tests for globulin (which was precipitated out indistinguishably in the usual albumin tests) were described.[118] These globulin tests were not strictly quantitative, the results were given by one or more plus signs or in such terms as absent or weak or strongly positive. In 1927 a truly quantitative test for globulin in the CSF was described.[119] In the mid-1920s authorities still found confusion in the literature over the significance of the relative quantities of albumin and globulin present. In 1925 the authors of the first specialized book published in Britain on the CSF observed that as a result of work using the globulin test a "general impression seems to have arisen . . . that globulin preponderates over albumen in the protein increase, whereas the reverse is always the case."[120] Interestingly chemical pathology texts tend to confirm this judgement, clinical ones do not. Some biochemistry texts did not even deign to mention albumin. Both clinicians and chemical pathologists agreed, however, that there was a great increase in globulin in proportion to albumin in neurosyphilis. A fairly simple test carried out in the Pathology Department in Edinburgh was Lange's colloidal gold test in which the CSF was mixed with varying proportions of colloidal gold, producing characteristic "curves" of colour change in various pathological conditions. Although proteins were held to cause the reaction the exact mechanisms at work were not agreed in the 1920s.

What was widely agreed from quite early on was that concentrations of most substances in the CSF—urea being a notable exception—did not simply mirror those in the blood. Glucose, for example, in normal CSF was found at about half its blood level. Decrease in glucose was regarded as "one of the cardinal signs of acute meningitis."[121] Like glucose, chlorides were also held to diminish in meningitis and all authors held that a level below 0.6 per cent constituted a diagnostic sign of tuberculous meningitis in children.[122] Overwhelmingly during the decade the tests most consistently and frequently requested of the Edinburgh lab were for glucose, chlorides, and various forms of protein. In 1921 the lab received one specimen of CSF (source unknown, but not Bramwell) on which three unspecified tests were performed. Figures for all CSF tests from all sources rose slowly until 1926 when the number leaped to 105. They fell again after this and by 1930 had climbed to ninety-one. The peak in 1926 suggests a TB meningitis outbreak although Bramwell had only two cases that year.[123] Perhaps a research interest accounted for the sudden rise. By 1930 the range of tests on the CSF offered by the lab had expanded to include estimations of urea nitrogen, NPN, creatinine, bile pigments, cholesterol, lactic acid, haemoglobin, albumin, globulin, total nitrogen, and inorganic phosphates. Some of these tests were done in very small numbers (only one lactic acid was ever requested). The significance of changes in the level of some of these substances was far from agreed.

Bramwell sent his first CSF specimen to the lab in August 1922, for a chloride estimation in a case of suspected TB meningitis. He sent a further two specimens from another patient that year. The following year he sent five. In 1925 he sent none. In 1930, seventeen specimens were sent. These were scarcely large numbers for a neurologist. Bramwell, of course, examined samples of CSF in the side room and sent them to the Pathology Department or the College of Physicians before the biochemistry lab existed. For example, on December 10, 1919, the 22-year-old Elizabeth R., from Lasswade and of unrecorded occupation, was admitted.[124] She had a two-week history of pain in the arm, twitching of limbs, difficulty with speech, and headache. Twenty-four hours before admission she lost her speech completely and developed left-sided weakness. On admission she had a temperature of 99.2 °F. She was suspected of having TB meningitis. A lumbar puncture was performed. The CSF was examined microscopically in the side room and sent to the Pathology Laboratory of the Infirmary, which reported: "Marked increase of lymphocytes. No pus cells. No TB or other organisms were found on the films. There has been no growth in the special media and for meningococcus." Elizabeth slipped into coma and died on December 22. A post-mortem report indicated TB meningitis. An estimation of CSF chloride, a low reading of which was very good guide to the condition, does not seem to have been an option at this time.

Bramwell had cases of TB meningitis on the ward in 1921 but the biochemistry of their CSF was not studied. This was also true of 1922 until Lizzie N., a 16-year-old from Portobello, was admitted on August 5.[125] Lizzie had a one-week history of headache and vomiting. On examination she was restless and groaning, and a characteristic sign of meningitis (Kernig's sign) was elicited. The CSF showed increased tension. The notes (there is no biochemistry form) record: "chlorides diminished, being 0.6%." Presumably this test was done in the lab. A diagnosis of TB meningitis was made, although whether before or after this test was done is unclear. Lizzie died on August 14, 1922, and a post-mortem report indicated cerebral TB. After this, estimations of chlorides in meningitis became more frequent in Bramwell's patients, although not invariable. Shortly after Lizzie's death, on September 2, 1922, Isabella S., aged 12 years, from Annandale, was admitted with a one-week history of severe pain in the head, drowsiness, and talking nonsense. Kernig's sign was positive.[126] A lumbar puncture on admission produced blood-stained fluid under pressure. The chlorides at 0.6 per cent were, the notes state: "suggestive of TB meningitis." Doubt over the diagnosis obviously remained and four days later a second puncture was done. The chlorides were 0.65 per cent. Isabella died eight days later. A post-mortem showed: "Cerebral Haemorrhage (old and recent)." The five CSF tests done in 1923 were also for chlorides in suspected TB. In at least three of these cases, CSF from Bramwell's patients was sent to the Pathology Department for globulin tests. The reason for this was not stated nor can it easily be guessed at.

In 1930, although there were cases of TB meningitis on the ward, none had their chlorides estimated. Curiously all except one of the seventeen CSF examinations done in that year were carried out after October 3. The exception was Thomas L., a 64-year-old lodging house manager from Edinburgh, admitted on May 8, 1930.[127] Thomas had a 24-hour history of shivering, headache, and drowsiness. On admission he was extremely ill, cyanosed, confused with a rapid, irregular pulse, and a temperature of 101.4 °F. The next day CSF was sent to the lab with a tentative diagnosis of acute encephalitis lethargica. A sugar content was requested, and it was reported as 102 mg per cent. This was markedly raised. One authority noted "the mass of evidence shows that readings [of sugar] above the normal are the rule in encephalitis lethargica."[128] The Wassermann reaction of the fluid was negative. On the morning after admission Thomas developed quite marked signs of left lower lobar pneumonia and three days later he was dead. There is no record of an X-ray in the notes. The final diagnosis was lobar pneumonia (confirmed by post-mortem) and auricular fibrillation.

The sixteen CSF examinations performed after October 3, 1930 may have been carried out with some project in mind (although Bramwell published nothing related to them) since fourteen of them had requests for protein estimation in some form or other (most notably total protein). Yet, except in bacterial meningitis, when protein was always raised (because of the numbers of white cells, pus, and dead and living bacteria), protein showed no consistent change in any condition. Estimating it in meningitis was hardly regarded as routinely necessary; the symptoms, signs, and the microscopic presence of white cells and bacteria in the CSF usually made the diagnosis easy. The sixteen cases themselves had little in common although five were suspected instances of cerebral tumour, but the remainder included cerebral thrombosis, Pott's disease, chronic meningitis, and hypertension. What fourteen of the patients did have in common, however, was the signature of G. M. Greig on the biochemistry form, and perhaps all these requests stemmed from an enthusiastic resident.

The first patient to have a lumbar puncture in the cluster of cases just described was Patrick M., a 49-year-old miner from Lumphinans, Fifeshire, who was admitted on October 3, 1930.[129] Patrick was one of the least typical of the group in that he was not considered to have a primary neurological disorder at all. Patrick had a three-week history of behaving strangely and had had a fit a week prior to admission. On examination he was in a stupor. A lumbar puncture was done. Renal failure was obviously suspected since the urea content of the CSF was asked for as well as the urea and NPN of the blood. These were all more or less normal. Patrick continued to have fits and died three days later. The pathologist reported marked oedema of the brain at post-mortem. What is odd here is that urea levels in both the CSF *and* blood were estimated whereas either one would have been sufficient to establish that there was no chronic renal disease. Yet the CSF was apparently not sent to pathology for microscopy or a Wassermann reaction. Like so many other tests carried out on Bramwell's patients there is no access to the clinical reasoning that initiated the requests. The sense that these tests were called for by a relatively inexperienced clinician is hard to resist.

Another patient admitted in this cluster was Joseph R., a 54-year-old patternmaker from Edinburgh. He entered hospital on September 25, 1930.[130] Joseph had a two-month history of muscular weakness and slowness of intellectual reaction. Six days prior to admission he had developed headache and vomiting, and two days later drowsiness. On examination he could not be roused. He had a right-sided positive Babinski sign (an extension reflex of the great toe), very suggestive of serious neurological mischief. CSF was sent to the Pathology Department but revealed nothing significant. Two weeks after admission he became incontinent of faeces and urine. This continued for three weeks, during which time a second lumbar puncture was done and the CSF was sent to the biochemistry lab for total protein estimation with a tentative diagnosis of "Cerebral Tumour." A reading of 18 mg per cent was probably considered within the normal range. Since, in the words of one authority, the "examination of the cerebro-spinal fluid in cases of tumour of the brain gives, in the majority of cases, negative results" it is hard to see why the protein was estimated.[131] A second CSF Wassermann was negative. A skull X-ray revealed nothing. He was finally discharged two months after admission with a diagnosis of "Encephalitis." Similarly Isabella M., a 49-year-old from Bo'ness, on the ward at the same time as Joseph R., had a CSF total protein estimation (nothing else was asked for) for a suspected spinal tumour.[132] The level was a little abnormal but the specimen was slightly contaminated with blood and this could have accounted for the result. Again, however, the notes reveal nothing of the reasoning behind the test. As with blood sugar estimations and BMRs, biochemical examination of the CSF did not figure significantly in Bramwell's investigative arsenal.

Nor did the lab feature prominently in Bramwell's investigation of renal disease. Richard Bright's description, in 1827, of the association of albumin in the urine with dropsy and other symptoms and the presence at post-mortem of changes in the kidney led quite rapidly to the recognition of a new disease—Bright's disease. The condition was acknowledged from the beginning, however, to comprehend a number of different disorders. Soon after Bright's publication it was agreed that the disease was usually associated with raised levels of urea in the blood and decreased amounts in the urine. Research into kidney disease in the nineteenth and early twentieth centuries generated new tests of function, histological findings, and, most significant, various competing classifications of renal disease (both morphological and functional). The variety of these in use by the early 1920s indicated that consensus over the nature of "Bright's disease" (a term falling into disuse) had not been reached.[133] By this time the biochemistry of the blood in renal disease was the object of considerable research, notably in America, because of the kidney's role in what was one of the hottest biochemical topics of the day: acid–base balance.

Bramwell saw quite a lot of people with renal disease and numbers admitted over the decade remained fairly constant—about twenty patients a year.[134] Cases were labelled in morbid anatomical terms either simply as nephritis or with a qualifier: acute, sub-acute, chronic, chronic interstitial etc.[135] This was a commonly employed classification. Sometimes added to the diagnosis was "and uraemia." At least two cases in the decade were labelled "scarlatina nephritis." Patients with renal disease were generally monitored by side room testing of the urine.

Bramwell's very first use of the laboratory was probably in a case of nephritis. Jessie P., a 42-year-old housewife from Edinburgh, was admitted on March 7, 1921.[136] She had a six-month history of shortness of breath and facial and ankle swelling. On admission she was oedematous, with a raised systolic blood pressure (a recognized accompaniment of chronic renal disease). Albumin was present in the urine and a quantitative estimation of it was made in the side room. At some point (probably shortly after admission) a diagnosis of chronic parenchymatous nephritis was made on ward findings alone. As far as can be understood from the notes the urine was monitored for albumin daily, although the blood pressure was seemingly not regularly checked. No blood count appears to have been done. She deteriorated and developed Cheyne-Stokes respiration, an ominous clinical sign. Three weeks (an astonishingly long period) after admission the urea content of a 24-hour urine sample was estimated in the side room. This was measured at 7 g. Since the normal range was 20 g to 40 g the result presumably confirmed a diagnosis of severe although not fulminating renal failure (that is, the low level in her urine indicated she was retaining urea). For reasons not made clear on, May 11, 1921—nine weeks after admission—her blood urea was measured in the lab.[137] It was raised from the normal of around 30 mg to 128 mg. This was certainly high, although much higher levels were on record. On the same day a urea concentration test was carried out—a test of the kidneys' capacity to excrete a fixed dose of ingested urea solution. The urea content of two samples of urine was measured in the urine in the side room. At 2 per cent the result was low (the normal was at least 3 per cent) but not grossly abnormal. From about this time, clinically, Jessie deteriorated rapidly. No further lab tests were done. She was treated with digitalis, diuretics (not named), hot air baths, Southey's tubes (to alleviate oedema), and paraldehyde. She died on May 30, 1921. The notes do not record whether it was considered that the lab added anything either to diagnosis or to management. It is hard to see how it did. Indeed her obvious clinical condition was far worse than her biochemical one.

Contrast this with the case of the 15-year-old laboratory assistant William R. from Edinburgh.[138] William was admitted on May 31, 1921, and remained in hospital for nearly three and a half months. He had acute nephritis, confidently diagnosed from his generalized oedema and the blood cells and albumin in the urine. At no time, including the five days in June when he had what were recognized as uraemic convulsions, was blood or urine biochemistry requested of the lab. Indeed it was about sixteen cases of nephritis later and September 1922 before Bramwell's staff next requested a blood urea test. Another was done the same month. The next nine cases of renal disease had no tests then, suddenly, beginning in late March 1923, eight successive patients with nephritis had NPN estimations carried out, sometimes more than once. It is likely that these tests were done on the initiative of George Malcolm-Smith, Clinical Tutor and a registered lab user with a research interest in nephritis. Quite why Malcolm-Smith preferred NPN to urea estimation is not clear. Both were measures of retained nitrogen and therefore of renal function. Contemporary texts saw no value in one over the other except that urea estimations were easier.[139] Perhaps it was a research interest. It is impossible to say, but the investigations indicate the difficulties of referring to the clinical care of these cases as though Bramwell personally managed them all.

The status quo in testing was then resumed. Of the following eleven admissions with nephritis in 1923 only three had NPN estimations and there is evidence that none of these was initiated by Malcolm-Smith.[140] No great recourse to testing was apparent in 1925, when twenty patients with renal disease were admitted. Only three had blood tests (one on two occasions), all of which were for urea. All three of these cases are puzzling. The first was Charles L., a 46-year-old "Railway surface man" from Edinburgh, admitted on October 29, 1925.[141] He had a ten-day history of breathlessness and four days prior to admission he had had swelling of the legs and face. Examination confirmed oedema and his urine contained albumin and, on microscopic examination, red blood cells were found. The concentration of urea in the urine was measured in the side room and recorded as 1.5 per cent. A figure of 2 per cent was generally taken as the lower limit of normal. This would lead the clinician to expect the blood urea to be raised, and no doubt in accordance with this logic, on the day after admission Charles had a blood urea estimated. The lab reported it as 25 mg per cent, a figure well within the normal range. Charles gradually improved with bed rest and was discharged three weeks after admission with his urine completely free of albumin. The final diagnosis was chronic interstitial nephritis. In this condition the kidney's ability to excrete urea was said to be almost invariably decreased with a consequent rise in blood urea levels. The clinical account here (including the urine tests) fitted this picture but the lab report did not. Presumably this was either ignored or explained away (the notes offer no comment). Whatever, it would be hard to find a more obvious example of the priority given to clinical experience over laboratory findings. The case of Charles M. was even more striking.[142] This 61-year-old retired marine engineer was admitted on November 12, 1925. He had a history of breathlessness and ankle swelling and while in hospital was "passing large quantities of albumin in the urine, with a low urea concentration" (there is no quantitative record). A blood urea estimation four days after admission was reported (on a biochemistry form) as 36 mg per cent—well within the normal range. This was clearly not taken into the clinical reckoning. He died in what was diagnosed as uraemic coma and the post-mortem showed "what one had suspected, that [the] patient was suffering from chronic glandular kidneys."

It was not as though the lab had unique biochemical standards. In 1930, Alexander S., a 30-year-old locomotive fireman from Bathgate was admitted with obvious nephritic symptoms and signs. He had, as might be expected, a markedly raised blood urea level of 162 mg per cent two days after admission.[143] It is impossible to tell whether the reporting of low blood urea levels in the face of clinical evidence discouraged lab usage but certainly no great demands were put on the lab in 1930 in the management of renal cases. Of the twenty-two patients treated by Bramwell for renal disease in that year, eight had blood specimens sent to the lab (only one specimen in every case save one). All specimens were accompanied by requests for urea estimation and five also had requests for creatinine. Some authorities claimed a high creatinine level indicated a poor prognosis.[144]

Occasionally the use of the lab is inexplicable and is illustrated by the case of Isabella A., a 34-year-old "clerkess" from Edinburgh admitted on November 9, 1930.[145] She had a two-week history of headache, facial swelling, and general malaise. Side room examination showed her urine to contain pus and a great deal of albumin. Acute nephritis was diagnosed and the day after admission the resident sent blood to the lab requesting estimations of NPN, chlorides, and urea. This was probably the only esti-mation of chloride in a nephritic patient of Bramwell's in ten years. Texts of the day considered blood chloride estimation in nephritis of little value and the request is a mystery. She recovered and her summary notes stated: "On discharge there was still a trace of albumin in the urine. She was advised to keep to a diet for some time and to guard herself against damp."

Throughout the decade Bramwell (or his staff) availed himself occa-sionally of some of the less commonly performed tests, in addition he (or his staff) sometimes used the lab in an idiosyncratic way. A good exam-ple of the latter occurred six months after the lab opened and suggests that in this case the initiative for biochemical testing came from the res-ident. Elizabeth H., a 68-year-old from Penicuik, was admitted on May 30, 1921.[146] Five days before admission she had severe chest pain, and developed breathlessness. On clinical examination she was found to have a right-sided pleural effusion. Her (systolic) blood pressure was esti-mated by touch alone and was determined to be about 120. Side room testing of urine proved normal, but on the day after admission urine was sent to biochemistry. The request form, signed by the resident, had no provisional diagnosis but a note requesting "examination for abnormal constituents, specially sugar." The reports states "urine gives no reduction of Benedict's reagent, therefore no sugar. The reduction of Fehling's solu-tion is probably due to creatinin [sic] which is present in moderate amounts. Indican is present. No acetone bodies present." This is a puz-zling case. It is hard to see why a urine sample was sent to the lab at all and the blunderbuss approach can scarcely have been initiated by Bramwell. In any event Elizabeth improved and was discharged two weeks after admission with the diagnosis of pleurisy with effusion.

Such a use of the lab was not a measure of its novelty value. Ten years later, on October 10, 1930, Alfred W., a 44-year-old electrical engineer from East Lothian was admitted.[147] He had had malarial treatment for disseminated sclerosis at a hospital in Bradford three months prior to admission. A week prior to admission he was given a further malarial injection. The case notes summary states: "patient was admitted as [i.e. because] a therapeutic malarial infection was expected to begin." Three days after admission he developed a high temperature, followed by rigors which continued for the next ten days. He was treated with Plasmaquine (an anti-malarial) and suddenly became cyanosed. A biochemistry form accompanying blood, dated November 4, 1930, stated the diagnosis as "Disseminated Sclerosis: patient has a marked cyanosis without symptoms following plasmaquine used to stop malarial rigors induced therapeutically." Investigation required was "Whatever is thought useful." The lab searched for methaemoglobin (a substance found in various forms of poisoning) but none was discovered. The request was made by the resident, Greig, and its idiosyncratic nature, coupled with the fact that it was Greig who asked for all the CSF protein tests in late 1930, suggests that a puzzled resident could initiate biochemistry requests.

Suspicions about Greig's idiosyncrasies seem to be confirmed by the case of Agnes C., aged 63 years, from Bo'ness.[148] Agnes was admitted on December 10, 1930. She had pain, pulsation in the abdomen, and was ceasing to pass urine. The diagnosis of a leaking aneurysm of the abdominal aorta was scarcely difficult. On the day after admission what can only be called an academic (or perhaps moral) Wassermann test was done (it was negative). Four days after admission Agnes was unconscious, pulseless, and passing no urine at all. On the following day at 3:00 p.m. a blood specimen was sent to the lab by Greig, and not surprisingly in a patient with total renal shut-down it showed vastly increased levels of sugar, NPN and creatinine (the specimen was sent "too late" for urea—and for the patient it might be said). For some reason which again can only be called academic, a cholesterol level was requested (it was normal).

Two conditions in which Bramwell had a particular interest and on which he published were lead poisoning and myopathy. Thomas A., a 37-year-old lead smelter from Stanlochead, Dumfrieshire, was admitted at the end of 1921, with an eight-year history of vomiting after meals.[149] On examination his gums showed "a slight suggestion of a blue line," a clinical sign of lead poisoning. A week after admission a urine sample was sent to the lab by the resident for detection of lead, the form having on it the diagnosis of gastritis and the request "Is lead being eliminated?" The report stated "Lead is present but in minute traces, only just sufficient for detection."[150] Two weeks later a diagnosis of lead colic was made. It was known that lead was not always detectable in the urine in lead poisoning and the negative result was ignored. A positive result would, presumably, have clinched the diagnosis.[151] Urine lead content was again requested in 1925 in a case of progressive muscular atrophy. This looked rather like a shot in the dark, based on the fact that the patient was a painter, since none of the symptoms pointed to classic lead poisoning. The urine showed only a trace of lead and "progressive muscular atrophy" stuck as the diagnosis (a negative Wassermann ruled out syphilis).[152]

Bramwell, as noted, was also interested in the muscular dystrophies and published on the subject. Theories of the causes of these diseases were many and implicated different systems, notably the muscles themselves, the voluntary nervous system, the sympathetic system, and pertinent here, the endocrine glands. Bramwell considered disturbances of pituitary function were too frequent in cases of muscular dystrophy to "be accounted for by coincidence."[153] He utilized the lab in many cases of muscular dystrophy to investigate endocrine function. In particular he investigated blood sugars, since changes in sugar tolerance were known to be associated with pituitary disorders. James Y., a 56-year-old farm worker from Gorebridge, was admitted at the end of 1921 with a long history of increasing weakness.[154] On examination there was evidence of atrophy of leg muscles. He had no sugar in his urine but two months after admission his fasting blood sugar was measured (it was normal). This looks very much like a search for evidence of pituitary abnormality rather than an attempt to diagnose diabetes. Little or no change was observed in his three-month stay and he left with a diagnosis of myopathy.

In 1925 Bramwell published on two cases of pseudohypertrophic muscular paralysis in which he had found evidence of pituitary disorder. Both had their fasting blood sugars investigated. One of these cases also had a brother who was admitted at the same time. He was similarly afflicted and had a full tolerance test.[155] In fact the brothers were quite extensively investigated, having their oxygen consumption and carbon dioxide output estimated in the lab (by breathing methods, not blood tests). These were used to arrive at figures for their basal metabolic rates and respiratory quotients (also a measure of metabolism). Since they had previously been admitted in 1923 and no lab tests had been done then, and since nothing could be done for their condition, the flurry of tests suggests that Bramwell had publication in mind (the tests were done in October 1925 and Bramwell's paper appeared in late November). In the same year, in a case of suspected suprarenal disease, the blood sugar was investigated again to determine the presence of endocrine imbalance rather than specifically to detect diabetes. This patient (who was obese) also had her total blood fat and cholesterol measured.[156]

The use of the lab by the surgeons is much more briefly dealt with. In 1925 John Fraser succeeded Harold Stiles in the Chair of Clinical Surgery. Fraser admitted about 1,000 patients per annum. By the time he occupied the Chair, Fraser was a regular lab user in specific circumstances. Whether Fraser initiated usage because of his own enthusiasm for lab tests or whether by 1925 peer pressure dictated that he do so is not clear. At St. Thomas' Hospital, London, in the early 1920s some of the surgeons were reluctant to employ laboratory facilities as an aid to clinical practice, believing in the superiority of their bedside judgement. Hugh MacLean, St. Thomas' Hospital's medical professor, was insisting on renal function tests before prostate operations, but in 1923 Pearce reported that "At first the Surgeons did not conform and insisted that they could tell clinically whether a patient would stand the operation."[157] In Edinburgh at this time, fragmentary evidence suggests surgeons had a similar faith in their bedside acumen. In July 1922 the surgeon Henry Wade read a paper on the surgical diagnosis of renal disease. He acknowledged the value of blood biochemistry. It was reported in discussion, however, that Wade considered that "in recognising when a patient was really ill, or when his general health was good, the clinical instinct of the medical man of experience was seldom at fault."[158] By 1925 Fraser was requesting pre-operative tests for all patients with enlarged prostates and retention of urine. They had routine testing of blood urea, NPN, and very often creatinine before any bladder or prostate operation. Many patients also had these tests done after operation.[159] The other patients for whom Fraser utilized the lab were sufferers from thyroid disease with any hint of toxicity. These patients had their BMR estimated and if it was excessively high they were sent to a medical ward to get it reduced prior to any thyroid operation. Only rarely were other lab tests utilized. On the surgical wards, as opposed to the medical ones, tests had become highly routinized. This difference requires explanation, but the large numbers of very similar surgical cases certainly facilitated the introduction of routine examination of blood. Among patients admitted for surgery there were fewer possibilities for idiosyncratic testing than existed on the medical wards.

Notes

1. Andrew Doig, Edited transcript of interview with Helen Coyle, November 20, 1997.

2. Exact quantification is impossible. I have included diagnoses such as neurasthenia, giddiness, neurosis etc. in this group.

3. For example RIE, "Case notes of medical patients under the care of Edwin Bramwell," 1919–1935, vol. 5, case 160, LHB1, CC/37a, LHSA, EUL. All of Bramwell's cases that follow are archived at this reference.

4. Ibid., vol. 5, case 162.

5. Ibid., vol. 6, case 182.

6. Ibid., vol. 5, case 159.

7. There are no records at the College of the tests having been done there. The notes state: "a similar set of estimations were made on another jaundiced patient" (whose notes in fact contain no record of this). Ibid., vol. 5, case 164.

8. It comprised 9.7 per cent of the total nitrogen.

9. The writer apparently reasoned that the liver was unable to carry out properly the conversion of ammonia salts into urea, hence their excess. A reading of contemporary texts suggests that this was well recognized. The writer's suggestion that acidosis secondary to liver failure was regarded as a more common cause does not seem to be substantiated. See James Campbell Todd, *Clinical Diagnosis: A Manual of Laboratory Method,* 4th ed. (Philadelphia: W. B. Saunders, 1918), 146; Andrew Watson Sellards, *The Principles of Acidosis and Clinical Methods for its Study* (Cambridge, MA: Harvard University Press, 1917), 49. Indeed, except in terminal liver conditions, that jaundice might be a cause of acidosis is nowhere described in the literature. The only suggestion that acidosis was considered in Elizabeth C.'s case was the quantitative assessment of urine acidity but this was hardly regarded as a pathognomonic sign of acidosis.

10. RIE, "Case notes of medical patients under the care of Edwin Bramwell," vol. 13, case 467.

11. N. W. Janny and V. I. Isaacson, "A Blood Sugar Tolerance Test," *JAMA* 70 (1918): 1131–34. The authors pressed the value of the test in endocrine disorders.

12. RIE, "Case notes of medical patients under the care of Edwin Bramwell," vol. 24, case 869.

13. Crude averaging for this year would suggest that specimens were sent from one in seven of Bramwell's patients but the mathematics would not quite reflect the reality since specimens were sent from only seventy-five patients. As in 1920, some patients came in for more intensive examination than others did, so in fact the number is slightly more than one in eight.

14. Robert A. Fleming, *A Short Practice of Medicine*, 3rd ed. (London: J. & A. Churchill, 1919) 132–40. There was of course a technological point here. Measuring blood sugars was laborious at this period.

15. D. Murray Lyon and Jonathan Meakins, "The Treatment of Diabetes Mellitus," *Edinburgh Medical Journal* 27 (1921): 270–85.

16. Michael Bliss, *The Discovery of Insulin* (Houndmills, Basingstoke: Macmillan, 1987), 33.

17. Hugh MacLean, "On the Present Position of Diabetes and Glycosuria with Observations on the New Insulin Treatment," *The Lancet* 1 (1923): 1039–46.

18. Murray Lyon and Meakins, "The Treatment of Diabetes Mellitus," 275, my emphasis.

19. Ibid. Not everyone agreed. See Janny and Isaacson, "A Blood Sugar Tolerance Test."

20. Murray Lyon and Meakins, "The Treatment of Diabetes Mellitus."

21. See R. B. Tattersall, "The Quest for Normoglycaemia: A Historical Perspective," *Diabetic Medicine* 11 (1994): 618–35.

22. "The advent of insulin has permitted no relaxation of these [dietary] rules," John Eason and D. M. Murray Lyon, "High Carbohydrate Diets in Diabetes," *The Lancet* 1 (1933): 743–45.

23. There were also two cases of renal glycosuria.

24. RIE, "Case notes of medical patients under the care of Edwin Bramwell," vol. 17, case 622.

25. Ibid., vol. 28, case 1026.

26. I suggest this was a student's record because nowhere in the nowhere in the notes except for the initial admission are urine sugar levels given and the first sugar plotted on the curve is different from this.

27. Ibid., vol. 27, case 993.

28. Ibid., vol. 32, case 1307.

29. "Quantitative estimation by Benedicts reveals 2.27% of sugar. There is a trace of diacetic acid present." Ibid.

30. Harry Rainy, "The Significance and Treatment of Glycosuria," *The Transactions of the Medico-Chirurgical Society of Edinburgh* 36 (1922): 47–69.

31. There were several methods available. Rainy's preference was for a "micromethod," in which only small amounts of blood were needed, although "great attention" to technique was required. Rainy had been performing estimations of blood sugar since at least 1916. Ibid., 51.

32. Rainy devoted much space to the prevention and treatment of acidosis. In the instance of diabetics needing surgery, he noted that the surgeon who operates without testing the urine for sugar and in ordinary cases without a thorough course of treatment "incurs a serious responsibility." Ibid.

33. Ibid., 61–66.

34. D. Murray Lyon, "Prognosis in Diabetes Mellitus," *The Lancet* 1 (1922): 1043–45. This *seems* strikingly at variance with the views of MacLean a year later. MacLean, "On the Present Position of Diabetes," 1042.

35. D. Murray Lyon, "Insulin Therapy," *Edinburgh Medical Journal* 30 (1923): 565–87.

36. Murray Lyon, "Prognosis in Diabetes Mellitus," 1043. Although he did not say why this was so.

37. RIE, "Case notes of medical patients under the care of Edwin Bramwell," vol. 38, case 1588.

38. Ibid., vol. 39, case 1660.

39. See Bliss, *Discovery*; for Britain see R. B. Tattersall, "A Force of Magical Activity: The Introduction of Insulin Treatment in Britain 1922–1926," *Diabetic Medicine* 12 (1995): 739–55.

40. Martin Edwards, "Good, Bad or Offal? The Evaluation of Raw Pancreas Therapy and the Rhetoric of Control in the Therapeutic Trial, 1925," *Annals of Science* 61 (2004): 79–98.

41. Bliss, *Discovery*, 125.

42. Meakins to Macleod, June 17, 1922, UTA, A82–0001/005(12), Records of the Board of Governors, Insulin Committee, File: Great Britain-General.

43. Macleod to Meakins, July 8, 1922, UTA, A82–0001/005(12), Records of the Board of Governors, Insulin Committee, File: Great Britain-General.

44. J. Meakins, "Autobiography," 107–8, 867/51, OLHM.

45. See Rae Murray Lyon, "The Early Days of Insulin Use in Edinburgh," *British Medical Journal* 2 (1990): 1452–54.

46. Meakins to Fletcher, July 25, 1922, FD1/913, 49222, PRO.

47. In 1923 Meakins addressed the Pharmaceutical Society of Great Britain in Edinburgh on insulin therapy. Barger proposed the vote of thanks noting their departments "were brought into intimate contact to a greater extent than any other two departments in the Faculty of Medicine." Jonathan Campbell Meakins, "Insulin in the Treatment of Diabetes: Science, Empiricism and Superstition. Inaugural Sessional Address Delivered at the Scientific Evening Meeting of the North British Branch of the Pharmaceutical Society in Edinburgh on November 23 1923," *Pharmaceutical Journal* 57 (1923): 567–70.

48. Meakins to Fletcher, July 25, 1922, FD1/913, 49222, PRO.

49. Macleod to Meakins, August 21, 1922, UTA, A82–0001/005(12), Records of the Board of Governors, Insulin Committee, File: Great Britain-General.

50. J. G. Fraser to Macleod, September 10, 1922, UTA, A82–0001/005(12), Records of the Board of Governors, Insulin Committee, File: Great Britain-General.

51. Macleod to Fraser, September 22, 1922, UTA, A82–0001/005(12), Records of the Board of Governors, Insulin Committee, File: Great Britain-General.

52. Meakins to Fletcher, October 17, 1922, FD1/913, 49222, PRO.

53. "The New Treatment of Diabetes by Insulin," *The Lancet* 2 (1922): 1086.

54. Fletcher to Meakins, November 10, 1922, FD1/913, 49222, PRO.

55. Meakins to Fletcher, November 15, 1922, FD1/913, 49222, PRO.

56. Fletcher ember 22, 1922, FD1/913, 49222, PRO.

57. Meakins to Fletcher, November 22, 1922, FD1/913, 49222, PRO.

58. Fletcher to Meakins, November 25, 1922, FD1/913, 49222, PRO. Emphasis mine.

59. Meakins, "Autobiography," 125.

60. Meakins to Fletcher, December 6 and 7, 1922, FD1/913, 49222, PRO.

61. Meakins to Fletcher, January 30, 1923, FD1/913, 49222, PRO.

62. "The Treatment of Diabetes by Insulin," *The Lancet* 1 (1923): 391–92.

63. Meakins to Fletcher, March 5, 1923, FD1/913, 49222, PRO.

64. Fletcher to Meakins, March 17, 1923, FD1/913, 49222, PRO.

65. Meakins to Fletcher, March 26, 1923, FD1/913, 49222, PRO.

66. "Insulin and the Treatment of Diabetes," *The Lancet* 2 (1923): 824–25; "The Manufacture of Insulin," ibid., 861. On the standardization of insulin see, Christiane Sinding, "Making the Unit of Insulin: Standards, Clinical Work, and Industry, 1920–1925," *Bulletin of the History of Medicine* 76 (2002): 231–70.

67. Jonathan Liebenau, "The MRC and the Pharmaceutical Industry: The Model of Insulin," in *Historical Perspectives on the Role of the MRC: Essays in the History of the Medical Research Council of the United Kingdom and its Predecessor, the Medical Research Committee, 1913–1953*, ed. Joan Austoker and Linda Bryder (Oxford: Oxford University Press, 1989), 163–80.

68. Fletcher to Meakins, April 14, 1923, FD1/913, 49222, PRO.

69. Meakins to Macleod, April 30, 1923, UTA, A82–0001/005(12), Records of the Board of Governors, Insulin Committee, File: Great Britain-General.

70. Macleod to Meakins, May 2, 1923, UTA, A82–0001/005(12), Records of the Board of Governors, Insulin Committee, File: Great Britain-General.

71. "Treatment of Diabetes with Insulin," *British Medical Journal* 1 (1923): 857.

72. J. Meakins et al., "The Treatment of Diabetes with Insulin," *Edinburgh Medical Journal* 30 (1923): 127–39.

73. "Insulin and the Treatment of Diabetes: Some Clinical Results," *The Lancet* 1 (1923): 905–8.

74. H. Whitridge Davies et al., "The Influence of Insulin upon Acidosis and Lipaemia in Diabetes," *British Medical Journal* 1 (1923): 847–57. In cases I and II the results of the first hours of treatment were shown graphically. In case III the results of the first eight days and in case IV tests done in the first twenty-four hours were plotted. Something between five and nine tests of each type were done on all the patients. A total of twenty-six estimations of bicarbonate reserve were done. As noted, reports

for 1923 state that in the whole year the laboratory carried out eighteen estimations of alkali reserve.

75. "The Supply of Insulin," *The Lancet* 1 (1923): 1066.

76. MacLean, "On the Present Position of Diabetes."

77. RIE, "Case notes of medical patients under the care of Edwin Bramwell," vol. 43, case 1897.

78. Murray Lyon, "Insulin Therapy."

79. A guinea was worth 21*s*.—£1.05 in decimal currency.

80. Tattersall, "A Force of Magical Activity," note 62.

81. RIE, "Case notes of medical patients under the care of Edwin Bramwell," vol. 43, case 1898.

82. Ibid., vol. 43, case 1902.

83. Ibid., vol. 46, case 2100.

84. Fletcher to Meakins, September 15, 1923, FD1/913, 49222, PRO.

85. Meakins to Fletcher, September 19, 1923, FD1/913, 49222, PRO.

86. Meakins to Fletcher, November 9, 1923, FD1/913, 49222, PRO.

87. Dale to Fletcher, November 13, 1923, FD1/913, 49222, PRO.

88. MacLean, "On the Present Position of Diabetes."

89. George Graham, "The Treatment of Diabetes Mellitus with Insulin," *The Lancet* 1 (1923): 1150–53. These regimes were to be challenged, notably by Robin Lawrence, physician at King's College Hospital, London, who, in his book for patients, considered: "The attempt to keep the blood sugar constantly normal may be ideal in theory, but in practice it is very difficult to achieve and makes the diabetic life unnecessarily hard without adequate benefit." R. D. Lawrence, *The Diabetic Life: Its Control by Diet and Insulin. A Concise Practical Manual for Practitioners and Patients*, 3rd ed. (London: J. & A. Churchill, 1927), 66.

90. "Discussion on Diabetes and Insulin," *British Medical Journal* 1 (1923): 445–51.

91. Murray Lyon, "Insulin Therapy," 595. The first aim of treatment, Murray Lyon observed, was to "enable the patient to make use of all the carbohydrate ingested and to avoid glycosuria," ibid., 566. Normoglycaemia was not in the first rank of practical requirements.

92. Chris Feudtner, "The Want of Control: Ideas, Innovations, and Ideals in the Modern Treatment of Diabetes Mellitus," *Bulletin of the History of Medicine* 69 (1995): 66–90. This paper is illuminating on the uses of the word "control" in this period.

93. Murray Lyon, "Insulin Therapy."

94. K. S. Hetzel and B. S. Adelaide, "The Diet During Insulin Treatment of Diabetes Mellitus," *British Medical Journal* 1 (1924): 230–31.

95. "Scotland," *The Lancet* 1 (1924): 460–61.

96. D. Murray Lyon, "Observations on the Use of Insulin," *The Lancet* 1 (1924): 158–62. The effects of ten units of insulin lasted eight hours or more but time was required for the greater part of the insulin to come into action. This fact had to be taken into account when giving the food the insulin was designed to "cover."

97. Ibid. In severe long-standing cases the plan might need to be varied when hypoglycaemia had been "found" to occur (presumably clinically, initially, whence his earlier comment about experience).

98. See p. 246.

99. D. Murray Lyon and R. Pybus, "A Table of Standard Diets for Use in Diabetes," *British Medical Journal* 2 (1924): 326–29. Emphasis mine. They published four dietary tables containing differing proportions of protein, carbohydrate, and fat to be employed according to the category of diabetic to be treated.

100. RIE, "Case notes of medical patients under the care of Edwin Bramwell," vol. 62, case 2938.

101. Ibid., vol. 63, case 2967.

102. Ibid., vol. 65, case 3251. The reading was 235 mg per cent.

103. Ibid.

104. Ibid., vol. 77, case 3534.

105. Ibid., vol. 72, case 3316.

106. Ibid., vol. 152, case 6555. As described by his general practitioner.

107. Ibid., vol. 150, case 6456.

108. J. Meakins and H. W. Davies, "Basal Metabolic Rate: Its Determination and Clinical Significance," *Edinburgh Medical Journal* 28 (1922): 1–15.

109. F. Eugene DuBois, *Basal Metabolism in Health and Disease* (Philadelphia: Lea & Febiger, 1924).

110. All the estimations on these 28 cases were done in 1921 and in total amounted to 64 tests and, presumably, were included in the 101 reported that year.

111. Meakins and Davies, "Basal Metabolic Rate."

112. RIE, "Case notes of medical patients under the care of Edwin Bramwell," vol. 30, case 1180. For Bramwell on the relation between muscular dystrophies and the endocrine system see Edwin Bramwell, "The Muscular Dystrophies, Sympathetic System, and Endocrine Glands," *The Lancet* 2 (1925): 1103–9.

113. RIE, "Case notes of medical patients under the care of Edwin Bramwell," vol. 31, case 1224.

114. Ibid., vol. 69, case 3225.

115. Some controversy surrounds priority. See J. A. N. Frederiks and P. J. Koehler, "The First Lumbar Puncture," *Journal of the History of the Neurosciences* 6 (1997): 147–53.

116. Including the famous neurologist Sir William Gowers who, it is said, would not permit it at the National Hospital, Queen Square, where it only made an appearance after his retirement in 1910. See ibid. In the same year Thomas Horder noted "with what difficulty this useful procedure … gained a foothold." *Clinical Pathology in Practice* (London: H. Froude, 1910), 90.

117. The standard urine tests for albumin: heat and acetic acid, and Esbach's method (if sufficient protein were present for quantification) were easily performed on CSF. Horder, *Clinical Pathology*.

324 Rockefeller Money, the Laboratory, and Medicine in Edinburgh

118. On separating globulin from albumin see, J. A. Milroy and T. H. Milroy, *Practical Physiological Chemistry*, 3rd ed. (Edinburgh: William Green & Son 1921), 334–36; William Mestrezat, *Le liquide céphalo-rachidien, normal et pathologique: valeur clinique de l'examen chimique; syndromes humoraux dans les diverses affections* (Paris: A. Maloine, 1912), 15; James Purves-Stewart, *The Diagnosis of Nervous Diseases*, 5th ed. (London: Edward Arnold, 1920), 418.

119. Leslie Frank Hewitt, "Proteins of the Cerebro-Spinal Fluid," *The British Journal of Experimental Pathology* 8 (1927): 84–92. On the difficulties of CSF analysis at this time see Naomi Rogers, *Dirt and Disease: Polio before FDR* (New Brunswick, NJ: Rutgers University Press, 1992).

120. J. Godwin Greenfield and E. Arnold Carmichael, *The Cerebro-Spinal Fluid in Clinical Diagnosis* (London: Macmillan, 1925), 62. In acute meningitis the authors reckoned there was a high proportion of albumin to globulin (12 to 1) and in general paralysis and spinal tumor a much lower proportion (7 to 3 and 2 to 1).

121. Ibid., 73.

122. Ibid., 77; Mestrezat, *Céphalo-rachidien, normal et pathologique*, 322.

123. RIE, "Case notes of medical patients under the care of Edwin Bramwell," vol. 84, case 3819, and vol. 89, case 4031.

124. Ibid., vol. 4, case 131.

125. Ibid., vol. 35, case 1437.

126. Ibid., vol. 36, case 1469.

127. Ibid., vol. 155, case 6670.

128. Greenfield and Carmichael, *The Cerebro-Spinal Fluid,* 177. See also R. Coope, "The Sugar Content of the Cerebro-Spinal Fluid and its Diagnostic Value Especially in Encephalitis Lethargica," *The Quarterly Journal of Medicine* 15 (1921–22): 1–8.

129. RIE, "Case notes of medical patients under the care of Edwin Bramwell," vol. 163, case 6969.

130. Ibid., vol. 162, case 6951.

131. Greenfield and Carmichael, *The Cerebro-Spinal Fluid*, 187.

132. RIE, "Case notes of medical patients under the care of Edwin Bramwell," vol. 163, case 6958.

133. Steven J. Peitzman, "From Bright's Disease to End-Stage Renal Disease," in *Framing Disease: Studies in Cultural History*, ed. Charles E. Rosenberg and Janet Golden (New Brunswick: Rutgers University Press, 1992), 3–19.

134. In 1920 there were nineteen, there were twenty in 1925 and twenty-two in 1930.

135. There were also cases labelled acute parenchymatous, sub-acute parenchymatous, chronic parenchymatous, and chronic glomerular (rarely used).

136. RIE, "Case notes of medical patients under the care of Edwin Bramwell," vol. 20, case 724.

137. The notes contain no official form, only a hand-written record.

138. RIE, "Case notes of medical patients under the care of Edwin Bramwell," vol. 23, case 834.

139. Hugh MacLean, *Modern Methods in the Diagnosis and Treatment of Renal Disease* (London: Constable, 1921), 40.

140. The request forms were not signed by him.

141. RIE, "Case notes of medical patients under the care of Edwin Bramwell," vol. 74, case 3426.

142. Ibid., vol. 75, case 3455.

143. Ibid., vol. 152, case 6542.

144. MacLean, *Modern Methods*, 41.

145. RIE, "Case notes of medical patients under the care of Edwin Bramwell," vol. 165, case 7036.

146. Ibid., vol. 23, case 831.

147. Ibid., vol. 163, case 6983.

148. Ibid., vol. 166, case 7101.

149. Ibid., vol. 29, case 1105.

150. Curiously no lead urine was returned in the lab statistics for that year but there was one in 1923.

151. See Edwin Bramwell, "Remarks on some Clinical Pictures Attributable to Lead Poisoning," *British Medical Journal* 2 (1931): 87–92.

152. RIE, "Case notes of medical patients under the care of Edwin Bramwell," vol. 73, case 3364.

153. Bramwell, "The Muscular Dystrophies."

154. RIE, "Case notes of medical patients under the care of Edwin Bramwell," vol. 28, case 1070.

155. Ibid., vol. 74, cases 3408 and 3409.

156. Ibid., vol. 75, case 3473.

157. Pearce to Vincent, January 28, 1923, folder 333, box 26, series 401A, RG 1.1, Rockefeller Foundation Archive, RAC.

158. Henry Wade, "The Choice of Methods Employed in the Surgical Diagnosis of Renal Disease," *Edinburgh Medical Journal* 29 (1922): 169–83.

159. See case notes of John Fraser, 1925–1946, GB239, LHB1, CC/29, LHSA, EUL.

10

CONCLUSION: MODERN TIMES

After assisting the reconstruction of the Medical Department, the RF pulled out of all further projects related to teaching and research in medicine in Edinburgh. This was a policy decision made before Pearce's death and which he talked about with Fletcher who agreed with it.[1] The decision seems to have resulted from a combination of factors, notably experience and general policy change. At the end of the 1920s at the Foundation headquarters the Division of Medical Education was dissolved and a new Medical Sciences division was created. Policy was changed from supporting schools to assisting individual research projects. Psychiatry, worldwide, came in for a great deal of support. North American research received extensive aid. None of the Edinburgh medical professors (Bramwell, Murray Lyon, and Ritchie) were undertaking the sort of studies that would appeal to the RF (in no case was extensive laboratory work involved and, anyhow, personal factors came into play).

Alan Gregg, Pearce's successor, persisted with attempts to assist the Medical Faculty, which in 1931 he still regarded as "the most important . . . in the British Empire in point of influence, rigorousness of standards, influence upon teaching, and research work, and intelligence and effectiveness of inner organization." Its weaknesses, he considered, were "in Physiology" and "in the division of its clinical resources over too large a number of uncorrelated teachers at the Infirmary."[2] In the light of his continuing optimism, Gregg was disposed to help the clinical professors in "the creation and maintenance of a thorough record system at the Royal Edinburgh Infirmary."[3] This proposition was said by Pearce to have been initiated by Wilkie in 1929 but apparently Murray Lyon considered it his "creation" (a point Gregg was inclined to dismiss).[4] At any rate Gregg backed it not only for its own merits but for what was described as a "byproduct" of the initiative—something the RF had wanted all along. It was hoped that by supporting the proposal there would be a *"considerable likelihood that collaborating professors, especially in the Department of Medicine, will be brought together on a much more satisfactory basis."*[5] Gregg's optimism was bolstered at the sight of "the rather unusual co-operation offered by the Royal Infirmary management."[6] In March 1931, the Rockefeller Trustees allocated $25,000 to the University for the project.[7]

New initiatives notwithstanding, in 1933 a foundation officer, R. A. Lambert, visiting Edinburgh for the first time confessed himself "a little disappointed" in what he had found. However, he admitted that he had not "read over carefully our dossier" on the Medical School beforehand. Had he done so, he confessed, he might have been less disillusioned. The "Edinburgh tradition", he wrote, still required the admission of large classes, there were not enough teachers, facilities were inadequate, and research was carried on under "a serious handicap." None the less he considered "great progress has been made in the past five years." Most important was "the development of a unifying spirit, exemplified by multiple examples of cooperation."[8] Most of Lambert's examples were culled from non-clinical departments. Clinical medicine still had some way to go in Rockefeller eyes.

After the mid-1930s the Department of Therapeutics was to return to the trajectory the RF and Meakins had planned for it in the early 1920s. Following Lambie's departure in 1930, Dunlop and Gilchrist remained the department's prize pupils and after Dunlop's accession to the Chair in 1936 the lab went through something of a golden age. Its young stars included John McMichael and Melville Arnott, both of whom were to have distinguished careers in academic medicine after the Second World War. John McMichael was knighted and made an FRS.

In the foregoing chapters I have tried to deal with three main subjects, only aspects of which have received serious attention by historians. All, however, except perhaps one, have been appreciated in a general way as issues requiring extensive research. I have used them as structuring themes. The first theme is the variety of the culture of medicine—medical difference—in the twentieth century. For years medical historians have made their livelihood in demonstrating the varieties of medicine in the past, even if scholars confined themselves to orthodoxy. The myriad schools and practices of the seventeenth and eighteenth centuries in particular have been a gold mine. Until recently the rhetoric of progress has merged twentieth-century medicine into a monolith in which every practitioner is infused with the same ideology, body of knowledge (more or less), and method of practice. Historians, however, have now started to become sensitive to the complementary and conflicting issues in twentieth-century medicine. They have started to explore the relative emphases laid on hospital and home care, art and science, different sciences, holism and reductionism, technology and human contact, individual attention and teamwork, surgery and internal medicine, mind and matter, the clinical art and the laboratory, and so on. It is to an understanding of this latter dyad—bedside and bench, as they were often called—that I hope this book makes a particular contribution. Another type of medical difference apparent in the twentieth century—at least in hospital practice and teaching—is regional or national, in this case that between Scottish and southern English and a particular sort of American medicine. Although there are many good regional studies of medicine, a specific *comparative* investigation within Britain has not been the source of publications.[9] I claim to have made no great inroads into this: it would have required researching other archives and, indeed, necessitated another book or at least a long academic paper. However, I do hope I have indicated that there were regional differences and that they were very visible to those who lived in the 1920s.

The second theme that structures this book relates to the last point: it is Scottish culture in general. Although Scottish twentieth-century cultural history has lived somewhat in the shadow of studies of the Celts and the Highland Clearances, it has been sufficiently well investigated for historians to demonstrate striking differences, particularly as evidenced in law, religion, and education, between the cultures north and south of the

Border. No one so far as I know has attempted to map out the medical ideologies of the elite doctors of the two nations and certainly not to relate these to broader cultural differences. But why should medicine be different from education, religion, or the law?

My third structuring theme has been modernization, a subject that has long been under intense historical scrutiny. In the case of this book the wider focus has been on the American, or the perceived American, presence in British life. This was a necessary part of my explanation for dealing with a narrower question: the move to academic medicine and the growth of the medical laboratory in Britain. This I have dealt with through Rockefeller involvement with a single institution (the RIE and the UE can be counted as one for present purposes).

To return to my first structuring theme: the varieties of medicine, two of which are particularly important for this book. The first is the calls upon and use of different types of science as the basis of medicine. These were by no means mutually exclusive but for analytical purposes can be separated out and the pay-off can be seen in actual work done and in the politics of promotions and appointments. It has long been recognized that pathological anatomy was *the science* of nineteenth-century medicine and that at the turn of the nineteenth–twentieth century a few clinicians endeavoured to bring to the wards a method of physiological problem solving based on experimental animal studies in the laboratory. There is abundant and much excellent historical work on experimental physiology and a few studies of the use of approaches derived from this on the wards. There are no accounts of how these approaches cohabited or conflicted in a single institution. Edinburgh clinicians were proud of the pathological–anatomical approach to disease and embedded it in Edinburgh tradition and reproduced it in training and research. New physiological approaches as embodied by Meakins were both welcomed and yet not fully embraced for they brought with them not only a new pedagogy and research style but a new organization of work, one which was not conducive to all Edinburgh clinicians or hospital governors. I embed these differences in tradition and the self-perceptions of the role of the Scottish elite clinician.

A second dichotomy within my first structural theme is in many ways one of the major statements of this book. Some years ago historians began to uncover the fact that the new nineteenth-century sciences not only changed the practices of early twentieth-century medicine (not necessarily by improving therapeutic efficiency) but pointed out that the language of science was an important resource for improving the status of medicine in the public eye. This use of scientific rhetoric was then placed by historians in the wider context of public endorsement of science as a force for social advance in all realms.[10] For Walter Morley Fletcher laboratory science was not only a force for a better medicine but a power to analyse and alleviate the ills of industrial society.

The historical understanding of science in this way seems to me an extremely rich historical vein to have mined. None the less I have been concerned for some years that this development directed attention away from clinicians who valued the clinical art, individual judgement, and tacit knowledge.[11] I have been frequently misinterpreted in this respect. It has often been said to me that the clinicians I write about were anti-science. They were not. They praised science but they resisted attempts to reduce clinical medicine to a science and they stood out against what they saw as the new organizational forms (notably division of labour) that they perceived modern laboratory science to bring. The clinicians I have studied from this perspective were elite hospital practitioners—patricians I have called them. In this respect I have found no marked differences between English practitioners and their Scottish counterparts. What this book has enabled me to do is go beyond rhetoric and look at how views of laboratory science were cashed out in practice. Here the case notes of Edwin Bramwell seem to show that laboratory science was but a minor resource for use in patient management and it was not necessarily employed in the way lab workers decreed (or indeed senior clinicians expected). The rhetoric of Bramwell and others about the value of laboratory medicine and its use at the bedside were largely at one. I have tried in other work to show how these perceptions and uses of science can be understood in terms of the social relations and interests of patrician physicians. This takes me back to my second structuring theme: English–Scottish differences.

My initial work on elite twentieth-century physicians was centred on men based at the great London hospitals. I sketched out what I considered a roughly coherent ideology that enabled these men to identify themselves as a natural ruling order of clinicians. They were committed to clinical individualism as well as individualism in the political sphere.

Their reservations about science were rooted in its presumed threat to this position. In characterizing their charitable hospital work the concept of bourgeois *noblesse oblige* proved useful. These descriptions and explanatory tools seemed to carry over to the Edinburgh elite with little difficulty. In order to explain this ideology among the English I resorted to a model of aristocratic patronage and an image the patricians constructed of the doctor as a member of the gentry in a rural, long gone (non-existent even), village-based hierarchical society.[12] Aware, as I hope I was, of the differences between Scottish and English culture, letting medicine take predominance, I initially—unwittingly—carried this explanation over the Border to the Lothians. I hope it was a combination of detailed empirical work and even wider reading into Scottish culture that disabused me of this prejudice. As I have argued in Chapter 5, although many Scottish and English clinicians shared an ideology of clinical medicine, the social roots that sustained this were different. In Scotland they lay not in the country and with the aristocracy but in the city and the university and were closely linked to those of the other professional classes. This if correct needs far more exploration but I hope it is fertile ground for the future.

I carried another prejudice into this book which I hope I have rectified and it is one which relates to my third structuring theme: modernization. Part of the English suspicion about science was a wariness of standardization and what was seen as the erosion of individualism. Some of the cautious approach to the new or academic medicine stemmed, I argued, not just from critical appraisal of the medicine itself but from a wider distrust of things perceived as American: mass production, mass consumption, and the whole new world of popular entertainment. Such suspicions fitted well into the rural ideology of the English doctors. Although the evidence is thinner the Scots too had doubts about transatlantic culture. This was my first serious work on Rockefeller, however. When confronted by an extremely slick, intelligent, wealthy piece of medical modernizing machinery (the RF) I bought their ideology hook, line, and sinker. Unthinkingly I took the approach that modernizing on Rockefeller lines was inevitable and that the Edinburgh Medical School was easily manipulated to transform itself through promises of money and images of a new modern medicine. It took me quite a time to figure out that while Rockefeller had its allies in Edinburgh, there were also

Edinburgh ways of doing things that seemed to many far better than the wholesale adoption of a transatlantic *modus operandi*. I eventually killed two birds with one stone. First, medicine did not have to change the way it did, a banality perhaps for the historian of other ages but not always so easy to recognize for the twentieth century. Indeed twentieth-century medicine did not take on the all the characteristics advocated by the most radical academic reformers. Second, I cured myself of the conflation of Rockefeller, modernity, and inevitability. I was slowly able to apprehend why Edinburgh doctors perceived their school as having rich traditions and why those traditions were seen as invaluable as a basis for teaching, practice, and research. If anything this book has been a salutary lesson for me in how easy it is to preach about the indeterminacy of the past without seeing it in the present.

Notes

1. R. M. Pearce, "Edinburgh, W. Fletcher talking to RMP, Aug. 27, 1929," folder 10, box 1, series 405, RG 1.1, Rockefeller Foundation Archives, RAC.

2. Alan Gregg, "Edinburgh—Record System," February 13, 1931, folder 10, box 1, series 405, RG 1.1, Rockefeller Foundation Archives, RAC.

3. Ibid.

4. R. M. Pearce, "Edinburgh, RMP's diary, Oct. 15, 1929," folder 10, box 1, series 405, RG 1.1, Rockefeller Foundation Archives, RAC; "Record system, University of Edinburgh," March 21, 1931," folder 10, box 1, series 405, RG 1.1, Rockefeller Foundation Archives, RAC.

5. Ibid.

6. Alan Gregg, "Edinburgh—Record System."

7. Minutes of Rockefeller Foundation, March 20, 1931, folder 10, box 1, series 405, RG 1.1, Rockefeller Foundation Archives, RAC.

8. R. A. Lambert, "Edinburgh Medical Faculty—Impressions of a Visit July 6–8, 1933," July 18, 1933, folder 18, box 2, series 405, RG 1.1, Rockefeller Foundation Archives, RAC.

9. Mike Barfoot and Steve Sturdy are the two historians I know who are acutely aware of this distinction in the case of Engand and Scotland. John Pickstone has emphasized the importance of regionality in John V. Pickstone, *Medicine and Industrial Society: A History of Hospital Development in Manchester and its Region, 1752–1946* (Manchester: Manchester University Press, 1985).

10. On this point see John Harley Warner, "The History of Science and the Sciences of Medicine," *Osiris*, 2nd ser., 10 (1995): 164–93.

11. Christopher Lawrence, "Incommunicable Knowledge: Science, Technology and the Clinical Art in Britain 1850–1914," *Journal of Contemporary History* 20 (1985): 503–20; "Still Incommunicable: Clinical Holists and Medical Knowledge in Interwar Britain," in *Greater than the Parts: The Holist Turn in Biomedicine 1920–1950*, ed. Christopher Lawrence and George Weisz (New York: Oxford University Press, 1998), 94–111.

12. Christopher Lawrence, "Edward Jenner's Jockey Boots and the Great Tradition in English Medicine 1918–1939," in *Regenerating England: Science, Medicine and Culture in Inter-War Britain*, ed. Christopher Lawrence and Anna-K. Mayer (Amsterdam. Rodopi, 2000), 45–66.

BIBLIOGRAPHY

Allbutt, Sir Clifford. "Modern Therapeutics." *The Practitioner* (September 1920): 157–63.

Alter, Peter. *The Reluctant Patron: Science and the State in Britain 1850–1920*. Oxford: Berg, 1987.

Amsterdamska, Olga. "Chemistry in the Clinic: The Research Career of Donald Dexter Van Slyke." In *Molecularizing Biology: New Practices and Alliances, 1910s–1970s*, edited by Soraya de Chadarevian and Harmke Kamminga, 47–82. Amsterdam: Harwood Academic, 1998.

Anderson, Benedict. *Imagined Communities: Reflections on the Origin and Spread of Nationalism*. London: Verso, 1983.

Ashworth, Bryan. *The Bramwells of Edinburgh: A Medical Dynasty*. Edinburgh: The Royal College of Physicians of Edinburgh, 1986.

Astrup, Poul, and John W. Severinghaus. *The History of Blood Gases, Acids and Bases*. Copenhagen: Munksgaard, 1986.

Austoker, Joan, and Linda Bryder, eds. *Historical Perspectives on the Role of the MRC: Essays in the History of the Medical Research Council of the United Kingdom and its Predecessor, the Medical Research Committee, 1913–1953*. New York: Oxford University Press, 1989.

Balinska, Marta Aleksandra. "The Rockefeller Foundation and the National Institute of Hygiene, Poland, 1918–45." *Studies in History and Philosophy of Biological and Biomedical Sciences* 31 (2000): 419–32.

Barcroft, J., J. Meakins, H. W. Davies, J. M. Duncan Scott, and W. J. Fetter. "On the Relation of External Temperature to Blood Volume." Appendix to Peru Report. *Philosophical Transactions of the Royal Society* series B, 211 (1923): 455–64.

Barker, Lewellys F. "The Organization of the Laboratories in the Medical Clinic of The Johns Hopkins Hospital." *Bulletin of The Johns Hopkins Hospital* 18 (1907): 193–98.

Bartholomew, Michael. *In Search of H.V. Morton*. London: Methuen, 2004.

Bédarida, François. *A Social History of England 1851–1990*. London and New York: Routledge, 2004.

Beit Memorial Trustees. *The Beit Memorial Fellowships for Medical Research 1909–1959*. [London]: Privately Printed for the Trustees, 1960.

Berliner, Howard S. *A System of Scientific Medicine: Philanthropic Foundations in the Flexner Era*. New York: Tavistock, 1985.

Birn, Anne-Emanuelle. "Wa(i)ves of Influence: Rockefeller Public Health in Mexico, 1920–50." *Studies in History and Philosophy of Biological and Biomedical Sciences* 31 (2000): 381–95.

Bliss, Michael. *The Discovery of Insulin*. Houndmills, Basingstoke: Macmillan, 1987.

Bonner, Thomas Neville. *Becoming a Physician: Medical Education in Britain, France, Germany, and the United States, 1750–1945*. New York: Oxford University Press, 1995.

Bramwell, Edwin. "A Plea for Accuracy in Therapeutic Deduction." *The Lancet* 1 (1925): 265–68.

———. "The Muscular Dystrophies, Sympathetic System, and Endocrine Glands." *The Lancet* 2 (1925): 1103–9.

———. "The Undergraduate Training in Medicine." *Edinburgh Medical Journal* 34 (1927): 746–53.

———. "Remarks on some Clinical Pictures Attributable to Lead Poisoning." *British Medical Journal* 2 (1931): 87–92.

Bright, Richard. *Reports of Medical Cases, Selected with a View of Illustrating the Symptoms and Cure of Diseases by a Reference to Morbid Anatomy*. 2 vols. London: Longman, Rees, Orme, and Green, 1827–31.

Brown, E. Richard. "Public Health in Imperialism: Early Rockefeller Programs at Home and Abroad." In *The Cultural Crisis of Modern Medicine*, edited by John Ehrenreich, 252–70. London: Monthly Review Press, 1978.

———. *Rockefeller Medical Men: Medicine and Capitalism in America*. Berkeley: University of California Press, 1979.

Brown, Walter Langdon. "Changing Standpoints in Metabolic Diseases: Diabetes, Nephritis, Jaundice." *British Medical Journal* 2 (1924): 1119–22.

———. *Thus We are Men*. London: Kegan Paul, 1938.

Bynum, W. F. "Sir George Newman and the American Way." In *The History of Medical Education in Britain*, edited by Vivian Nutton and Roy Porter, 37–50. Amsterdam: Rodopi, 1994.

Cannadine, David. *The Rise and Fall of the British Aristocracy*. New Haven, Conn., London: Yale University Press, 1990.

Cantor, David. "Between Galen, Geddes, and the Gael: Arthur Brock, Modernity, and Medical Humanism in Early-Twentieth-Century Britain." *Journal of the History of Medicine and Allied Sciences* 60 (2005): 1–41.

Carnegie, Andrew. *The Gospel of Wealth and other Timely Essays*. New York: Doubleday, Page & Co., 1905.

Christie, R. V., H. W. Davies, and C. P. Stewart. "Studies in Blood Coagulation and Haemophilia. II. Observations on Haemic Functions in Haemophilia." *Quarterly Journal of Medicine* 20 (1927): 481–98.

Clayson, Christopher. "Some Glimpses of Medicine Seventy Years Ago." *University of Edinburgh Journal* 39 (1999): 92–95.

Cole, Sydney W. *Practical Physiological Chemistry*. 6th ed. Cambridge: Heffer, 1920.

Colley, Linda. *Britons: Forging the Nation 1707–1737*. Yale: Yale University Press, 1992.

Collini, Stephan. *Public Moralists: Political Thought and Intellectual Life in Britain 1850–1930*. Oxford: Clarendon Press, 1991.

Comrie, John Dixon. "The Faculty of Medicine." In *The History of the University of Edinburgh 1883–1933*, edited by A. Logan Turner, 100–163. Edinburgh: Oliver and Boyd, 1933.

Conybeare, J. J. "Diseases of Metabolism." In *A Textbook of Medicine*, edited by J. J. Conybeare, 284–327. Edinburgh: E. & S. Livingstone, 1929.

Coope, R. "The Sugar Content of the Cerebro-Spinal Fluid and its Diagnostic Value Especially in Encephalitis Lethargica." *The Quarterly Journal of Medicine* 15 (1921–22): 1–8.

Corr, Helen. "Where is the Lass o' Pairts?: Gender, Identity and Education in Nineteenth Century Scotland." In *Image and Identity: The Making and Re-making of Scotland Through the Ages*, edited by Dauvit Broun, R. J. Finlay and Michael Lynch, 220–28. Edinburgh: John Donald, 1988.

Craig, Jessie McCririe, and Robert Harington. "Disturbances in Metabolism. I. Variations in Protein Metabolism as Indicated by Sulphur Excretion." *The Biochemical Journal* 18 (1924): 85–92.

Craig, W. S. *History of the Royal College of Physicians of Edinburgh*. Oxford: Blackwell Scientific Publications, 1976.

Crenner, Christopher. "Organisational Reform and Professional Dissent in the Careers of Richard Cabot and Ernest Amory Codman." *Journal of the History of Medicine and Allied Sciences* 56 (2001): 211–37.

Crookshank, Francis. *The Mongol in our Midst*. 3rd ed. London: Kegan, Paul, Trench, Trubner, 1931.

Cushny, Arthur R. *The Action and Uses in Medicine of Digitalis and its Allies*. London: Longmans, Green, 1925.

Dautrebande, Lucien. "Blood and Circulatory System: The Acid Base Equilibrium of the Blood in Circulatory Stasis." Ph.D. thesis, University of Edinburgh, 1925.

Dautrebande, L., and H. W. Davies. "Variations in Respiratory Exchange with Masks of Different Types." *Edinburgh Medical Journal* 29 (1922): 127–35.

———. "A Study of the Chlorine Interchange between Corpuscles and Plasma." *Journal of Physiology* 57 (1923): 36–46.

Dautrebande, L., H. W. Davies, and J. Meakins. "The Influence of Circulatory Changes on the Gaseous Exchanges of the Blood. III. An Experimental Study of the Circulatory Stasis." *Heart* 10 (1923): 133–52.

Davidson, L. Stanley P. "The Evolution of Modern Medicine, with Special Reference to Medical Research." *Edinburgh Medical Journal* 38 (1931): 113–25.

Davidson, Roger. *Dangerous Liaisons: A Social History of Venereal Disease in Twentieth-Century Scotland.* Amsterdam: Rodopi, 2000.

Davie, George Elder. *The Democratic Intellect. Scotland and her Universities in the Nineteenth Century.* Edinburgh: Edinburgh University Press, 1961.

———. *The Crisis of the Democratic Intellect. The Problem of Generalism and Specialisation in Twentieth-Century Scotland.* Polygon: Edinburgh, 1986.

Davies, H. W. "Methods for the Therapeutic Administration of Oxygen." *Edinburgh Medical Journal* 29 (1922): 161–68.

Davies, H. W., and John Eason. "The Relation between the Basal Metabolic Rate and the Pulse-Pressure in Conditions of Disturbed Thyroid Function." *Quarterly Journal of Medicine* 18 (1924): 36–61.

Davies, H. W., and A. R. Gilchrist. "A New Outfit for Oxygen Administration." *The Lancet* 1 (1925): 916–17.

———. "Oxygen Therapy: Indications, Principles and Methods." *Edinburgh Medical Journal* 32 (1925): 225–44.

———. "Observations upon the Circulation Rate in Man by the Ethyl Iodide Method." *Quarterly Journal of Medicine* 20 (1927): 245–64.

Davies, H. W., George. R. Brow, and Carl A. L. Binger. "The Respiratory Response to Carbon Dioxide." *Journal of Experimental Medicine* 41 (1925): 37–52.

Davies, H. W., Jonathan Meakins, and Jane Sands. "The Influence of Circulatory Disturbances on the Gaseous Exchange of the Blood. V. The Blood Gases and Circulation Rate in Hyperthyroidism." *Heart* 11 (1924): 299–307.

Davies, H. W., Charles G. Lambie, D. Murray Lyon, Jonathan Meakins, and William Robson. "The Influence of Insulin upon Acidosis and Lipaemia in Diabetes." *British Medical Journal* 1 (1923): 847–57.

"Discussion on Diabetes and Insulin." *British Medical Journal* 1 (1923): 445–51.

DuBois, F. Eugene. *Basal Metabolism in Health and Disease.* Philadelphia: Lea & Febiger, 1924.

Dunlop, D. M., and R. M. Lyon. "A Study of 523 Cases of Obesity." *Edinburgh Medical Journal* 38 (1931): 561–77.

Eason, John. *Exophthalmic Goitre.* Edinburgh: Oliver and Boyd, 1927.

Eason, John, and D. M. Lyon. "High Carbohydrate Diets in Diabetes." *The Lancet* 1 (1933): 743–45.

Eason, J., and G. L. Malcolm-Smith. "Hereditary and Familial Nephritis." *The Lancet* 2 (1924): 639–46.

Edinburgh Pathological Club. *An Inquiry into the Medical Curriculum.* Edinburgh: W. Green & Son, 1919.

Edwards, Martin. "Good, Bad or Offal? The Evaluation of Raw Pancreas Therapy and the Rhetoric of Control in the Therapeutic Trial, 1925." *Annals of Science* 61 (2004): 79–98.

Fedunkiw, Marianne. "'German Methods,' 'Unconditional Gifts,' and the Full-Time System: The Case of the University of Toronto, 1919–23." *Canadian Bulletin of Medical History* 21 (2004): 5–39.

Feudtner, Chris. "The Want of Control: Ideas, Innovations, and Ideals in the Modern Treatment of Diabetes Mellitus." *Bulletin of the History of Medicine* 69 (1995): 66–90.

Fisher, Donald. "The Rockefeller Foundation and the Development of Scientific Medicine in Britain." *Minerva* 16 (1978): 20–41.

Fleming, Robert A. *A Short Practice of Medicine*. 3rd ed. London: J. & A. Churchill, 1919.

Fletcher, Maisie. *The Bright Countenance. A Personal Biography of Walter Morley Fletcher*. London: Hodder and Stoughton, 1957.

Fletcher, Walter Morley. *Medical Research: The Tree and the Fruit*. British Science Guild, The Norman Lockyer Lecture. London: MRC, 1929.

―――. "University Ideals and the Future of Medicine." *JAMA* 19 (1930): 1389–93.

―――. *Biology and Statecraft*. The Seventh of the National Lectures Delivered on 23 January 1931. London: The British Broadcasting Corporation, 1931.

―――. "An Address on the Scope and Needs of Medical Research." *British Medical Journal* 2 (1932): 42–47.

Flexner, Abraham. *Medical Education in the United States and Canada*, Bulletin no. 4. New York: Carnegie Foundation for the Advancement of Teaching, 1910.

―――. *Medical Education in Europe*, Bulletin no. 6. New York: Carnegie Foundation for the Advancement of Teaching, 1912.

―――. *Medical Education. A Comparative Study*. New York: The Macmillan Company, 1925.

Folin, O., and H. Wu. "A System of Blood Analysis." *Journal of Biological Chemistry* 38 (1919): 81–110.

Fosdick, Raymond B. *The Story of the Rockefeller Foundation*. New York: Harper and Brothers, 1952.

Foster, W. D., and J. L. Pinniger. "History of Pathology at St Thomas's Hospital, London." *Medical History* 7 (1963): 330–47.

Frederiks, J. A. N., and P. J. Koehler. "The First Lumbar Puncture." *Journal of the History of the Neurosciences* 6 (1997): 147–53.

Fulton, John F. *Harvey Cushing: A Biography*. Springfield, IL: C. C. Thomas, 1946.

Garrod, Archibald E. "The Laboratory and the Ward." In *Contributions to Medical and Biological Research Dedicated to Sir William Osler*, 59–69. New York: Paul B. Hoeber, 1919.

Gee, Samuel. "Sects in Medicine." In *Medical Lectures and Aphorisms*, edited by Samuel Gee. London: Smith Elder & Co., 1902.

Gilchrist, A. R. "Novasurol: A New Diuretic." *The Lancet*, 2 (1925): 1019–23.

————. "The Use of Massive Doses of Digitalis." *Edinburgh Medical Journal* 33 (1926): 65–73.

Gradwohl, R. B. H., and A. J. Blaivas. *The Newer Methods of Blood and Urine Chemistry.* 2nd ed. London: Henry Kimpton, 1920.

Graham, George. "The Treatment of Diabetes Mellitus with Insulin." *The Lancet* 1 (1923): 1150–53.

————. "The Formation of the Medical and Surgical Professorial Units in the London Teaching Hospitals." *Annals of Science* 26 (1970): 1–22.

Greenfield, J. Godwin, and E. Arnold Carmichael. *The Cerebro-Spinal Fluid in Clinical Diagnosis.* London: Macmillan, 1925.

Gulland, G. Lovell. "The Teaching of Medicine." In Edinburgh Pathological Club, *An Inquiry into the Medical Curriculum*, 185–89. Edinburgh: W. Green & Son, 1919.

Guthrie, D. *Extramural Medical Education in Edinburgh and the School of Medicine of the Royal Colleges.* Edinburgh and London: Livingstone, 1965.

Haldane, J. S., J. G. Priestley, and H. W. Davies. "The Response to Respiratory Resistance." *Journal of Physiology* 53 (1919): 60–69.

Harvie, Christopher. *No Gods and Precious Few Heroes: Twentieth-Century Scotland.* 3rd ed. Edinburgh: Edinburgh University Press, 1998.

Heaman, E. A. *St. Mary's: The History of a London Teaching Hospital.* Montreal & Kingston, London, Ithaca: Liverpool University Press, McGill–Queen's University Press, 2003.

Hetzel, K. S., and B. S. Adelaide. "The Diet During Insulin Treatment of Diabetes Mellitus." *British Medical Journal* 1 (1924): 230–31.

Hewat, Andrew Fergus. *Examination of the Urine and other Clinical Side-Room Methods.* 6th ed. Edinburgh: E. & S. Livingstone, 1921.

Hewitt, Leslie Frank. "Proteins of the Cerebro-Spinal Fluid." *The British Journal of Experimental Pathology* 8 (1927): 84–92.

Holland, Thomas H., introduction to *The History of the University of Edinburgh 1883–1933*, edited by A. Logan Turner, xiii–xiv. Edinburgh: Oliver and Boyd, 1933).

Honigsbaum, Frank. *The Division in British Medicine: A History of the Separation of General Practice from Hospital Care 1911–1968.* London: Kogan Page, 1979.

Horder, Mervyn. *The Little Genius: A Memoir of the First Lord Horder.* London: Gerald Duckworth and Co., 1966.

Horder, Thomas. *Clinical Pathology in Practice.* London: H. Froude, 1910.

————. "Clinical Medicine as an Aid to Pathology: A Criticism." *St. Bartholomew's Hospital Journal* 19 (1911–12): 192–95.

————. *Health and a Day.* London: J. M. Dent and Sons Ltd., 1937.

Howell, Joel D. *Technology in the Hospital: Transforming Patient Care in the Early Twentieth Century.* Baltimore: The Johns Hopkins University Press, 1995.

Howkins, Alun. *The Death of Rural England: A Social History of the Countryside since 1900.* London: Routledge, 2003.

Hutchison, Robert and Harry Rainy. *Clinical Methods: A Guide to the Practical Study of Medicine*. London: Cassell, 1897.

————. *Clinical Methods: A Guide to the Practical Study of Medicine*. 6th ed. London: Cassell, 1916.

"Insulin and the Treatment of Diabetes." *The Lancet* 2 (1923): 824–25.

"Insulin and the Treatment of Diabetes: Some Clinical Results." *The Lancet* 1 (1923): 905–8.

Isaacs, Raphael, and David S. Hachen. "Chemistry of the Blood." In *Clinical Laboratory Diagnosis: Designed for the Use of Students and Practitioners of Medicine*, edited by Roger Morris, 367–405. New York and London: D. Appleton, 1923.

Jacyna, L. S. "Science and Social Order in the Thought of A. J. Balfour." *Isis* 71 (1980): 11–34.

Janny, N. W., and V. I. Isaacson. "A Blood Sugar Tolerance Test." *JAMA* 70 (1918): 1131–34.

Jonas, Gerald. *The Circuit Riders: Rockefeller Money and the Rise of Modern Science*. New York, London: W. W. Norton and Company, 1989.

Kavadi, Shirish N. *The Rockefeller Foundation and Public Health in Colonial India 1916–1945. A Narrative History*. Pune/Mumbai: Foundation for Research in Community Health, 1999.

Kermack, W. O., C. G. Lambie, and R. H. Slater. "Studies in Carbohydrate Metabolism. IV. Action of Hydroxymethylglyoxal upon Normal and Hypoglycaemic Animals." *The Biochemical Journal* 23 (1929): 410–15.

————. "Studies in Carbohydrate Metabolism. V. The Effect of Administration of Dextrose and Dihydroxyacetone upon the Glycogen Content of Muscle in Depancreatised Cats." *The Biochemical Journal* 23 (1929): 416–21.

Kininmonth, J. G. "The Circulation Rate in some Pathological States, with Observations on the Effect of Digitalis." *Quarterly Journal of Medicine* 21 (1928): 277–96.

Kohler, Robert E. "Walter Fletcher, F. G. Hopkins, and the Dunn Institute of Biochemistry: A Case Study in the Patronage of Science." *Isis* 69 (1978): 331–35.

————. *From Medical Chemistry to Biochemistry: The Making of a Biomedical Discipline*. Cambridge: Cambridge University Press, 1982.

Lambie, C. G. "Insulin and Glucose Utilization: Effects of Anaesthetics and Pituitrin." *The British Journal of Experimental Pathology* 7 (1926): 22–32.

Lambie, C. G., and Frances Agnes Redhead. "Studies in Carbohydrate Metabolism. III. The Influence of Dihydroxyacetone upon the Respiratory Metabolism and upon the Inorganic Phosphate of the Blood." *The Biochemical Journal* 21 (1927): 549–59.

————. "Studies in Carbohydrate Metabolism. VI. The Antagonistic Action of Pituitrin and Adrenaline upon Carbohydrate Metabolism with Special Reference to the Gaseous Exchange, the Inorganic Blood-Phosphate and the Blood-Sugar." *The Biochemical Journal* 23 (1929): 608–23.

Lambie, C. G., W. O. Kermack, and W. F. Harvey. "Effect of Parathyroid Hormone on the Structure of Bone." *Nature* 1234 (1929): 348.

Lawrence, Christopher. "Incommunicable Knowledge: Science, Technology and the Clinical Art in Britain 1850–1914." *Journal of Contemporary History* 20 (1985): 503–20.

———. "Moderns and Ancients: The New Cardiology in Britain 1800–1930." In *The Emergence of Modern Cardiology*, edited by W. F. Bynum, Christopher Lawrence, and V. Nutton. *Medical History*, Supplement 5 (1985): 1–33.

———. "Still Incommunicable: Clinical Holists and Medical Knowledge in Interwar Britain." In *Greater than the Parts: The Holist Turn in Biomedicine 1920–1950*, edited by Christopher Lawrence and George Weisz, 94–111. New York: Oxford University Press, 1998.

———. "A Tale of Two Sciences: Bench and Bedside in Twentieth-Century Britain." *Medical History* 43 (1999): 421–49.

———. "Edward Jenner's Jockey Boots and the Great Tradition in English Medicine 1918–1939." In *Regenerating England: Science, Medicine and Culture in Inter-War Britain*, edited by Christopher Lawrence and Anna-K. Mayer, 45–66. Amsterdam: Rodopi, 2000.

Lawrence, Christopher, and Anna-K. Mayer, eds. *Regenerating England: Science, Medicine and Culture in Inter-War Britain*. Amsterdam: Rodopi, 2000.

Lawrence, R. D. *The Diabetic Life: Its Control by Diet and Insulin. A Concise Practical Manual for Practitioners and Patients*. 3rd ed. London: J. & A. Churchill, 1927.

Liebenau, Jonathan. "The MRC and the Pharmaceutical Industry: The Model of Insulin." In *Historical Perspectives on the Role of the MRC: Essays in the History of the Medical Research Council of the United Kingdom and its Predecessor, the Medical Research Committee, 1913–1953*, edited by Joan Austoker and Linda Bryder, 163–80. Oxford: Oxford University Press, 1989.

Löwy, Ilana, and Patrick Zylberman. "Medicine as a Social Instrument: Rockefeller Foundation, 1913–45." *Studies in History and Philosophy of Biological and Biomedical Sciences* 31 (2000): 365–79.

Lyon, D. M. "Blood Viscosity and Blood-Pressure." *Quarterly Journal of Medicine* 14 (1921): 398–408.

———. "Prognosis in Diabetes Mellitus." *The Lancet* 1 (1922): 1043–45.

———. "Xanthoma Diabeticorum: With Report of a Case." *Edinburgh Medical Journal* 28 (1922): 168–73.

———. "Does the Reaction to Adrenaline Obey Weber's Law?" *Journal of Pharmacology and Experimental Therapeutics* 21 (1923): 229–35.

———. "Insulin Therapy." *Edinburgh Medical Journal* 30 (1923): 565–87.

———. "The Absorption of Adrenaline." Journal of Experimental Medicine 38 (1923): 655–65.

———. "The Influence of the Thyroid Gland on the Response to Adrenaline." British Medical Journal 1 (1923): 966–67.

———. "The Reaction to Adrenaline in Man." Quarterly Journal of Medicine 17 (1923): 19–33.

————. "Observations on the Use of Insulin." *The Lancet* 1 (1924): 158–62.

Lyon, D. M., and W. L. Lamb. "Difficulties in Comparing Methods of Treatment for Lobar Pneumonia." *Edinburgh Medical Journal* 36 (1929): 79–92.

Lyon, D. M., and Jonathan Meakins. "The Treatment of Diabetes Mellitus." *Edinburgh Medical Journal* 27 (1921): 270–85.

Lyon, D. M., and R. Pybus. "A Table of Standard Diets for Use in Diabetes." *British Medical Journal* 2 (1924): 326–29.

Lyon, D. M., and F. A. Redhead. "Synthetic Thyroxine—Clinical Tests." *Edinburgh Medical Journal* 34 (1927): 194–99.

Lyon, D. M., and Jane Sands. "Studies in Pulse Wave Velocity. IV. Effect of Adrenaline on Pulse Wave Velocity." *The American Journal of Physiology* 71 (1925): 534–42.

Lyon, D. M., D. M. Dunlop, and C. P. Stewart. "The Effect of Acidic and Basic Diets in Chronic Nephritis." *Edinburgh Medical Journal* 38 (1931): 87–108.

————. "The Alkaline Treatment of Chronic Nephritis." *The Lancet* 2 (1931): 1009–13.

Lyon, D. M., W. Robson, and A. C. White. "The Use of Intarvin in Diabetes Mellitus." *British Medical Journal* 1 (1925): 207–10.

Lyon, Rae Murray. "The Early Days of Insulin Use in Edinburgh." *British Medical Journal* 2 (1990): 1452–54.

Lyons, J. B. "Irish Medicine's Appeal to Rockefeller." In *Rockefeller Philanthropy and Modern Biomedicine: International Initiatives from World War I to the Cold War*, edited by William H. Schneider, 61–86. Bloomington: Indiana University Press, 2002.

Mackie, T. J. *Medical Education: An Evaluation*, Promoter's Address. Edinburgh: University of Edinburgh, 1929.

MacLean, Hugh. *Modern Methods in the Diagnosis and Treatment of Renal Disease*. London: Constable, 1921.

————. "On the Present Position of Diabetes and Glycosuria with Observations on the New Insulin Treatment." *The Lancet* 1 (1923): 1039–46.

Macleod, J. J. R. *Physiology and Biochemistry in Modern Medicine*. 3rd ed. London: Henry Kimpton, 1921.

Maier, Charles S. *Recasting Bourgeois Europe. Stabilization in France, Germany and Italy in the Decade after World War I*. Princeton: Princeton University Press, 1975.

Marks, Harry M. *The Progress of Experiment: Science and Therapeutic Reform in the United States, 1900–1990*. Cambridge: Cambridge University Press, 1997.

Matheson, A. R., and S. E. Ammon. "Observations on the Effect of Histamine on the Human Gastric Secretion." *The Lancet* 1 (1923): 482–83.

Mathews, Albert P. *Physiological Chemistry: A Textbook and Manual for Students*. London: Baillière, Tindall and Cox, 1916.

McCrone, David. "Towards a Principled Elite: Scottish Elites in the Twentieth Century." In *People and Society in Scotland. III 1914–1990*, edited by Tony Dickson and James H. Treble, vol. 3, 174–200. 3 vols. Edinburgh: John Donald, 1992.

————. *Understanding Scotland: The Sociology of a Stateless Nation*. London and New York: Routledge, 1992.

———. "We're A' Jock Tamson's Bairns: Social Class in Twentieth-Century Scotland." In *Scotland in the Twentieth Century*, edited by T. M. Devine and R. J. Finlay, 102–21. Edinburgh: Edinburgh University Press, 1996.

Meakins, J. "Observations on the Gases in Human Arterial Blood in Certain Pathological Pulmonary Conditions, and their Treatment with Oxygen." *Journal of Pathology and Bacteriology* 34 (1921): 79–90.

———. "Observations on the Duodenal Tube in the Diagnosis and Treatment of Biliary Diseases." *British Medical Journal* 1 (1922): 483–87.

———. "Oxygen-Want: Its Causes, Signs and Treatment." *Edinburgh Medical Journal* 29 (1922): 142–61.

———. "Some Chemical Influences in Regard to the Endocrine Glands and the Central Nervous System." *Journal of Mental Science* 68 (1922): 367–74.

———. "Insulin in the Treatment of Diabetes: Science, Empiricism and Superstition." *Pharmaceutical Journal* 57 (1923): 567–70.

Meakins, J., and H. W. Davies. "Observations on the Gases in Human Arterial and Venous Blood." *Journal of Pathology and Bacteriology* 23 (1920): 451–61.

———. "Basal Metabolic Rate: Its Determination and Clinical Significance." *Edinburgh Medical Journal* 28 (1922): 1–15.

———. "The Influence of Circulatory Disturbances on the Gaseous Exchange in the Blood. II. A Method of Estimating the Circulation Rate in Man." *Heart* 9 (1922): 191–98.

———. *Respiratory Function in Disease*. Edinburgh: Oliver and Boyd, 1925.

Meakins, J., and C. R. Harington. "The Relation of Histamine to Intestinal Intoxication. I. The Presence of Histamine in the Human Intestine." *Journal of Pharmacology and Experimental Therapeutics* 18 (1921): 455–65.

———. "The Relation of Histamine to Intestinal Intoxication. II. The Absorption of Histamine from the Intestine." *Journal of Pharmacology and Experimental Therapeutics* 20 (1923): 45–64.

Meakins, J., Lucien Dautrebande, and W. J. Fetter. "The Influence of Circulatory Disturbances on the Gaseous Exchange of the Blood. IV. The Blood Gases and Circulation Rate in Cases of Mitral Stenosis." *Heart* 10 (1923): 153–78.

Meakins J., W. Robson, C. G. Lambie, and H. W. Davies. "The Treatment of Diabetes with Insulin." *Edinburgh Medical Journal* 30 (1923): 127–39.

Medical Research Council, *The Acid–Base Equilibrium of the Blood*. London: HMSO, 1923.

Mestrezat, William. *Le liquide céphalo-rachidien, normal et pathologique: valeur clinique de l'examen chimique; syndromes humoraux dans les diverses affections*. Paris: A. Maloine, 1912.

Milroy, J. A., and T. H. Milroy. *Practical Physiological Chemistry*. 3rd ed. Edinburgh: William Green & Son 1921.

Morris, Roger. *Clinical Laboratory Diagnosis: Designed for the Use of Students and Practitioners of Medicine*. New York and London: D. Appleton, 1923.

Morton, Graeme. "What if? The Significance of Scotland's Missing Nationalism in the Nineteenth Century." In *Image and Identity: The Making and Re-making of Scotland Through the Ages*, edited by Dauvit Broun, R. J. Finlay and Michael Lynch, 157–76. Edinburgh: John Donald, 1998.

Murad, Lion, and Patrick Zylberman. "Seeds for French Health Care: Did the Rockefeller Foundation Plant the Seeds between the Two World Wars?" *Studies in History and Philosophy of Biological and Biomedical Sciences* 31 (2000): 463–75.

Nicholas, Siân. "Being British: Creeds and Cultures." In *The British Isles: 1901–1951*, edited by Keith Robbins, 103 35. Oxford: Oxford University Press, 2002.

O'Shea, Alan. "English Subjects of Modernity," in *Modern Times: Reflections on a Century of English Modernity*, edited by Mica Nava and Alan O'Shea, 7–37. London: Routledge, 1996.

Osler, William, and Thomas McCrae. *The Principles and Practice of Medicine*. 9th ed. New York, London: D. Appleton and Company, 1920.

Overy, R. J. *The Inter-War Crisis 1919–1939*. Harlow: Pearson Education Limited, 1994.

Palló, Gábor. "Rescue and Cordon Sanitaire: The Rockefeller Foundation in Hungarian Public Health." *Studies in History and Philosophy of Biological and Biomedical Sciences* 31 (2000): 433–45.

Panton, P. N. *Clinical Pathology*. London: J. & A. Churchill, 1913.

Paterson, H. M. "Incubus and Ideology: The Development of Secondary Schooling in Scotland." In *Scottish Culture and Scottish Education 1800–1980*, edited by Walter M. Humes and Hamish M. Paterson, 197–215. Edinburgh: John Donald, 1983.

"Pathological Chemistry Technique." *The Laboratory Journal* 10 (1929): 271.

"Pathological Departments." *The Lancet* 2 (1923): 522.

Peitzman, Steven J. "From Bright's Disease to End-Stage Renal Disease." In *Framing Disease: Studies in Cultural History*, edited by Charles E. Rosenberg and Janet Golden, 3–19. New Brunswick: Rutgers University Press, 1992.

Percival, G. H., and C. P. Stewart. "A Note on Renal Function in Scarlet Fever." *Edinburgh Medical Journal* 33 (1926): 53–57.

———. "Pathological Variations in the Serum Calcium." *Quarterly Journal of Medicine* 19 (1926): 235–48.

Phillipson, Nicholas. "Towards a Definition of the Scottish Enlightenment," in *City and Society in the Eighteenth Century*, edited by P. Fritz and D. Williams, 125–47. Toronto: Hakkert, 1973.

———. "Culture and Society in the Eighteenth-Century Province: The Case of Edinburgh and the Scottish Enlightenment," in *The University in Society*, edited by Lawrence Stone, 2 vols., vol. 2, 407–48. Princeton, NJ: Princeton University Press, 1975.

Picard, Jean-François, and William H. Schneider. "From the Art of Medicine to Biomedical Science in France: Modernization or Americanization?" In *Rockefeller Philanthropy and Modern Biomedicine: International Initiatives from World War I to the Cold War*, edited by William H. Schneider, 106–24. Bloomington: Indiana University Press, 2002.

Pickstone, John V. *Medicine and Industrial Society: A History of Hospital Development in Manchester and its Region, 1752–1946*. Manchester: Manchester University Press, 1985.

Potter, Dorothy G. E. "Changes in the Blood in Anaesthesia." *Quarterly Journal of Medicine* 18 (1925): 261–73.

Purves-Stewart, James. *The Diagnosis of Nervous Diseases*. 5th ed. London: Edward Arnold, 1920.

Rabinbach, Anson, *The Human Motor: Energy, Fatigue and the Origins of Modernity*. Berkeley: University of California Press, 1992.

Rainy, Harry. "The Significance and Treatment of Glycosuria." *The Transactions of the Medico-Chirurgical Society of Edinburgh* 36 (1922): 47–69.

Royal Infirmary of Edinburgh, *Reports Regarding the Affairs of the Royal Infirmary of Edinburgh from 1st October 1919 to 1st October 1920*. Edinburgh: The Darien Press, n.d.

Ritchie, John. *History of the Laboratory of the Royal College of Physicians of Edinburgh*. Edinburgh: Royal College of Physicians, 1953.

Ritchie, W. T. "Medicine in Edinburgh." *Edinburgh Medical Journal* 35 (1928): 665–73.

Robson, W. "Protein Metabolism in Cystinuria." *The Biochemical Journal* 23 (1929): 138–48.

Robson, William. "The Metabolism of Tryptophane. I. The Synthesis of Racemic Bz-Methyltryptophane." *Journal of Biological Chemistry* 62 (1924): 495–514.

Rodgers, Daniel T. *Atlantic Crossings: Social Politics in a Progressive Age*. Cambridge, MA: The Belknap Press, 1998.

Rogers, Naomi. *Dirt and Disease: Polio before FDR*. New Brunswick, New Jersey: Rutgers University Press, 1992.

Rosenfeld, Louis. *Four Centuries of Clinical Chemistry*. Amsterdam: Gordon and Breach Science Publishers, 1999.

Royal Commission on University Education in London, *Final Report*. Cd. 6718. 1913. Parliamentary Papers, vol. xxiii.

Royal Society, The. "Charles Robert Harington, 1897–1972." *Biographical Memoirs of Fellows of the Royal Society* 18 (1972): 267–308.

Sands, Jane. "Studies in Pulse Wave Velocity. III. Pulse Wave Velocity in Pathological Conditions." *The American Journal of Physiology* 71 (1925): 519–33.

Savill, Thomas Dixon. *A System of Clinical Medicine*. 5th ed. London: Edward Arnold, 1919.

Schneider, William H. "The Men who Followed Flexner: Richard Pearce, Alan Gregg, and the Rockefeller Foundation Medical Divisions, 1919–1951." In *Rockefeller Philanthropy and Modern Biomedicine: International Initiatives from World War I to the Cold War*, edited by William H. Schneider, 7–60. Bloomington: Indiana University Press, 2002.

"Scotland." *The Lancet* 1 (1924): 460–61.

"Scotland: Clinical Meeting of the Edinburgh Branch." *British Medical Journal* 2 (1922): 368.

Sellards, Andrew Watson. *The Principles of Acidosis and Clinical Methods for its Study*. Cambridge, MA: Harvard University Press, 1917.

Shannon, Richard. *The Crisis of Imperialism 1865–1915*. Frogmore: Paladin, 1976.

Siegmund-Schultz, Reinhard. *Rockefeller, and the Internationalization of Mathematics between the Two World Wars: Documents and Studies for the Social History of Mathematics in the 20th Century*. Science Networks Historical Studies 25. Basel: Birkhäuser, 2001.

Simpson, Elliot. *People who Made Scottish Clinical Biochemistry*. Airdrie: Sponsored by Mannheim Boehringer Diagnostics, 1995.

Sinding, Christiane. "Making the Unit of Insulin: Standards, Clinical Work, and Industry, 1920–1925." *Bulletin of the History of Medicine* 76 (2002): 231–70.

Slyke, Donald Dexter Van, and Glenn E. Cullen. "Studies of Acidosis. I The Bicarbonate Concentration of the Blood Plasma; Its Significance and its Determination as a Measure of Acidosis." *Journal of Biological Chemistry* 30 (1917): 289–346.

Smith, Charles J. *Edinburgh's Contribution to Medical Microbiology*. Glasgow: Wellcome Unit for the History of Medicine, 1994.

Smout, T. C. *A Century of the Scottish People 1830–1950*. New Haven and London: Yale University Press, 1986.

Solomon, Susan Gross. " 'Through a Glass Darkly': the Rockefeller Foundation's International Health Board and Soviet Public Health." *Studies in History and Philosophy of Biological and Biomedical Sciences* 31 (2000): 409–18.

Stevens, Marianne Pauline Fedunkiw. "Dollars and Change; The Effect of Rockefeller Foundation Funding on Canadian Medical Education at the University of Toronto, McGill University, and Dalhousie University." Ph.D. thesis, University of Toronto, 2000.

Stevens, Rosemary. *American Medicine and the Public Interest: A History of Specialization*. Berkeley: University of California Press, 1971.

Stewart, C. P. "Studies on the Metabolism of Arginine and Histidine. Part II. Arginine and Histidine as Precursors of Purines." *The Biochemical Journal* 19 (1925): 1101–10.

Stewart, C. P., and William Archibald. "The Estimation of Phosphorus and Magnesium." *The Biochemical Journal* 19 (1925): 484–91.

Stewart, C. P., and D. M. Dunlop. *Clinical Chemistry in Practical Medicine*. Edinburgh: E. & S. Livingstone, 1930.

Stewart, C. P. and A. C. White. "The Estimation of Fat in Blood." *The Biochemical Journal* 19 (1925): 840–44.

Stone, Willard J. *Blood Chemistry, Colorimetric Methods for the General Practitioner: With Clinical Comments and Dietary Suggestions*. New York: Paul B. Hoeber, 1923.

Sturdy, Steve. "Biology as Social Theory: John Scott Haldane and Physiological Regulation." *British Journal for the History of Science* 21 (1988): 315–40.

———. "From the Trenches to the Hospitals at Home: Physiologists, Clinicians and Oxygen Therapy, 1914–30." In *Medical Innovations in Historical Perspective*, edited by John V. Pickstone, 104–23. Basingstoke, Hampshire: Macmillan, in association with the Centre for the History of Science, Technology, and Medicine, University of Manchester, 1992.

———. "The Political Economy of Scientific Medicine: Science, Education and the Transformation of Medical Practice in Sheffield, 1890–1922." *Medical History* 36 (1992): 125–59.

———. "Medical Chemistry and Clinical Medicine: Academics and the Scientisation of Medical Practice in Britain, 1900–1925." In *Medicine and Change: Historical and Sociological Studies of Medical Innovation*, edited by Ilana Löwy, 371–93. Paris: Montrouge, 1993.

———. "Hippocrates and State Medicine: George Newman Outlines the Founding Policy of the Ministry of Health." In *Greater than the Parts: The Holist Turn in Biomedicine 1920–1950*, edited by Christopher Lawrence and George Weisz, 112–34. New York: Oxford University Press, 1998.

———. "War as Experiment: Physiology, Innovation and Administration in Britain, 1914–1918: The Case of Chemical Warfare." In *War, Medicine and Modernity*, edited by Roger Cooter, Mark Harrison and Steve Sturdy, 63–84. Stroud: Sutton, 1998.

Sturdy, Steve, and Roger Cooter. "Science, Scientific Management and the Transformation of Medicine in Britain c.1870–1950." *History of Science* 36 (1998): 421–66.

Tattersall, R. B. "The Quest for Normoglycaemia: A Historical Perspective." *Diabetic Medicine* 11 (1994): 618–35.

———. "A Force of Magical Activity: The Introduction of Insulin Treatment in Britain 1922–1926." *Diabetic Medicine* 12 (1995): 739–55.

Taylor, Frederick. *The Practice of Medicine.* 11th ed. London: J & A Churchill, 1918.

Taylor, W. W. *Practical Chemical Physiology.* London: Edward Arnold, 1922.

"The Introductory Address." *British Medical Journal* 2 (1885): 655.

"The Manufacture of Insulin." *The Lancet* 2 (1923): 861.

The Medical Who's Who, 8th ed. London: Grafton, 1927.

"The New Treatment of Diabetes by Insulin." *The Lancet* 2 (1922): 1086.

"The Supply of Insulin." *The Lancet* 1 (1923): 1066.

"The Treatment of Diabetes by Insulin." *The Lancet* 1 (1923): 391–92.

Thomson, A. Landsborough. *The Medical Research Council: Half a Century of Medical Research.* 2 vols. London: HMSO, 1973–1975.

Todd, James Campbell. *Clinical Diagnosis: A Manual of Laboratory Methods.* 4th ed. Philadelphia, London: W. B. Saunders, 1918.

"Treatment of Diabetes with Insulin." *British Medical Journal* 1 (1923): 857.

Turner, A. Logan, ed. *The History of the University of Edinburgh 1883–1933.* Edinburgh: Oliver and Boyd, 1933.

———. *Story of a Great Hospital. The Royal Infirmary of Edinburgh 1729–1929.* Edinburgh: Oliver and Boyd Ltd., 1937.

Turner, A. Logan, J. Davidson, and A. C. White. "Xanthomatosis: Some Aspects of its Blood Chemistry and Pathology." *Edinburgh Medical Journal* 32 (1925): 153–74.

University of Edinburgh, *Edinburgh University Calendar, 1920–1921*. Edinburgh: James Thin, 1920.

University of Edinburgh, Faculty of Medicine. *Bicentenary of the Faculty of Medicine 1726–1926. Records of the Celebrations*. Edinburgh: James Thin, 1926.

University of Edinburgh Journal (Autumn 1927).

Waddington, Keir. *Medical Education at St Bartholomew's Hospital 1123–1995*. Woodbridge, Suffolk: The Boydell Press, 2003.

Wade, Henry. "The Choice of Methods Employed in the Surgical Diagnosis of Renal Disease." *Edinburgh Medical Journal* 29 (1922): 169–83.

Wailoo, Keith. *Drawing Blood: Technology and Disease Identity in Twentieth-Century America*. Baltimore: The Johns Hopkins University Press, 1997.

Warner, John Harley. "The History of Science and the Sciences of Medicine." *Osiris*, 2nd series, 10 (1995): 164–93.

Weatherall, Mark W. *Gentlemen, Scientists and Doctors: Medicine at Cambridge 1800–1940*. Woodbridge, Suffolk: The Boydell Press in Association with Cambridge University Library, 2000.

Weindling, Paul. "Public Health and Political Stabilisation: The Rockefeller Foundation in Central and Eastern Europe between the Two World Wars." *Minerva* 31 (1993): 253–67.

Wesselow, O. L. V. De. *The Chemistry of the Blood in Clinical Medicine*. London: Ernest Benn, 1924.

White, A. C. "The Bicarbonate Reserve and the Dissociation Curve of the Oxyhemoglobin in Febrile Conditions." *Journal of Experimental Medicine* 41 (1925): 315–26.

Wilkinson, Lise, and Anne Hardy. *Prevention and Cure: The London School of Hygiene & Tropical Medicine: A 20th Century Quest for Global Public Health*. London: Kegan Paul, 2001.

INDEX

George Barger and, 111, 113, 117,
    119, 174
Arthur Cushny and, 111, 113
Howard Davies and, 233
death, 4, 28
on Edinburgh University Medical
    Faculty, 88n9, 88n11, 88n14,
    90n64, 110, 111–12,
    113–17, 118–31, 134n61,
    134n62, 141, 152–60,
    161–62, 179n5, 182n52, 327
David Edsall and, 94–95, 96
J. Alfred Ewing and, 110, 119, 121,
    122, 126, 130, 144, 145,
    149, 154, 155, 156, 173–74
Walter Morley Fletcher and,
    33–34, 42–43, 110–11, 121,
    159, 161–62, 172–73, 178,
    254
Francis Fraser and, 156–57
Alan Gregg and, 45, 119, 174
David Murray Lyon and, 129–30,
    156, 159, 162, 175, 254
Jonathan Meakins and, 111, 113,
    114, 115, 118, 119, 120–22,
    123–24, 126, 141, 142, 143,
    145–46, 157–58
on medical education, 113–14
on RIE, 113, 127–28
on William Ritchie, 174–75
James Lorrain Smith and, 96, 111,
    113, 117, 119, 145, 155
Harold Stiles and, 110, 113, 114,
    115, 116–17, 119, 122, 125,
    126–27, 128, 141, 142–43,
    144, 146, 148, 154
St Thomas's Hospital, London and,
    45–47, 111
George Vincent and, 39, 40,
    43–44, 119
David Wilkie and, 147, 148,
    149–50, 155, 156, 157,
    158–59, 173, 174

Peitzman, Steven J., 324n133
Percival, G. H., 222n86, 256
pernicious anaemia, 16
Peru High Altitude Committee,
    232
pharmaceutical companies, 227, 289
    insulin sales, 290
Pharmaceutical Society of Great Britain,
    320n47
pharmacology, 66, 77, 78
philanthropy, 19, 20–21, 22, 24n15. *See
    also* medical funding
Philip, Robert Wilson, 88n18, 117,
    122
Phillipson, Nicholas, 104
philosophy, as an academic subject, 105,
    106
physiology, 14, 23, 35–36, 37, 41, 45,
    80, 83, 99, 329
    biochemistry and, 187
    in Edinburgh, 64, 65–66
    Walter Morley Fletcher on, 16,
        51–52
    Jonathan Meakins on, 229, 329
    respiratory, 80–81, 230, 231–32,
        233, 243, 258
Picard, Jean-François, 57n18
Pickstone, John V., 332n9
Pinniger, J. L., 218n5
pituitary disorder, 273, 274, 316–17
pneumonia, 257–58
    lobar, 309
Poland, 32
political issues, 107
    in medical reform, 8, 52–53
the poor
    dispensary system for, 96
    hospital treatment for, 12, 13, 35,
        49, 54
post-mortems. *See* morbid anatomy
Potter, Dorothy, 210, 249
poverty, disease and, 29
Priestly, John Gillies, 81, 261n15

Lightning Source UK Ltd.
Milton Keynes UK
UKHW021041290822
407896UK00009B/993